KU-504-721

LIBRARY
AND
INFORMATION
SERVICES
CAERLEON

# DOWN SYNDROME

## VISIONS FOR

## THE 21ST CENTURY

EDITED BY

**WILLIAM I. COHEN**
Child Development Unit
Children's Hospital of Pittsburgh

**LYNN NADEL**
Department of Psychology
University of Arizona

**MYRA E. MADNICK**
National Down Syndrome Society

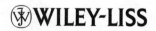WILEY-LISS

A JOHN WILEY & SONS, INC., PUBLICATION

This book is printed on acid-free paper. ∞

Copyright © 2002 by Wiley-Liss, Inc., New York. All rights reserved.

Published simultaneously in Canada.

No part of this publication may be reproduced, stored in a retrieval system or transmitted in any form or by any means, electronic, mechanical, photocopying, recording, scanning or otherwise, except as permitted under Sections 107 or 108 of the 1976 United States Copyright Act, without either the prior written permission of the Publisher, or authorization through payment of the appropriate per-copy fee to the Copyright Clearance Center, 222 Rosewood Drive, Danvers, MA 01923, (978) 750-8400, fax (978) 750-4744. Requests to the Publisher for permission should be addressed to the Permissions Department, John Wiley & Sons, Inc., 605 Third Avenue, New York, NY 10158-0012, (212) 850-6011, fax (212) 850-6008, E-Mail: PERMREQ@WILEY.COM.

For ordering and cutomer service information please call 1-800-CALL-WILEY.

*Library of Congress Cataloging-in-Publication Data:*
Down syndrome: visions for the 21st century / edited by William I. Cohen, Lynn Nadel, Myra E. Madnick.
    p.   ;   cm.
Includes bibliographical references.
    ISBN 0-471-41815-3 (alk. paper)
1. Down syndrome.
    [DNLM: 1. Down Syndrome—rehabilitation.   2. Community Mental Health Services—trends.   3. Education, Special—trends.   4. Interpersonal Relations.   5. Patient Advocacy—trends.   6. Patient Participation—trends.   WM 308 D751 2002]   I. Cohen, William I.   II. Nadel, Lynn.   III. Madnick, Myra E.
    RC571  .D694  2002
    616.85'8842—dc21

                                                                2002001890

Printed in the United States of America.

10 9 8 7 6 5 4 3 2 1

*The National Down Syndrome Society would like to dedicate this book to the real experts—the individuals with Down syndrome and their families who are in the forefront of the Down syndrome movement. Their insight, passion, and dedication have greatly enhanced the lives of all people with Down syndrome.*

# Contents

# PREFACE

*Down Syndrome: Visions for the 21st Century* grew out of the NDSS conference of the same name held July 27–29, 2000 in Washington, DC. A major goal of this conference was to create a dynamic vision for the new century by asking the more than 650 participants to share their ideas and priorities in education, research, and advocacy. This book encompasses that theme and the mission of NDSS: to ensure that all individuals with Down syndrome are provided the opportunity to achieve their potential in community life.

*Visions* is designed to explore the highlights of the conference through chapters submitted by many of the presenters. This book will be most valuable to several different groups of people including parents and family members of individuals with Down syndrome, expectant parents of children with Down syndrome, educators, physicians, and health care professionals as well as the interested public.

The book is divided into ten sections that include specific chapters on topics of interest to both parents and professionals. The first three sections, Self-Determination, Self-Advocacy, and Advocacy, address the issues of how individuals with Down syndrome and their families can play a greater role in how the person with Down syndrome optimally leads his/her life. This material is augmented by a number of accounts written by young adults with Down syndrome.

The next section, Role of the Family, includes personal reflections by parents of children with Down syndrome as well as chapters on siblings and life planning. The following section, Health and Clinical Care, is comprehensive, covering such topics as pediatrics, gross motor development, behavior, adult health care, and the recently updated Healthcare Guidelines for Individuals with Down Syndrome (1999).

The Research section includes in-depth discussions of the sequencing of chromosome 21, alternative therapies, and recent advances in research. Psycho-Social Issues are the theme of the next section, which includes chapters on relationships, sexuality, healthy lifestyles, and autism and Down syndrome.

One of the most important topics for people with Down syndrome, their families, and professionals is addressed in the Education/Inclusion section. Such topics as the philosophy of inclusion, positive behavioral supports, postsecondary education, and assistive technology and computers are discussed. Another aspect of education is detailed in the Communication, Math, and Language Skills section. This section includes discussions of speech and language for infants, toddlers, children, and adolescents as well as the teaching of reading and math to children with Down syndrome.

The book concludes with a section entitled Turning the Vision into Reality, which examines the significant changes that have occurred for people with Down syndrome and the many challenges that lay ahead.

This book will assist the reader in obtaining a better grasp of the present and an understanding of what the future could hold for individuals with Down syndrome if we work collectively to make positive changes across all disciplines.

William I. Cohen, M.D.
Lynn Nadel, Ph.D.
Myra E. Madnick, M.Ed.

# ACKNOWLEDGMENTS

The National Down Syndrome Society wishes to acknowledge our editors, William I. Cohen, M.D., Lynn Nadel, Ph.D., and Myra E. Madnick, M.Ed., for all their efforts in bringing this book to fruition. Additionally, NDSS greatly appreciates the efforts of our contributing authors, who put aside their busy schedules to meet publication dates. The result of their combined effort is a current, comprehensive, and very relevant book on all aspects of Down syndrome.

# CONTRIBUTORS

GILLIAN BARLOW, PH.D.
Cedars-Sinai Medical Center

MARTHA BECK, PH.D.
Phoenix, AZ

PRANAY BHATTACHARYYA, B.S.
Cedars-Sinai Medical Center

CHRIS BURKE
National Down Syndrome Society,
New York, NY

GEORGE T. CAPONE, M.D.
Department of Pediatrics, Johns
Hopkins University School of
Medicine, Baltimore, MD, and
Division of Neurology and
Developmental Medicine, Kennedy
Krieger Institute, Baltimore, MD

XIAO-NING CHEN, M.D.
Associate Professor of
Pediatrics, UCLA
UCLA School of Medicine
Cedars-Sinai Medical Center

BRIAN A. CHICOINE, M.D.
Adult Down Syndrome Center of
Lutheran General Hospital,
Park Ridge, IL

WILLIAM I. COHEN, M.D.
Down Syndrome Center,
Children's Hospital of Pittsburgh,
Pittsburgh, PA

W. CARL COOLEY, M.D.
Department of Pediatrics,
Dartmouth Medical School,
Hanover, NH, and Crotched
Mountain Rehabilitation Center,
Greenfield, NH

HANK EDMONSON, M.ED.
Loyola University, Chicago, IL

TERRY HASSOLD, PH.D.
Department of Genetics and The
Center for Human Genetics, Case
Western Reserve University and
The University Hospitals of
Cleveland, Cleveland, OH

JOHN PETER ILLARRAMENDI
Bethesda, MD

PHYLLIS JACKS, ED.D.
Chapel Haven, New Haven, CT

JULIE R. KORENBERG, PH.D., M.D.
Professor of Pediatrics & Human
Genetics, UCLA
Brawerman Chair of Molecular
Genetics, Vice Chair for Pediatrics,
Research Cedars-Sinai Medical
Center

LIBBY KUMIN, PH.D., CCC-SLP
Speech-Language Pathology
Audiology Department, Loyola
College in Maryland, Graduate
Center, Columbia, MD

ANDREA LACK, M.S.W., C.S.W.
National Down Syndrome Society,
New York, NY

LEN LESHIN, M.D., FAAP
Corpus Christi, TX

SUSAN P. LEVINE, M.A., C.S.W.
FRA, Shrewsbury, NJ

GARY E. LYONS, PH.D.
Associate Professor,
Anatomy/Pediatrics,
University of Wisconsin Medical
School, Madison, WI

JEFFERY MATTSON
Monarch Beach, CA

KATHLEEN H. MCGINLEY, PH.D.
Health Care and Housing Policy,
The Arc of the United States,
Washington, DC

DENNIS E. MCGUIRE, PH.D.
Adult Down Syndrome Center of
Lutheran General Hospital,
Park Ridge, IL

JOAN E. MEDLEN, R.D., L.D.
Disability Solutions
Portland, OR

MICHAEL MORRIS
Community Options, Inc.,
Washington, DC

THOMAS NERNEY
Center for Self Determination,
Ann Arbor, MI

JOSHUA G. O'NEILL
Fort Wayne, IN

THOMAS J. O'NEILL
Admetco, Fort Wayne, IN

PATRICIA LOGAN OELWEIN, M.ED.
Bellevue, WA

BONNIE PATTERSON, M.D.
Cincinnati Center For
Developmental Disorders,
University of Cincinnati,
Cincinnati, OH

DAVID PATTERSON, PH.D.
The Eleanor Roosevelt Institute,
Denver, CO

MIA PETERSON
National Down Syndrome Society,
Cincinnati, OH

SIEGFRIED M. PUESCHEL, M.D.,
PH.D., J.D., M.P.H.
Child Development Center, Rhode
Island Hospital, Providence, RI

LORA S. SALANDANAN, B.S.
Cedars-Sinai Medical Center

STEPHANIE SHERMAN
Department of Genetics, Emory
University School of Medicine,
Atlanta, GA

STEPHANIE SMITH LEE
National Down Syndrome Society,
Oakton, VA

JACQUELINE THOUSAND, PH.D.
College of Education, California
State University, San Marcos,
San Marcos, CA

ANN TORNBILL, ED.D.
University of Kansas,
Lawrence, KS

RICHARD A. VILLA, ED.D.
Bayridge Consortium, Inc.
San Marcos, CA

LESLIE WALKER-HIRSCH, M.ED.
Moonstone Group, Yorktown
Heights, NY

JOSEPH F. WALLACE, PH.D.
Virginia Assistive Technology
System, Richmond, VA

DAVID A. WEINGARTEN
Wealth Advisory Group LLC,
New York, NY

PATRICIA C. WINDERS, PT
North East, MD

# Self-Determination

# Understanding Self-Determination

## Thomas Nerney

### Introduction

The new century offers the possibility of unparalleled opportunities for individuals with Down syndrome. It offers as well the hazard of rising skepticism concerning the value of individuals with cognitive and intellectual disabilities.

The enormous gains made in the last third of the twentieth century in education, employment, and community living for these individuals can be further broadened. For this to occur, society must change the terms and rationale for obtaining necessary supports to those based on freedom and equality rather than paternalism and professional domination. As well, support for long-term care will falter without a better grounding in public policy, law, and ethics that is more widely shared by the larger society.

Individuals with Down syndrome today are benefiting from so much that has been learned from the fields of medicine, education, and rehabilitation that it would not be too optimistic to predict further gains if structural reforms of the present human service system are implemented quickly and carefully. These reforms would place the authority for controlling individual budgets needed for support with the individual, family, and close allies. Information and data garnered to date from the self-determination movement demonstrate the cost-effectiveness of this approach and the improvements in quality.

*Down Syndrome*, Edited by William I. Cohen, Lynn Nadel, and Myra E. Madnick.
ISBN 0-471-41815-3   Copyright © 2002 by Wiley-Liss, Inc.

However, the backlash occurring throughout this country over special education spending seems likely to move into the field of long-term care sooner rather than later. The strain on state Medicaid budgets will be exacerbated as America ages and the population over 65, and especially over 85, increases dramatically. A new utilitarian agenda arising from the field of bioethics is beginning to call into question the value of any public expenditure that purports to serve those who cannot "benefit"—those with cognitive and intellectual disabilities (Nerney, 1999). This recent assault on the value of individuals with intellectual disabilities can be traced to Drs. Duff and Campbell, who wrote one of the first articles to be published in the *New England Journal of Medicine*. In 1973 they revealed that they did not treat many babies born with disabilities at Yale New Haven Hospital (Duff and Campbell, 1973). These decisions were based on "quality of life" criteria. Life-long disability was now a subject for debate.

But the debate soon moved from quality of life considerations to considerations regarding the cost to society. A group of doctors and social workers published a seminal article in *Pediatrics*, the journal of the American Academy of Pediatrics, in 1983 explaining that they made decisions not to treat infants born with spina bifida based on both quality of life criteria and the resources available to families as well as from society (Gross et al., 1983). Contemporary discussions in the bioethical literature point out the lack of "benefit" for providing needed supports to individuals with cognitive disabilities (Buchanan and Brock, 1992; Walker et al., 1984; Hardwig, 1997). Individuals with cognitive or intellectual disabilities are no longer seen, according to this literature, as worthy of society's resources. The Australian ethicist Peter Singer has been calling into question the value of individuals with Down syndrome since 1979 (Singer, 1979; 1984; 1991; 2000). Long considered by many to be outside the mainstream of contemporary philosophy, Singer was recently appointed to an endowed chair at Princeton University.

This tension, then, will mark the early decades of the twenty-first century. Our response to it may very well determine whether continued commitment to individuals with these disabilities receives widespread support from elected and appointed officials as well as ordinary citizens across the country.

## BACKGROUND

In the early 1990s a small group of people in southeastern New Hampshire asked the following question: "What would the human service system for individuals with cognitive disabilities look like, how would it perform, if those with disabilities, their families and allies controlled the resources?" This fundamental attempt to both question the foundation for the current system and suggest a fundamental realignment of power and control arose from a systematic evaluation of policies and practices in what was arguably one of the finest systems in the United States. Visitors from across the country and from other lands came to Monadnock Developmental Services to observe. Group homes averaged fewer than three individuals. Everyone lived in the community. New Hampshire was touted for its efforts in supported employment. Nonetheless, this small group raised serious questions about just how far off the rhetoric of human services was from the reality of those being served.

People with disabilities were far from fully participating members of their communities. Few had any say about where or even with whom they would live. Average wages and hours in supported employment were close to negligible. Individual service plans focused on goals and activities not germane to a meaningful life in the community. Many individuals merely remained "supervised" during the day. Few had keys to their homes or ready access to transportation. In fact, some individuals were not safe. The current system had unintentionally relegated them to second-class citizenship.

On the basis of these analyses and the initial experience of what was later to be called "self-determination," the first monograph was produced calling for a fundamental overhaul in the system. Entitled "An Affirmation of Community: A Revolution of Vision and Goals" (Nerney and Crowley, 1993), it systematically laid out the vision necessary to meet the rhetorical goals of real community inclusion, real choice and freedom, and meaningful membership in one's community. The publication of this document was meant to articulate for all community members that individuals with disabilities in southeastern New Hampshire had a right to fully participate in society, not as clients of a human service system, but as ordinary citizens with the supports in place to help them accomplish these and other highly personal goals.

## THE "EXPERIMENT"

A demonstration involving 45 persons with disabilities, including those with very significant disabilities, was launched in 1993 with the assistance of a grant from the Robert Wood Johnson Foundation. In that grant request the authors stated that the present human service system was so ". . . outmoded, so disenfranchising and so costly that radical departures must be demonstrated and evaluated immediately." The simple premise was that as individuals and their allies gained control of the resources, quality would improve and costs would be better managed (Conroy, 1996).

Patty, a young lady with Down syndrome, was one of the early participants. Patty had an extraordinary personal relationship with two direct support workers who were about to be married. All three joined forces to buy a house together and create a new life in their community. Patty became involved with a town softball league as assistant manager and today lives in a home she now owns.

Sean lay in a coma for five years in a hospital and nursing home in a nearby state as a result of an acquired brain injury that occurred in high school. The professionals had given up on him after that length of time. His mom and dad wanted to bring him back to his home community. With fewer resources than the nursing home used for custodial care, Sean moved into his own home with support staff hired by his family and a budget developed by them. Sean's improvements have been slow but very noticeable. Today he frequently accompanies his parents on the lecture circuit.

Julie was in the last stages of a degenerative disease. She had no family involvement but did have some committed friends who all worked in the human service system. Her dream, they all knew from the years when she used speech, had been to move out of the group home and into her own place with staff who had exhibited real interest and love for Julie. With her individual budget completed, Julie moved to her own place and lives there today in defiance of her prognosis.

Cathy was a woman with very significant disabilities who was continually found to be unsafe in a variety of community placements. There was evidence of abuse. By researching her records and speaking carefully with family and others, it was discovered that she and her twin sister, who lived in another state, had long ago dreamed of living together. Typical human service systems neither recognized nor supported these arrangements. Soon, Cathy with her case manager got into a car and drove to a nearby state to the home of her sister. Funds from her budget had been used to make the house accessible, and her budget just happened to be enough to cover the lost salary her sister would experience from leaving her job as a nurse.

Individuals began to think of what has now become the hallmark of self-determination: looking at public dollars as an investment in the lives of individuals with disabilities. One-time investments and small, creative purchases were tried as well.

Ron was a middle-aged man who always wanted to get a job. Agencies had been paid for years to accomplish this task. One day a commitment of $500 was put on the table for *anyone* who could get Ron a job he liked. A few weeks later, a staff member from his group home came in to collect. Ron then demonstrated the power of small, creative purchases. He used $200 from his budget to help a local experimental theatre group rent space to practice. Ron became a member and today lives in a life-sharing arrangement with another member of the troupe.

Rethinking current expenditures, addressing system change issues, and listening more deeply to individuals with disabilities, family members, and close allies (including direct support staff) from both the human service system and the wider community became a new way of doing business. At the end of two years, the results were startling. Change was so positive that it was palpable and measurable. It was measured independently by a Robert Wood Johnson Foundation contract (Conroy, 1996). The costs for a few individuals went up because they had been so poorly served in the past. Many remained the same. Some decreased considerably. At the end of the "experiment" the annualized savings in this resource rich state amounted to $300,000.

This was an unusual experiment. For the first time individuals with disabilities were not asked to change. The "experiment" was on those who managed and worked in human services to see if *they* could change. The essential goal of self-determination had become clear. It was to change the human service system from one in which individuals gave up their freedom in favor of professionally directed services to one in which individuals could craft a meaningful and unique life deeply embedded in their communities.

## NATIONAL INITIATIVE

The Robert Wood Johnson Foundation then moved to set up a national program office at the University of New Hampshire and sent out a request for proposals (RFP) to increase the number of demonstration sites across the country. Five million dollars was made available for this effort. Thirty-five states and the District of Columbia responded—one of the largest state responses to an RFP in the history of the Foundation.

Nineteen states received grants ranging from $100,000 to $400,000. The following year another, smaller technical assistance fund allocated dollars to an additional 10 states. Interest in self-determination spread rapidly throughout the country and has been featured in countless meetings, trainings, and national and international self-determination conferences. In 1996 self-determination was articulated as a series of principles to give greater clarity to the demonstration sites and to keep the original vision alive:

*Freedom:* the ability for persons with a disability to choose where to live and with whom as well as to choose what important activities would be features of their lives.

*Authority:* the ability of a person with a disability to control necessary and sufficient resources with the assistance of valued friends, family, and allies. This would be accomplished with the development of a highly unique individual budget with the assistance of a fiscal intermediary to handle disbursement and tax and benefit issues.

*Support:* the creation of highly personal and unique support plans that reflected the dreams and ambitions of the person with a disability.

*Responsibility*: the mandate for the wise use of public dollars and for the ability of each person with a disability to contribute to the community (Nerney and Shumway, 1996).

Following the advice and input of the national self-advocacy organization SABE, the Center for Self-Determination added the following fifth principle in 2000:

*Confirmation*: recognition of the major role that individuals with disabilities must play in the redesign of the human service system and recognition of the importance of supporting the self-advocacy movement.

## EXPERIENCE OVER FIVE YEARS OF DEMONSTRATIONS

The demonstrations and pilots carried out in the ensuing five years ranged from small, local or county-based ones to statewide reform efforts. Some abandoned the goals of the initiative early on, all struggled with complex system issues, and, with small successes in a variety of urban and rural areas, some committed to real change in their systems to make self-determination a reality for all those served. These latter projects realized that this kind of system and cultural change would require many years to implement. Self-determination is an ongoing proposition in demonstrations large and small in over 30 states today.

Two relatively innovative assumptions began to undergird the self-determination movement for all individuals with disabilities. One is that all persons should "have their own place," and, two, that virtually all individuals can work in meaningful employment and/or produce income through the development of microenterprises. Individuals with disabilities may indeed want to live with another person, but that is always a freely chosen situation and one susceptible to renegotiation when necessary. More and more projects across the country are gradually changing the goal from "getting a job" to one of "producing income." This enables everyone to understand that there are many ways to secure employment or to start a very small business. In the future, if reform is to be successful, individuals within their budgets may (with assistance from a variety of sources) contract directly with employers for coworker support, transportation, and even training. Individual budgets then may also be used to help secure or pay down the cost of equipment necessary for a microenterprise (Nerney, 1998).

To accomplish the system changes necessary for successful self-determination, the following minimum structural changes must be implemented:

## INDIVIDUAL BUDGETS

Based on current best practice, individual budgets meet *ideal* requirements for self-determination when the budget is actually controlled by the person and their freely chosen allies. Public dollars are now seen as an ongoing investment in the person's life, and the obligation to be responsible as well as to contribute to one's community becomes part of the budget development. In many demonstrations these ideal standards are only partially reached, but this represents an important step in the right direction. This means that the following is in place:

## INDIVIDUALLY CREATED BUDGETS

The person with a disability and freely chosen family and friends create individual budgets. This includes the creation of unique line items that reflect the distinct dreams and ambitions of the person with a disability.

## AUTHORITY OVER PERSONNEL

Any person who works for the individual with a disability is hired and can be fired as well by that person with assistance when necessary. In fact, all employees and consultants work for the person and that person's social support network. Even if another organization assumes some legal responsibility, to become the employer of record, for example, all personnel and consultants work for the person with a disability.

## FLEXIBILITY

Within approved amounts, dollars can be reasonably moved from line item to line item as long as the essential supports are maintained. New line items may also be created as well as old ones being erased.

## INDEPENDENT SUPPORT COORDINATION

The linchpin to the success of creative, highly individual budgets and life plans is the function that is variously referred to as independent support coordination, "personal agents," or independent brokering. What is important with regard to this function is the potential for conflict of interest. This is a person who may help with plan development, assist in organizing the unique resources that a person needs, and even assist with ongoing evaluation of these supports. There are many ways that this function can be carried out, from family members doing it to case managers assuming new roles. In today's complex case management-dominated systems, there must be a retraining of case managers and, frequently, the addition of an independent broker as well. These brokers can be individuals who operate as independent contractors or an agency that specializes in providing only these kinds of individual supports. Ideally, individuals with disabilities and family members can govern these agencies. One creative project allows the person with a disability to select anyone they know and trust and to pay them separately if necessary. When ongoing and independent support coordination is also required, some individuals are including this cost in their individual budget because it can meet the test of a "service." The characteristics of an independent brokering function include the following.

## INDEPENDENCE FROM SERVICE PROVISION

It is important to keep this function separate from any form of service provision to avoid both the appearance and the reality of conflict of interest. Even those "brokers" who have great integrity should not be put in a position of divided loyalties. Current systems, which feature service provision and support coordination, may take years to accomplish the transition. Many individuals with disabilities and families have relationships and loyalties in place that must be respected while this transition proceeds.

## REAL AUTHORITY

Whether the person is an independent contractor or works for an independent agency, this function has to carry some state, county, or publicly sanctioned authority if he/she is to adequately represent the person with a disability. Again, it should be clear that the person who carries out this function works for the person with a disability.

## FISCAL INTERMEDIARIES

Fiscal intermediaries are simply organizations, places, really, where an individual budget gets "parked" or "banked." The functions carried out by a fiscal intermediary include, but are not limited to, check writing for all bills and personnel costs, tax withholding, and paying worker's compensation, health insurance, and other taxes and benefits that might be appropriate depending on the individual's budget. The fiscal intermediary works for the individual and remains accountable for ensuring compliance with all federal and state laws. In some localities, community banks are carrying out this function. New organizations are also springing up to provide this service. State-imposed Medicaid regulations frequently dictate which organizations or individuals can carry out this service. Minimum standards include the following.

## Individual Budget Isolation

This means that every person's individual budget is isolated from any other and certainly from traditional provider contracts. The money is available on receipt of an approved budget and is accounted for by the fiscal intermediary to the public funding authority as well as to the person with a disability.

## Free from Conflict of Interest

Fiscal intermediaries have no other duties that conflict with their role. This means that they are independent of service provision. If the fiscal intermediary is a government or quasi-government agency, there are specific rules that prohibit the use of this money for any other purpose. If a typical provider agency must perform this function, then that agency is prohibited from providing supports as well.

## Close to the Person and the Community

Fiscal intermediaries, to the extent possible, should be generic, neighborhood, community organizations that enable the person with a disability to create relationships with personnel who work there in regular community settings. The closer this function moves to a "neighborhood bank," the better for the person with a disability.

## IMPLICATIONS OF SELF-DETERMINATION

Self-determination requires that all of the assumptions and practices of the present system be thoroughly evaluated. It requires that a new analysis of the worth of current expenditures be made with the goal of increasing the value of those purchases. One of the results of this kind of analysis is the exposure of all of the unconscious assumptions that support the present service delivery system. These range from conflicts of interest over dollars spent (whose money is it, really?) to conflicts that assume incapacity and continued, almost total, dependence.

Conflicts of interest pervade the entire system from individual planning to state contracting provisions. Almost all of these revolve around the issue of ownership and traditional provider attitudes concerning their historical relationships with funding authorities. Individuals with disabilities become commodities in this arrangement. It is not unusual for the current system to place more emphasis on typical provider arrangements than on real freedom and choice for individuals with disabilities.

One of the major revelations of this kind of analysis is the pernicious effect of continued, enforced personal impoverishment of an entire group of individuals. The relationship between lack of real community participation and enduring relationships and personal poverty is an emerging issue in the self-determination movement. Freedom, without the means to exercise it, remains a hollow promise.

The arbitrary restrictions imposed by state policies and Medicaid waivers become clear when state Medicaid waiver implementation plans are examined. Despite an antiquated federal Medicaid statute, virtually all of the barriers to real implementation of self-determination remain state imposed. These include, among many others, arbitrary definitions of "qualified Medicaid provider" to burdensome regulations that define individual service plans as though the person with a disability had to remain in perpetual learning mode without ever experiencing the real world.

## AN AGENDA FOR THE FUTURE

Self-determination is still in its infancy. To grow and develop as the foundation for supporting individuals in the future, an ambitious policy agenda must be developed and carried out.

- The federal Medicaid statute that controls the majority of expenditures for long-term care in America must be revamped. This statute was enacted to provide medical care for indigent Americans and was amended many times to include, among other items, long-term care for the aging population as well as younger individuals with disabilities. This institutional bias is well known. However, the vast majority of younger individuals as well as older Americans with disabilities live in the community and intend to remain there. The institutional orientation continues to wag the community system. Additionally, the utter complexity of this system defies rational explanation and continues to withhold its mysteries from the very individuals who need most to understand it and change it: individuals with disabilities and their families.

- Quality assurance is still somewhat of an oxymoron in human services. Liability assurance has largely replaced any culturally sound notion of what constitutes "quality." Pretending that quality exists where there is no freedom is another indication of how paternalistic this system really is. In the future, individuals with disabilities, family members, and allies will largely determine what constitutes quality.

- Policy is largely developed in all 50 states and the District of Columbia without significant input from those most affected. In the future, all policy affecting individuals with disabilities and families must be developed in concert with them.

- The lack of equity in the present system remains largely unacknowl-edged. The distribution of public dollars across the country and even within individual states remains unfair and inequitable. Resources available to one person with a disability similar to another may vary by three or four hundred percent. Program models that feature con-gregation tend to be higher funded than those that emphasize indi-viduality. Massive waiting lists stand in silent judgment on the huge per-person expenditures in our public and private institutional system in most states. A more equitable system of allocating public dollars must be created.

- Poverty for those in the Medicaid system, both individuals with dis-abilities and direct support staff, is largely ignored. As the federal Medicaid statute gets re-evaluated, the time has come to create incentives for modest amounts of income for individuals with dis-abilities without jeopardizing essential benefits. A better fix between Supplemental Security Income (SSI), Social Security Disability Income (SSDI), and Medicaid must be developed that will encourage earnings and gradually reduce dependence on benefits only when income becomes significant enough. Recent federal legislation allow-ing states to dramatically allow significant earnings for those indi-viduals who have the ability to earn wages comparable to those without disabilities without losing Medicaid is an example. This kind of policy change needs to be brought to the population of individu-als who remain fiscally tied to SSI and SSDI.

- The crisis in hiring and retaining direct support workers is a direct result of low wages and lack of status for these individuals. New forms of compensation packages need to be piloted, and the status of these workers must be improved. Typical human service responses include "credentialing" and professionalizing these per-sonnel. This simply creates one more barrier between the person with a disability and the wider community, reinforcing the separa-tion from community so characteristic of contemporary human services.

- The imposition of guardianship, often accomplished to protect the person with a disability, results in loss of legal and ethical status. It not only labels the person as incompetent but frequently denies voting and marriage rights as well as depriving the person of the right to choose, with assistance when necessary, where and with whom that person will live. Moving from incompetence to "assisted competence" as a foundation for supporting individuals in decision making is more respectful and preserves citizenship as an inalienable right. A thorough review and recrafting of all guardianship statutes must be undertaken.

## NETWORK OF ADVOCATES AND ALLIES

As the self-determination movement grows from infancy to adulthood it will require nurturing by families and individuals with disabilities. Because self-determination is relatively new vis-à-vis the typical long-term care system, families may find it frustrating to access this new way of doing business. In some states like Michigan public policy has already been articulated and any individual or family who wants to secure an individual budget can do so. That said, as in most states, regional mental health boards are at various stages of implementation. In Ohio, 30 counties now offer some aspects of self-determination. In Hawaii, the only state with legislation that gives every eligible individual with a developmental disability the right to an individual budget, implementation is underway and the state is supportive of these efforts. The same is true in a host of other locations including Maryland, certain counties in Wisconsin and Minnesota, parts of New England, as well as certain sections of many other states including small demonstrations as well as larger ones.

To make information more accessible, create the opportunity to find out what is going on state by state, and foster dialogue among those interested, the Center for Self-Determination offers a website to allow family members and others to find out what they need to know and how to foster self-determination where they live (www.self-determination.com).

The Center is a place where individuals with disabilities, family members, and their allies can connect to support self-determination throughout their communities. In addition to this networking, the website will offer statewide summaries of activities, statistics and support for independent coordination and independent brokering, individual planning and budgeting, self advocacy, leadership, and other elements of self-determination as well as the opportunity to participate in learning activities. Through a broad network of members the Center offers training and technical assistance on all aspects of systems change and self-determination.

## A NEW LEGAL AND ETHICAL FOUNDATION

The current foundation for providing necessary resources for individuals with cognitive and intellectual disabilities is based on an ad hoc paternalistic notion that relies almost exclusively on appropriations on a state-by-state basis. Even when, rarely, resources are abundant, individuals with disabilities are expected to accept what is offered, surrender elementary freedoms, and, often, curtail burgeoning personal dreams and ambitions.

A new legal and ethical foundation based on equality and equal citizenship must be articulated in both law and legal policy. Only such a foundation will give rise to the broad support needed in the future, especially as utilitarian ethics move inexorably into public policy. Such a movement, founded on self-determination, will only succeed if it is led by individuals with disabilities and their close family and friends.

## REFERENCES

Buchanan AE, Brock DW (1992): Deciding For Others: The Ethics of Surrogate Decision Making. Cambridge University Press.

Conroy J (1996): Independent Evaluation of the Monadnock Self-Determination Demonstration. Ardmore, PA: Conroy Outcome Analysis.

Duff R, Campbell (1973)Moral and ethical dilemmas in the special care nursery. N Engl J Med 289:890.

Gross, Cox, Tatyrek, Pollay, Barnes (1983): Early management and decision making for the treatment of myelomeningocele. Pediatrics 72:450.

Hardwig J (1997): Is There a Duty to Die? Hastings Center Report 27, no 2

Nerney T, Crowley R (1993): An Affirmation of Community: A Revolution of Vision and Goals. University of New Hampshire, Institute on Disability.

Nerney T, Shumway D (1996): Beyond Managed Care, Vol. 1. University of New Hampshire, Institute on Disability.

Nerney T (1998): The Poverty of Human Services, University of New Hampshire, Institute on Disability.

Nerney (2002): Challenging incompetence. In: Self-Determination and Guardianship, University of New Hampshire, Institute on Disability. In Press.

Singer P (1983): Sanctity of Life or Quality of Life? Pediatrics 72:1.

Singer P (1979): Practical Ethics. Cambridge: Cambridge University Press.

Singer P (April 1991): On Being Silenced in Germany. The New York Review of Books.

Singer P (2000): Writings on an Ethical Life. New York, NY: The Ecco Press.

Walker, Feldman, Vohr, OH (1984): Pediatrics cost benefit analysis of neonatal intensive care for infants weighing less than 1000 grams at birth. Pediatrics 74:20.

# ECONOMIC INDEPENDENCE AND INCLUSION

## MICHAEL MORRIS

### INTRODUCTION

In the *Emerging Disability Policy Framework: A Guidepost for Analyzing Public Policy*,[1] Robert Silverstein, Director of the Center for the Study and Advancement of Disability Policy, provides an historical perspective on disability policy. Society has historically imposed attitudinal and institutional barriers that subject persons with disabilities to lives of unjust dependence, segregation, isolation, and exclusion. Attitudinal barriers are characterized by beliefs and sentiments held by nondisabled persons about persons with disabilities. Institutional barriers include policies, practices, and procedures adopted by entities such as employers, businesses, and public agencies.[2]

Sometimes, these attitudinal and institutional barriers are the result of deep-seated prejudice.[3] At times, these barriers result from decisions to follow the "old paradigm" of considering people with disabilities as

---

[1] Emerging Disability Policy Framework: A Guidepost for Analyzing Public Policy, 85 Iowa L. Rev. 1691 (2000); author: Robert Silverstein.
[2] *See* Americans with Disabilities Act of 1990 § 2(a), 42 U.S.C. § 12101(a) (1994) (listing congressional findings regarding Americans with disabilities); *see also* S. REP. NO. 101-116, at 5-20 (1989). Former Senator Lowell Weicker testified before Congress "that people with disabilities spend a lifetime 'overcoming not what God wrought but what man imposed by custom and law'." *Id.* at 11.
[3] S. REP. NO. 101-116, at 5-7.

---

*Down Syndrome*, Edited by William I. Cohen, Lynn Nadel, and Myra E. Madnick.
ISBN 0-471-41815-3   Copyright © 2002 by Wiley-Liss, Inc.

"defective" and in need of "fixing."[4] At other times, these barriers are the result of thoughtlessness, indifference, or lack of understanding.[5] It is often difficult, if not impossible, to ascertain precisely why the barriers exist.

In response to challenges by persons with disabilities, their families, and other advocates, our nation's policy makers have slowly begun to react over the past quarter of a century. They have begun to recognize the debilitating effects of these barriers on persons with disabilities and have rejected the "old paradigm."

A "new paradigm" of disability has emerged that considers disability as a natural and normal part of the human experience. Rather than focusing on "fixing" the individual, the "new paradigm" focuses on taking effective and meaningful actions to "fix" or modify the natural, constructed, cultural, and social environment. In other words, the focus of the "new paradigm" is on eliminating the attitudinal and institutional barriers that preclude persons with disabilities from fully participating in society's mainstream.

Aspects of the "new paradigm" were included in public policies enacted in the early 1970s.[6] Between the 1970s and 1990, lawmakers further defined society and further accepted the "new paradigm."[7] In 1990, the "new paradigm" was explicitly articulated in the landmark American with Disabilities Act (ADA)[8] and further refined in subsequent legislation.[9]

Despite changes in public policy, across this country, the typical working-age adult with a developmental disability is not employed, does not control an individual budget, does not choose who will provide supports

---

[4] *See* National Institute on Disability and Rehabilitation Research, 64 Fed. Reg. 68,576 (1999) (providing notice for the final long-range plan for fiscal years 1999-2003 and explaining that the new paradigm of disability is an expectation for the future).

[5] S. Rep. No. 101-116, at 5-7.

[6] *See* Education for All Handicapped Children Act of 1975, Pub. L. No. 94-142, 89 Stat. 773 (adding Part B to the Individuals with Disabilities Education Act, 20 U.S.C. ch. 33 (1994)). *See also* Rehabilitation Act of 1973, 29 U.S.C. ch. 16 (1994).

[7] Fair Housing Amendments Act of 1988, Pub. L. No. 100-430, 102 Stat. 1619; Developmental Disabilities Assistance and Bill of Rights Act Amendments of 1987, Pub. L. No. 100-146, 101 Stat. 840; Air Carrier Access Act of 1986, Pub. L. No. 99-435, 100 Stat. 1080; Rehabilitation Act Amendments of 1986, Pub. L. No. 99-506, 100 Stat. 1807; Education of the Handicapped Act Amendments of 1986, Pub. L. No. 99-457, 100 Stat. 1145.

[8] 42 U.S.C. ch. 126 (1994). President Bush signed the ADA into law on July 26, 1990. *Id.* Senator Tom Harkin (D. Iowa), the chief sponsor of the ADA, often refers to the legislation as the "20th century Emancipation Proclamation for persons with disabilities." 136 Cong. Rec. S9689 (daily ed. July 13, 1990).

[9] Ticket to Work and Work Incentives Improvement Act of 1999, Pub. L. No. 106-170, 113 Stat. 1860; Individuals with Disabilities Education Act Amendments of 1997, Pub. L. No. 105-17, 111 Stat. 37; Developmental Disabilities Assistance and Bill of Rights Act Amendments of 1994, Pub. L. No. 103-230, 108 Stat. 284; Rehabilitation Act Amendments of 1992, Pub. L. No. 102-569, 106 Stat. 4344.

and services for his/her benefit, and does not have access to all the information needed to consider ways to become more socially and economically independent.[10] An individual with a developmental disability is three times more likely to be in a sheltered workshop earning less than minimum wage or in a day activity program than earning better than minimum wage in a supported or competitive employment setting. Since 1975, children with disabilities have benefited from a "free appropriate public education" that must be tailored to individual needs. There is no corresponding entitlement to service and support for adults with disabilities. The world of adult services and the transition from school to work is to many families a bewildering maze of funding streams, differing rules of eligibility, and confusing rules of coverage and support. The purpose of this article is to share a conceptual framework to address these issues and to help accelerate participation in systems change activities that promote self-determination, economic independence, and inclusion.

## VALUES

A conceptual framework for economic independence and inclusion must be anchored by the values articulated in the Developmental Disabilities Act, which include:

- respect for individual capabilities and competencies;
- informed choice and decision making; and
- services, supports, and other assistance provided in a manner that demonstrates "respect for individual dignity, personal preferences, and cultural differences."[11]

Section 101(a) of the Developmental Disabilities Act clearly states that disability "is a natural part of the human experience" that does not diminish the right of individuals with developmental disabilities to "enjoy self-determination, make choices and experience full integration and inclusion in the economic, political and social mainstream of society."[12] Section 101(c) of the Act goes on to further state that individuals with developmental disabilities and their families are the *primary decision makers* regarding "the

[10] National Council on Disability. National Disability Policy: A Progress Report. (11/99-11/00) (In 1999, unemployment rate for people with disabilities exceeded 70%). *See also* Butterworth, J. and Kiernan, W. State Trends in Employment Services for People with Disabilities. Boston: Institute for Community Inclusion (1999); Nerney, T. "The Poverty of Human Service." *www.self-determination.com* ("almost 75% of people with disabilities remain unemployed today in an economy that has seen unemployment plummet for all other workers").

[11] Developmental Disabilities Act of 1984 (P.L. 98-527) (§101 (c)).

[12] Developmental Disabilities Act of 1984 (P.L. 98-527) (§101 (a)).

services and supports they receive . . . that responds to personal goals, and unique strengths and capabilities."[13]

A review and analysis of some 20 federal- and state-funded model programs and/or systems that have supported individuals with developmental disabilities in securing and retaining jobs in diverse business sectors has as a common operational philosophy the value of individual choice and self-determination. Although there is no definition of choice in the Rehabilitation Act or the Developmental Disabilities Act, Michael Collins, former Director of the Vermont Choice Project funded by the Rehabilitation Services Administration, breaks down the essential elements of "choice" into six components:

1. choice of actual services needed to reach the consumer's vocational goal;
2. choice of who will provide those services;
3. choice of how the services will be purchased and delivered;
4. a clear description of the components of the decision making process that takes into account individual values and cultural differences;
5. gathering and understanding information, active involvement in decision making, and following through with decision; and
6. active involvement in the negotiation and purchase of needed services including management of an individual budget.[14]

Thus a conceptual framework for an economic independence and inclusion ($EI^2$) model must start with a statement of values that defines the underlying program philosophy of consumer choice and control. As stated in the Vermont Self-Determination Project Mission Statement: "All people with developmental disabilities have the right to take control over their own lives and future." Thus the $EI^2$ model blends the lessons learned from a cadre of public and private self-determination initiatives nationwide with the best practices experiences and research findings of supported employment over the past 15 years.

The values foundation is also based on the following eight principles to guide decision making developed by Dakota County, Minnesota:

---

[13] Developmental Disabilities Act of 1984 (P.L. 98-527) (§101 (c)) (emphasis added).

[14] Collins, M. The Vermont Welfare-to-Work "Work First" Project. Burlington: University of Vermont Press (1999). Expanding on Collins' definition of choice, Michael Callahan advocates that "customers not only make individualized choices concerning their employment goals, the types of services received and the providers of those services, but that those choices . . . meet a higher standard—that is 'informed' choice." Callahan, M. "Advice, Information and Choice, Helping People to Become Informed and to Make Effective Decisions Concerning Employment" (1997).

1. **Relationship Principle:** People are able to plan with and be supported by those who know and care about them. Relationships provide the context for all of the other principles.

2. **Control and Authority Principle:** People are able to have authority over and control of the resources available for their support.

3. **Responsibility Principle:** People are able to take responsibility for their own support and well-being.

4. **Equity Principle:** People with similar needs have similar financial resources with which to obtain their support.

5. **Flexibility Principle:** People are able to design support in ways that best meet their needs.

6. **Health and Safety Principle:** Health and safety parameters are created within an individual context of reasonable risk and responsibility.

7. **Simplicity Principle:** Rules, regulations and funding streams are understandable to those who receive support from service systems.

8. **Information Principle:** Rules, regulations, and funding streams will address how people are informed about the contents therein.[15]

## CRITICAL DESIGN ELEMENTS OF THE FRAMEWORK

In addition to a solid values foundation, a conceptual model for economic independence and inclusion requires major changes in the relationship among public funder, providers, and the individual consumer of support and services. Such a framework must be able to operationalize the values foundation of informed choice, individual direction of resources, and respect for personal preferences and cultural differences in a way that is *flexible, supports existing and new relationships*, is *individualized and individually driven*, is *culturally competent* and is *outcome driven*. These characteristics comprise the critical design elements of a conceptual framework and can be defined as follows:

## FLEXIBLE AND ACCOUNTABLE

The framework must be flexible to respect individual differences and personal preferences.[16] The individual with a developmental disability has

---

[15] Dakota County Self-Determination Project, "Principles to Guide Decision-Making."

[16] Callahan, M.; Garner, B. Keys to the Workplace. (1999). *See also* Callahan, M. Final Report (UCPA's three-year demonstration project on supported employment) (1991); Brooke, V; Inge, K; Armstrong, A; Wehman, P. Supported Employment Handbook: A Customer-Driven Approach for Persons with Significant Disabilities (1997); Wehman, P; Revell, WG; Kregel, J. Supported Employment from 1986–1993: A National Program That Works (1995);

lifelong needs and requires supports that must respond regularly and be funded by multiple payers. Traditional funders must blend their public resources to flexibly meet the individualized needs of the consumer.[17] Accountability is based on the economic outcomes that define performance. Resources must be coordinated across traditional funding streams to achieve mutually beneficial outcomes for the individual, the microenterprise, the employer, and/or the community.[18]

## SUPPORTS EXISTING AND NEW RELATIONSHIPS

The individual with a developmental disability is free to choose who will assist him or her and to negotiate the terms of the relationship.[19] From natural supports in a workplace to new negotiated relationships with an employer, a job coach, a personal assistant, or a driver, the individual determines need and negotiates cost of the identified support.[20] Consumers have

Hammis, D; Griffin C. Employment for Anyone, Anywhere, anytime: Creating New Employment Options Through Supported Employment and Supported Self-Employment (1998); Arnold, N (ed.). Self-employment in Vocational Rehabilitation: Building on Lessons from Rural America (1996); Griffin, C. Rural Routes: Promising Supported employment practices in America's frontier (In press). The Monograph of the National Supported Employment Consortium (1999).

[17] See Dane County Department of Human Services. "Forging a Partnership: Individualizing Funding and Increasing Choices for People with Developmental Disabilities in Dane County Wisconsin" at 2 (1998). See also Callahan, M. Final Report: UCPA's Choice Access Project (1999); Cooper, A. Final Report: PEP Project. Seattle: Washington State Vocational Rehabilitation (1999); Skiba, J. Reaching the door to employment; Is it really open? Journal of Vocational Rehabilitation (in press) (2000); Callahan, M. Personal Budgets: The future of funding. Journal of Vocational Rehabilitation (in press) (2000).

[18] Butterworth, J. and Kiernan, W. State Trends in Employment Services for People with Disabilities. Boston: Institute for Community Inclusion. (1999). See also Griffin, C; Hammis, D. Streetwise Guide to Person-Centered Planning (1996); Griffin, C; Flaherty, M; Kriskovich, B; Shelley, R; Hammis, D; Katy, M. Bringing Home the Bacon: Inventive Self-Employment in rural America. Missoula: The Rural Institute (1999); Unger, D; Parent, W; Gibson, K; Kane-Johnston, K; Kregel, J. An Analysis of the Activities of the Employment Specialist in a Natural Support Approach To Supported Employment. (2000). Available at *www.worksupport.com*; Callahan, M. Common sense and quality: meaningful employment outcomes for persons with severe physical disabilities. Journal of Vocational Rehabilitation, 1(2) 21–28 (1991); Wehman, P; Kregel, J. At the crossroads: Supported employment a decade later. Journal of the Association for Persons with Severe Handicaps, 20(4) 286–299 (1995); Wehman, P; Kregel, J. More Than A Job. Baltimore: Paul H. Brookes Publishing. (1998); Brooke, V; Inge, K; Armstrong, A; Wehman, P. Supported Employment Handbook: A Customer-Driven Approach for Persons with Significant Disabilities. Richmond: VCU (1997).

[19] See, e.g.,Callahan, M; Garner, B. "Keys to the Workplace" (1999); Callahan, M. Final Report: UCPA's Choice Access Project (1999); Cooper, A. Final Report: PEP Project (1999).

[20] Wehman, P; Kregel, J. "At The Crossroads: Supported Employment a Decade Later." Journal of the Association for Persons with Severe Handicaps 20(4) 286–299 (1995).

direct relationships with their support providers, not with a third-party provider.[21]

## Individualized and Individually Driven

A person-centered plan defines economic goals based on consumer preferences and direction.[22] The consumer determines who is invited to be involved in the planning process. The plan presumes that the consumer is able to work.[23] Each person's individual budget is unbundled from other traditional provider contracts. The critical notion of ownership must be part of the plan development. Therefore, the individual with the developmental disability must decide and direct a) individual employment goals, b) the need for supports, c) how service needs are to be addressed, d) how providers are to be selected, e) how services are to be delivered, f) payments based on mutually agreed outcomes, g) how and when payment will be made, and h) how to resolve differences.[24]

## Culturally Competent

The system, agency, or professionals that provide services and supports have integrated and transformed what they know about individuals and groups of people into specific standards, policies, practices, and attitudes to

[21] Hagner, D. and DiLeo, D. *Working Together: Workplace Culture, Supported Employment and People with Disabilities.* Cambridge: Brookline Books. (1993). *See also* Bradley, VJ; Ashbaugh, JW; Blaney, BC. *Creating individual supports for people with developmental disabilities: A mandate for change at many levels.* Baltimore: Paul H. Brookes. (1994); Pearpoint, J; O'Brien, J; Forest, M. *PATH: A workbook for planning positive personal futures.* Toronto, Canada: Inclusion Press (1993); Perske, R. Circle of Friends: People with disabilities and their friends enrich the lives of others. Nashville: Abington Press (1989); Amado, AN. Friendships and community connections between people with and without developmental disabilities. Baltimore: Paul H. Brookes Publishing; Callahan, M. DOL- One Stop to success. Monograph. Gautier, MS. (2000).

[22] *See,* e.g., Callahan, M. Final Report: UCPA's Choice Access Project (1999); Cooper, A. Final Report: PEP Project (1999); Wehman, P; Kregel, J. "More Than A Job" (1998); Pearpoint, J; O'Brien, J; Forest, M. PATH: A Workbook for Planning Positive Personal Futures (1993); Perske, R. Circle of Friends: People with Disabilities and Their Friends Enrich the Lives of Others (1989).

[23] Wehman, P; Kregel, J. "At the Crossroads: Supported Employment A Decade Later." Journal of the Association for Persons with Severe Handicaps 20(4) 286–299 (1995); Callahan, M. Final Report (1991) (UCPA's three-year demonstration project on supported employment); Wehman, P; Revell, WG; Kregel, J. Supported Employment from 1986–1993: A National Program That Works (1995).

[24] Callahan, M; Garner, B. "Keys to the Workplace" (1999); Brooke, V; Inge, K; Armstrong, A; Wehman, P. Supported Employment Handbook: A Customer-Driven Approach for Persons with Significant Disabilities (1997); Skiba, J. "Reaching the Door to Employment: Is It Really Open?" Journal of Vocational Rehabilitation (in press) (2000); Callahan, M; Collins, M. and Cooper, A. "Advice, Information, and Choice." Washington, DC: United Cerebral Palsy Association (1997).

be used in specific cultural settings to increase the quality of services and produce better outcomes.[25] Four essential elements of such a system are a) value diversity, b) the capacity for cultural self-assessment, c) a consciousness of the dynamics inherent when cultures interact, and d) service delivery that is flexible and adaptable to reflect an understanding of cultural particularities.[26]

## Outcome Driven

Economic independence as an outcome must be achieved by earning more than minimum wage. It must be more broadly defined to include producing income from self-employment, sharing in the ownership of a business, and a change in status from an employee to employer. Self-employment is a viable vocational outcome in addition to other supported and competitive employment options.[27]

## Systems Design

The fundamental question for those concerned with high-quality services for people with significant disabilities is, How can we use our resources to assist the people who rely on us to live better lives as defined by increasing economic independence and inclusion? The answer lies in a test of leadership at the individual, family, community, and systems levels. Leadership is achieved when people mobilize their resources to make progress on difficult problems.

[25] Callahan, M. "Personal Budgets: The Future of Funding." Journal of Vocational Rehabilitation (in press) (2000); Callahan, M. "Common Sense and Quality: Meaningful Employment Outcomes for Persons with Severe Physical Disabilities." Journal of Vocational Rehabilitation (2) 21–28 (1991). See Kielson, J. "General Policy and Procedure for Family Governing Boards-DRAFT." (Guidelines for empowering cultural minority groups through family governing boards in Boston Metro Region); Massachusetts Metro Region Self-Determination Project.

[26] Isaacs, M; Benjamin, M. Towards a Cultural Competent System of Care (vol. II) (1991); Freedman, R; Fesko, S. "The Meaning of Work in the Lives of People with Significant Disabilities: Consumer and Family Perspectives." Journal of Rehabilitation 49-55 (1996); Levatt, S; Hueneman, J; Zukas, H. "Attending to America" (Monograph) Berkeley, CA: World Institute on Disability (1987); Russell, M; Toy, A; Malone, B. "A Community Divided." New Mobility Magazine (1996).

[27] Wehman, P; Kregel, J; Shofer, M. "Emerging Trends in the National Supported Employment Initiative: A Preliminary Analysis of Twenty-Seven States" Richmond: Rehabilitative Research and Training Center (1989); Seekins, T. "Rural Economic Development and Vocational Rehabilitation: Lessons From Analyses of Self Employment as a Vocational Outcome." On-line: *http://ruralinstitute.umt.edu/rtcrural/RuEcD/Switzer.htm*. Parent, W. Consumer Satisfaction and Choice at the Workplace: A Survey of Individuals with Severe Disabilities Who Receive Supported Employment Services. Richmond: VCU (1994).

Traditionally, human services have been managed as though they were factories, producing relationships that are ordered and in which bureaucratic authority structures and standardization are expected to produce reliable outcomes. However, in his article, "Discovering Community Living: Learning from Innovations in Services to People with Mental Retardation," John O'Brien concludes that "community cannot be manufactured; it is not a commodity or the reliable outcome of any professional activity. It arises when valued personal involvements with a network of others give rise to purposeful action and celebration."[28] The proposed EI$^2$ model seeks to move service delivery toward meaningful personal involvements with a focus on individual choice and direction. It represents a fundamental shift in the relationships among funder, provider, and consumer.

From an individual, family, and community perspective, six key systems are built on the values foundation of consumer choice and control.

## LEGAL AND POLICY STRUCTURE

With significant public policy developments at the federal level in the past five years (welfare reform, workforce development system, ticket to work, and work incentives), there is an unprecedented opportunity for new approaches to service delivery, interagency coordination, and blending of resources to support individualized, person-centered plans.

The policy framework to support the EI$^2$ model cuts across typical jurisdictional lines at federal and state levels. Policy and funding streams impacted include:

- Social Security and Supplemental Security Income (SSI) and (SSDI);
- Medicaid (ICF/MR and Home and Community-Based Waivers);
- Workforce development system and one-stop centers;
- Vocational rehabilitation and short-term interventions;
- Transition planning and the Individual with Disabilities Education Act (IDEA);
- Work incentives and the interrelationship among SSI, SSDI, and accessible health care.

No single federal agency has management authority over all of these policy and funding streams, and no single congressional committee has full authority and oversight over the full complement of effected policies. The new approach fostered by the EI$^2$ equation will need to embrace six critical shifts in current decision making:

[28] O'Brien, J. "Discovering Community Living: Learning from Innovators in Services to People with Mental Retardation." at 4 (1987).

1. All individuals with developmental disabilities (age 18–65)[29] are capable of work and/or production of income regardless of the nature or severity of disabilities.

2. Social Security and related Medicaid policies must shift determination of eligibility from an "inability to work" to "the level of supports needed to work and/or produce income."

3. Asset and resource limits that are now part of the eligibility requirements for Social Security maintenance payments (SSI, SSDI) must be significantly altered to encourage asset accumulation and a goal of self-sufficiency instead of forcing individuals to remain stuck at the poverty level to keep public benefits.

4. There must be incentives to work and/or produce income that encourage individual and employer risk-taking that is perceived as more valuable by the individual than remaining on public benefits.

5. There must be incentives for agency administrators, providers, and employers to pursue public-private sector partnerships and interagency collaboration (federal to state, state to local, and local to local agencies) that blend traditional lines of separate funding into a unified support plan customized to individual identified needs.

6. Direction of public resources blended into an individualized budget and person-centered plan must be led by the consumer.

## HUMAN RESOURCES

Under the proposed framework, persons with disabilities will receive consumer-directed services that meet their unique needs and preferences as specified in an individual service or personal support plan. The person or entity that delivers the services will not be limited to existing human service providers or traditional agencies. The person who will receive the services will select and direct the agent. Thus a friend, family member, employer, self-employed independent contractor, group, or organization may provide the consumer-chosen services. The role of the professional, then, must change from one of planning and making judgments to one of helping people understand a range of choices that match their personal preferences. The professional must shift his or her thinking and practices, renouncing his or her power over others. As a result, the new framework will increase the demand for employment specialists, job coaches, and individuals who can assist individuals explore self-employment options. Additionally, the framework will require new sustained approaches to expand the available pool of skilled

---

[29] *See* n. 34 herein. (successful employment facilitated by high school to work transition programs starting as early as age 14.)

individuals to implement community-support plans. It is likely that these individuals may not have skills that match any current, single-discipline, and professional training.

## Funding Mechanisms

Researchers have found there is no single funding stream that makes the EI$^2$ model feasible. In the case studies reviewed, individually directed budgets have relied on a flexible blending of multiple funding streams to include local tax dollars, federal Medicaid funds, and in the future, social security, labor, education, and rehabilitation funds. Several states have paved the way for a broader scope of Medicaid coverage to promote increased consumer control over resources, services, and supports funded by the Home and Community-Based Waivers. For example, the Wisconsin and Minnesota approaches to person-centered and directed community supports rely on a more flexible use of Medicaid Waiver funding and, therefore, provide critical foundations to the EI$^2$ model.

THE MINNESOTA MODEL. The Minnesota Department of Human Services received approval from the Health Care Finance Administration for amendments to their state Home and Community-Based Services Waiver Plan for Persons with Mental Retardation and Related Conditions.[30] A new set of guidelines was issued at a state level for the local county-based system of management of Waiver funds.[31] The guidelines explain that the new service options include consumer-directed community support services[32] and consumer training and education services.[33] The new services do not require licensing under Minnesota state law.[34] As a result, new providers will not need to be licensed.[35] Providers must be able to meet the service needs as documented in an individual service plan.[36]

THE WISCONSIN MODEL. Similarly, in Wisconsin, the local agency must have a memorandum of understanding with the state agency to demonstrate feasibility of a consumer-directed community support approach.[37] The local plan will:

[30] Minnesota FY 1998-2002 MR/RC Waiver Plan Minnesota Statutes, section 256B.092; Minnesota Rules parts 9525.1800-9525.1930 (hereafter "Minnesota MR/RC Waiver Plan").
[31] Minnesota Department of Human Services, "New Services Available Through the MR/RC Waiver." (July 1998) (hereafter "Minnesota MR/RC Waiver Guidelines").
[32] Developmental Disabilities Act of 1984 (P.L. 98-527) (§3-5).
[33] Developmental Disabilities Act of 1984 (P.L. 98-527) (§7-9).
[34] Minnesota MR/RC Waiver Plan. "New Services Implication."
[35] Developmental Disabilities Act of 1984 (P.L. 98-527)
[36] Minnesota MR/RC Waiver Guidelines at 4-5; 7.
[37] Amendment to Wisconsin's Home and Community Based Services Waiver (Section 0275.90) at 23o (May 1998).

1. Specify how consumers, families and other natural supports were involved in developing the plan and will be involved in ongoing oversight of the plan.

2. Specify how the local agency will provide information about consumer-directed support options to consumers, families, and other natural supports, guardians, and providers.

3. Specify how participating consumers and their families, guardians, and other natural supports will be supported: to know their rights as citizens and consumers, to learn about the methods provided by the consumer-directed supports plan to take greater control of decision-making, and to develop skills to be more effective in identifying and implementing personal goals.

4. Establish support for development of person-centered support plans that are based on individual goals and preferences and that allow the person with a disability to live in the community, establish meaningful community associations, and make valued contributions to his/her community.

5. Provide for mechanisms for consultation, problem solving, technical assistance, and financial management assistance to assist consumers in accessing and developing the desired support(s) and to assist in securing administrative and financial management assistance to implement the support(s).

6. Establish a mechanism for allocating resources to individuals for the purpose of purchasing consumer-directed community support services based on identified factors. These factors may include the person's functional skills, his/her environment, the supports available to the person, and the specialized support needs of the person.

7. Describe how the local agency will promote use of informal and generic sources of support.

8. Describe how the county will promote availability of a flexible array of services that is able to provide supports to meet identified needs and that is able to provide consumer choice as to nature, level, and location of services.

9. Describe how the local agency will ensure that consumer-directed community supports meet the person's health and safety needs.

10. Provide for outcome-based quality assurance methods.[38]

---

[38] Amendment to Wisconsin's Home and Community Based Services Waiver (Section 0275.90) at 23o–23p (May 1998).

The EI$^2$ model will increase collaboration at a local level among generic workforce development providers, vocational rehabilitation and education agencies, as well as state Medicaid and mental retardation and developmental disabilities agencies. These collaborations offer a new approach, one that supports individually directed budgets that define specific economic goals to produce income or become employed in a work setting that matches ability, interests, and personal preferences.

## Organizational Design

Model programs studied support three critical organizational elements:

1. Individual directed budget: With a presumption of a goal to produce income or become employed with the objective of enhanced economic self-sufficiency.

2. Independent support coordination: An individual or agency helps with plan development, organizing of resources needed, and evaluation of supports being provided. Such an individual or entity should be free of conflict of interest and should not provide the direct supports needed.[39]

3. Independent fiduciary agent: To oversee the management of public dollars. Public dollars are an investment in future independence and inclusion. The management of those public resources by an individual or entity must also be free of any potential conflict of interest.[40] The amount of resources expended per individual budget must be governed by the principles of equity and fairness. Accountability must result from a fee-for-service negotiated on the basis of competitive market forces and the achievement of agreed-to outcomes and milestones.

The following chart contrasts the traditional conceptual framework with the proposed EI$^2$ model:

---

[39] *See*, e.g., Wisconsin Self-Determination Learning Project (Dane County) (support brokers independent of both the county and service providers); Self-Determination Resources, Inc. (Portland, OR), (a consumer-directed, independent support brokerage); Human Services Research Institute (HSRI), The Robert Wood Johnson Foundation Self-Determination Initiative-Year One Impact Assessment Report (1999) (32.3% of sites surveyed offered independent support brokerage); Nerney, T. "Communicating Self-Determination: Freedom, Authority, Support and Responsibility" *www.self-determination.com* ("the linchpin to the success of . . . individual budgets . . . is . . . independent support coordination").

[40] Approximately 23% of sites surveyed by HSRI had created an independent fiscal intermediary. HSRI report at 39-40. Hawaii and Oregon are two sites specifically identified as having established a new and independent entity to serve in this capacity. Id at 39.

| | Traditional Framework | Proposed EI² Model |
|---|---|---|
| 1. | Professional-driven decision making | Informed choice and customer-directed |
| 2. | Process driven | Outcomes driven |
| 3. | Fee for service | Outcomes-based reimbursement |
| 4. | Provider-controlled funding | Consumer-controlled funding |
| 5. | Individualized plan for supports with limited expectation of employment outcome | Individualized plan with presumption of possibilities of employment outcome |
| 6. | Provider-controlled planning process based on available options | Person-centered and controlled planning process based on abilities, interests, and personal preferences |
| 7. | Agency/vendor/provider contracts | Individualized budgets controlled and directed by consumer |
| 8. | Case management | Independent service brokers |
| 9. | Provider-controlled funds | Independent fiduciary manager |
| 10. | Day activity, sheltered or supported employment options | Self-employment options added as alternative |
| 11. | Provider and public agency limitations on service and support options | Consumer-directed selection of providers and use of natural supports |
| 12. | Public agency rate setting | Consumer-directed and negotiated rate setting within limits of individualized budgets |
| 13. | Public agency-controlled hiring and firing of providers | Consumer-directed and control of hiring and firing of providers |
| 14. | Accountability focused on health and safety | Accountability driven by employment and revenue generation outcomes and customer satisfaction |
| 15. | A service philosophy | Commitment to self-determination PRINCIPLES |

## THE EMPLOYMENT PROCESS[41]

The conceptual framework also incorporates a process that has been refined during the past 15 years through supported employment, choice demon-

[41] As discussed herein, the focus of the Conceptual Framework is working-aged adults with developmental disabilities. However, a successful employment process for adults is clearly facilitated by high school-to-work transition programs that provide education and training and create career opportunities for students with developmental disabilities. Office of Inspector General, "Employment Programs for persons with Developmental Disabilities" Report # 0EI-

strations, and the use of natural supports for successful employment of individuals with disabilities.[42] The proposed process incorporates five core employment services:

1. a person-centered planning process called the *vocational profile*;
2. a meeting that links planning with job development called the *profile meeting*;
3. *individualized job development* that targets the type of job that the individual wants;
4. *a job/technology analysis* of the employment site and specific responsibilities; and
5. *an employer-directed support plan* that provides the individual with all the support he or she needs to successfully perform the job.[43]

For individuals who choose self-employment possibilities, the vocational profile provides an alternative course to move from an idea or concept to business plan development. The vocational profile begins with an expectancy of job placement or self-employment that builds on individual strengths, personal preferences, and individual and community natural supports already in place. There is a presumption that anyone who wishes to work can work. The profile moves away from traditional assessment models of standardized tests and time and productivity studies of ability to work. Through observation and structured interviews with the individual and others who know the individual, an individually selected employment specialist will capture the family support available, a description of typical

07-98-00260 (August 1999). *See* Coller-Klingenberg, Lana. "The Reality of Best Practices in Transition: A Case Study" 65 Exceptional Children at 67 (1998)("professional literature emphasizes the importance of transition planning and instruction"). Starting early increases the flexibility and options available to students and offers a larger variety of possible future career paths. Kiernan, W. "Moving On: Planning for the Future. On-line. www.childrenshospital.org. (transition process ideally should start at age 14). The concept of person-centered and person-directed planning is equally successful in transition programs. Id. *See also* Missouri Transition Alliance Partnership et al. "Fundamentals of Transition" On-line. www.coe.missouri.edu/mocise/pubs/fortrans/toc. htm#ack; Natural Transition Alliance. "NTA Transition Practices Framework—Categories, Elements, Practices." On-line. www.ed.edu/sped/pdk/categories.htm. *See also* Luecking, R; and Tilson, G. "Best and Effective Practices in School-to-Work Transition for Youths with Disabilities." Online.www.doe.state.de.us/exceptionalchild/tgmpublications.htm.

[42] Mank, D; Cioffi, A; and Yovanoff, P. The Consequences of Compromise: An Analysis of Natural Supports, Features of Supported Employment Jobs and Their Relationship to Wage and Integration Outcomes. Indiana: University of Indiana Press, 1996. Hagner, D; and DiLeo, D. Working Together: Workplace Culture, Supported Employment and People with Disabilities. Cambridge: Brookline Books, 1993. Callahan, M; Collins, M; and Cooper, A. *Advice*, Information, and Choice. Washington, DC: United Cerebral Palsy Association, 1997.

[43] Callahan, M. Garner, B. "Keys to the Workplace" (1999).

routines, friends, and social relationships, a description of the neighborhood, transportation available, employment options near home, work history, present activity levels, and interests, potential connections to employers, potential needs for flexibility or supports in the workplace, and other information that may be helpful. The profile should be written in positive language that reflects the individual's perspective.

After the development of the profile, a profile meeting should be held. Meeting attendance should include friends, family members, and others selected by the individual. The purpose of the meeting is to set out the future plan of action for job development or self-employment opportunities. The discussion includes perceived components of an ideal job, where such a job is found, and places the individual wants to avoid. The result of the discussion will be the development of a checklist of conditions, preferences, and contributions from which the individual can evaluate any job possibility found by the employment specialist.

A similar approach will be taken with ideas for producing income and self-employment. The job development and/or self-employment interests would form the basis for a prospecting list that details types of jobs and/or activities that could produce income. The outcome from the vocational meeting is a blueprint of the preferred kind of work/activity and a prospect list of employers who will be contacted.

The third critical step is individualized job development. Rather than calling on random employers to see whether a job exists, employment specialists target employers identified during the profile meeting and relate to them the individual's potential contributions. The $EI^2$ model proposes that the employment specialist be paid based on an outcome-based reimbursement system that rewards for timely performance. Payment for an acceptable job match within 60 days would be double that for similar results in 120 days.

A job development process includes an evaluation of work site quality. This evaluation will include the following factors:

1. interactions available with coworkers
2. wages
3. benefits
4. working conditions
5. terms of employment
6. any unique enhancing features
7. internal training and support
8. transportation availability
9. employer reputation
10. turnover rate

Before the individual with a disability starts a job, the job/technology analysis will be completed that will include identification of core and job-related routines, an explicit list of employer expectations, observations of the job performed by others, physical and communication demands, academic demands (reading, math, writing skills), work pace, possible natural informal and formal workplace supports, potential for use of adaptations or modifications in the work site, willingness of coworkers and/or supervisors to provide support and assistance, and any possible leaders or allies in the workforce.

The final key element is an employer-directed support plan. The plan is employer directed because the individual with a disability works for the employer, not a nonprofit service provider. The plan is signed by the employer and employee and details specific supports, who will provide them, how they will be provided, for what time period, and the estimated costs. The plan is reviewed weekly during the first month of employment and monthly thereafter. Changes are negotiated per discussion with employer and employee as well as support providers. The identification, negotiation, and refinement of supports needed and the provision of the supports by individual(s), agencies, coworkers, or others are critical elements of employment success.[44] As defined by Wehman, Revel, and Kregel in *An Analysis of the Activities of Employment Specialists in a Natural Support Approach to Supported Employment*, individual support needs are considered to include any type of assistance required or desired that aids or facilitates participation in the community and workplace environment of his or her choice. In ADD-funded Projects of National Significance to test and learn from natural support interventions in the workplace, over 57 different support needs were identified. These were broken into six categories: 1) finding a job, 2) assistance with completing the job tasks, 3) learning the job, 4) addressing other work-related issues, 5) addressing non-work-related issues, and 6) transportation.[45]

The proposed $EI^2$ model offers a conceptual framework in which the individual consumer directs an array of services and support that must be invented rather than simply selected from a menu of proven solutions. Whether the goal is supported employment or self-employment, the planning process is person centered and -directed and responsive to personal preferences. Resources and supports are configured to match individual needs and interests.

Support coordination must be independent of a fiduciary agent to avoid potential conflict of interest in the choice of provider or the amount to be

---

[44] Wehman, P; Kregel, J. and Shafer, M. eds. "Emerging Trends in the National Supported Employment Initiative: A Preliminary Analysis of Twenty-Seven States." Richmond: Rehabilitative Research and Training Center (1989).

[45] Hagner, D; Butterworth, J. and Keith, G. "Strategies and Barriers in Facilitating Natural Supports for Employment of Adults with Disabilities." 20 Journal of American People with Severe Handicaps, 110–120 (1995).

paid for identified needed supports. The independent support coordination must also recognize the value of benefits counseling to facilitate informed choice and risk-taking. Working and/or earning income has consequences from a benefits standpoint. Earning at or above the substantial gainful activity level (SGA) will impact on Social Security cash benefits and access to health care (Medicaid) and may affect other public benefits (food stamps, housing vouchers, personal assistance services). Understanding and managing the risk of a change in work and asset status must be an important part of the support coordination function. Peer and professional advice would be sought to consider best approaches to minimize risk and maximize benefits support and resource accumulation. The chart below recognizes the need for independence between support coordination and banking functions.

*EI² Model:* **Person-Centered and Directed Approach**

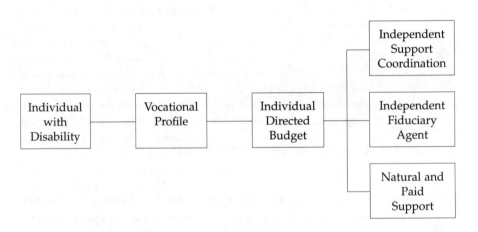

## Capacity Building

The development of a seamless workforce development system is in its early stages. States are at very different points of embracing and adopting the principles of self-determination. The process of change and capacity building to establish new relationships at a local community level is both a challenge and an opportunity for unprecedented inclusion of individuals with developmental disabilities in training, support ,and entry into the labor force.

At a local level, new agreements must be reached between potential partners (education, labor, vocational rehabilitation, mental retardation, Medicaid) and their representatives to serve on a "finance committee" to review and commit resources in support of individual personal budgets.

Agencies that agree to be independent of direct service provision need to be identified and selected as independent service coordinators. Generic agencies, such as local banks or credit unions, need to be identified for consideration as independent fiduciary agents.

A major training and education effort must be targeted to a) existing providers, b) consumers and families, and c) potential new support providers.[46] The concepts and methodologies of vocational profiles, business plan development, individualized job development, employer-directed support plans, personal budgets, and negotiated services and supports represent a new way of meeting the individualized needs of working-age adults with disabilities. For the traditional funder, the customer is no longer the nonprofit provider. The customer is the individual with developmental disabilities directing resources allocated within an approved personal budget.

Appendix I includes an annotated list of publications on employment initiatives for persons with disabilities, and Appendix II includes a list of websites of interest on employment initiatives for persons with disabilities. These documents include information on reports and publications, policies and procedures, and resources of public and private programs and services related to employment and related support services for youth and working-age adults with disabilities that is available on the Internet. The resources are not meant to be all-inclusive. However, the references will help to provide more detailed information on topics of relevance to the employment and support of persons with disabilities.

## ACKNOWLEDGMENT

Michael Morris is the Director of the U.S. Department of Education-funded Research and Training Center on Workforce Investment and Employment Policy for Persons with Disabilities. The Research was supported under a cooperative agreement with NIDRR #H133B980042-01 and a SBIR subcontract with DHHS #105-00-7000.

## APPENDIX I

This document includes information on reports and publications, policies and procedures, and resources on public and private programs and services related to employment and related support services for youth and working-age adults with disabilities that is available on the Internet. The following

---

[46] Please see appendices for a list of relevant publications and web sites to add further to understanding this shift in emphasis to a customer-driven system.

list is not meant to be all-inclusive. However, the references will help to provide more detailed information on topics of relevance to the employment and support of persons with disabilities.

## AMERICANS WITH DISABILITIES ACT

### ADA REGULATIONS AND TECHNICAL ASSISTANCE MATERIALS
*http://www.usdoj.gov/crt/ada/publicat.htm*

The U.S. Department of Justice provides free ADA materials. Printed materials may be ordered by calling the ADA Information Line [1-800-514-0301 (voice) or 1-800-514-0383 (TDD)]. Automated service is available 24 hours a day for recorded information and to order publications. Publications are available in standard print as well as large print, audiotape, Braille, and computer disk for people with disabilities. Many of these materials are available from an automated fax system that is available 24 hours a day. Access the website to view a list of the available materials.

### GENERAL ADA PUBLICATIONS AND MATERIALS

- *ADA Questions and Answers.* (Spanish, Chinese, Korean, Tagalog and Vietnamese editions available.) A 32-page booklet giving an overview of the ADA's requirements for ensuring equal opportunity for persons with disabilities in employment, State and local government services, public accommodations, commercial facilities, and transportation and requiring the establishment of TDD/telephone relay services. FAX #3106

- *ADA Information Services.* A 2-page list with the telephone numbers and Internet addresses of federal agencies and other organizations that provide information and technical assistance to the public about the ADA. FAX #3101

- *Enforcing the ADA. A Status Report from the Department of Justice.* A brief report issued by the Justice Department each quarter providing timely information about ADA cases and settlements, building codes that meet ADA accessibility standards, and ADA technical assistance activities. FAX #3102 (for the most current issue)

- *A Guide to Disability Rights Laws.* A 21-page booklet that provides a brief overview of eleven federal laws that protect the rights of people with disabilities and provides information about the federal agencies to contact for more information. (Spanish, Cambodian, Chinese, Hmong, Japanese, Korean, Laotian, Tagalog, Vietnamese editions available from the ADA Information Line.) FAX #3103

- *A Guide for People with Disabilities Seeking Employment.* A 2-page pamphlet for people with disabilities providing a general explanation of the employment provisions of the ADA and how to file a complaint with the Equal Employment Opportunity Commission. (Spanish edition available from the ADA Information Line.) FAX #3108

- *Learn About the ADA in Your Local Library.* An 10-page annotated list of 95 ADA publications and one videotape that are available to the public in 15,000 public libraries throughout the country. FAX #3104

- *Myths and Facts.* A 3-page fact sheet dispelling some common misconceptions about the ADA's requirements and implementation. This publication contains basic information for businesses and state and local governments. (Spanish edition available from the ADA Information Line.) FAX #3105

- *ADA Mediation Program.* A 6-page publication that provides an overview of the Department's Mediation Program and examples of successfully mediated cases. FAX #3107

## Reasonable Accommodation and The Americans with Disabilities Act

September 1999, No. 1
*http://www.worksupport.com/Topics/downloads/rrtcfactsheet2.pdf*

This fact sheet provides definitions of key terms and procedures related to job accommodations under the employment provisions (Title 1) of the ADA. The following questions are answered:

- Who is covered?
- Who is qualified applicant?
- What are essential functions?
- What are reasonable accommodations?
- What constitutes an undue hardship?
- What is the average cost of a reasonable accommodation?
- What should an employee do to request an accommodation?
- What should an employer do after a request for an accommodation?

## Disability Public Policy

### Emerging Disability Policy Framework: A Guidepost for Analyzing Public Policy
Robert Silverstein, J.D.
2000
*http://www.comop.org/rrtc/rrtc/Fed_Disability.htm*

The purpose of this article is to provide an Emerging Disability Policy Framework consistent with the "new paradigm" that can be used as a lens or guidepost to design, implement, and evaluate generic, as well as disability-specific, public policies and programs to ensure meaningful inclusion of people with disabilities in mainstream society.

To this end, this article is targeted to the needs of several audiences, including federal, state and local policymakers, as well as persons with disabilities, their families, and their advocates. For researchers, this article provides a benchmark for studying the extent to which generic and disability-specific policies and programs reflect the "new paradigm" and achieve its goals. For service providers, this article provides a lens for designing, implementing, and evaluating the delivery of services to persons with disabilities. Finally, for college and university professors teaching courses that include disability policy, this article provides a framework for policy analysis.

The research methodology applied in developing the Emerging Disability Policy Framework involved a comprehensive review and analysis of authoritative materials on disability policy, including statues, regulations, and legislative and regulatory histories. The purpose was to discern the fundamental values, principles, and policies inherent in these laws and the extent to which they are consistent with the fundamental goals of disability policy.

## EMPLOYMENT OF PERSONS WITH DISABILITIES

### BUSINESS TAX CREDITS & DEDUCTIONS FOR EMPLOYMENT OF PEOPLE WITH DISABILITIES
January 2000, No. 2
*http://www.worksupport.com/Topics/downloads/factsheet3.pdf*

This fact sheet describes three tax incentives available to help employers cover accommodation costs for employees and/or customers with disabilities, making their businesses accessible for everyone. The following tax credits and deductions are explained:

- Architectural/Transportation Tax Deduction: IR Code Section 190, Barrier Removal
- Small Business Tax Credit: IR Code Section 44, Disabled Access Credit
- Work Opportunity Tax Credit (WOTC)

### CHARACTERISTICS OF EFFECTIVE EMPLOYMENT SERVICES: THE CONSUMER'S PERSPECTIVE
Monograph (50 pp., 2001, $7.00, Order #MON31)
*http://www.childrenshospital.org/ici/publications/newpubs.htmol#rtp*

This monograph reports on a study investigating the characteristics of effective state service systems. Findings are based on the experiences of individuals with disabilities who have used a state agency (Vocational Rehabilitation, Department of Mental Retardation, Department of Mental Health, or One Stop Center) to find employment. Interviews were conducted to examine individuals' experiences with employment services including job search, job entry, strategies that facilitated involvement, supports provided, and barriers experienced. Findings indicated five key components to effective service delivery, including agency culture, consumer-directedness, access to resources, quality personnel, and coordinated services. Obstacles faced during the employment process and personal strategies used to overcome these barriers were also identified. These findings provide information about what job seekers and state systems can do to maximize their experience together. Recommendations for what both parties can do independently and collaboratively to achieve success are offered.

CHARTBOOK ON WORK AND DISABILITY IN THE UNITED STATES, 1998
Prepared by: Susan Stoddard, Lita Jans, Joan M. Ripple, Lewis Kraus
Prepared for: U.S. Department of Education, National Institute on Disability and Rehabilitation Research Washington, D.C. H133D50017-96
*http://www.infouse.com/disabilitydata/workdisability.pdf.html*
The Charbook on Work and Disability in the United States, 1998, is a reference on work and disability in the U.S. population, created for use by both nontechnical and technical audiences. The book is a resource for agencies, employers, organizations, policymakers, researchers, and others concerned with the relationship between disability and work. Each section addresses an aspect of work and disability. Each page within the section contains a topic question, explanatory text on the topic, and an explanatory graphic or table that provides data in an easy-to-read form.

ECONOMICS OF POLICIES AND PROGRAMS AFFECTING
THE EMPLOYMENT OF PEOPLE WITH DISABILITIES
Gina A. Livermore, David C. Stapleton, Mark W. Nowak, David C. Wittenburg, and Elizabeth D. Eiseman
Prepared by Cornell University
March 2000
*http://*
*www.ilr.cornell.edu/extension/files/download/Economics.policies.programs.pdf*
This paper presents the general economic framework in which the factors affecting the employment of people with disabilities will be identified and described and provides an overview of the major factors affecting the employment of people with disabilities. It includes discussion on specific factors and evidence of the importance of each factor for employment decisions. Recent initiatives are discussed along with their implications for employment of those with disabilities. The paper ends with a discussion of

key issues for public policy identified in the review and a discussion of gaps in existing research.

### Effective Customer Service Delivery in Employment Support: Finding a Common Ground Between Guided and Self-Directed Service Delivery

Research to Practice Brief (4 pp, May 2001, Vol. 7 No. 1, Order #RP26)
*http://www.childrenshospital.org/ici/publications/pdf/rp26.pdf*

Characteristics of effective employment services based on the experiences of individuals who successfully found jobs through agencies. Consumers were active recipients of services who shaped their own career searches to achieve a balance between support and independence. Describes characteristics of the guided and self-directed approaches and provides recommendations for agency staff.

### Employing People with Disabilities

August 1999, Vol. 1, No. 1
*http://www.worksupport.com/Topics/downloads/2dialoguenewsltr.pdf*

Inside this issue:

- Learning from the Best—Case Studies
- Reverse Funnel Approach—Manpower's Approach to Employment
- Manager's Corner—Ask the HR Expert . . . Question & Answers on Interviewing, Recruiting, Hiring, and Accommodation Cost
- Resources for Accommodations

Additional copies may be purchased: 25 newsletters/$9.95. For information on placing an order contact Roberta Martin at *rsmartin@atlas.vcu.edu* or (804) 828-1851.

### Getting Down to Business: A Blueprint for Creating and Supporting Entrepreneurial Opportunities for Individuals with Disabilities

*http://www.dol.gov/dol/odep/public/pubs/business/toc.htm*

This report discusses the current status of small business and self-employment opportunities for people with disabilities and offers recommendations for addressing barriers to business ownership. The findings in this report build on the proceedings of the National Blue Ribbon Panel on Self-Employment, Small Business and Disability, convened in July 1998 by the President's Committee on Employment of People with Disabilities (now the Office of Disability Employment Policy), with additional support from the Social Security Administration, the World Institute on Disability, and the Association for Enterprise Opportunity.

NATIONAL DAY AND EMPLOYMENT SERVICE TRENDS IN
MR/DD AGENCIES
Research to Practice Brief (4 pp, July 2001, Vol. 7 No. 3, Order #RP28)
*http://www.childrenshospital.org/ici/publications/pdf/rp28.pdf*

The past twenty years have seen an increasing emphasis on community-based services and equal access to employment for all individuals, including those with the most significant disabilities. The question is, To what extent have changes in philosophy translated into changes for state agencies and the people they serve? The brief analyzes MR/DD agencies day and employment service trends from 1988 to 1999 and discusses relevant trends in policy and legislation.

OFFICE OF DISABILITY EMPLOYMENT POLICY FOR THE DEPARTMENT
OF LABOR TECHNICAL ASSISTANCE MATERIALS
*http://www.dol.gov/dol/odep/public/pubs/publicat.htm*

Fact Sheets available on accommodations, barriers, employment rights, recruitment, business involvement, and many other relevant issues.

RECRUITING FROM NONTRADITIONAL SOURCES OF LABOR
April 2000, No. 3
*http://www.worksupport.com/Topics/downloads/factsheet4.pdf*

This fact sheet explains how to find nontraditional workers and the benefits to business and provides many resources for managers and HR staff. The following business issues are covered:

- How do I find nontraditional workers?
- Do many other businesses recruit nontraditional workers?
- What are the benefits or incentives to business?
- Do I need to change my recruitment strategy?
- Resource groups to contact for more information

WORKING AGE ADULTS WITH DISABILITIES: DEMOGRAPHICS,
ISSUES AND TRENDS
*http://www.comop.org/rrtc/rrtc/Work_age.htm*

- Background information on working-age adults with disabilities

The target population consists of working-age (18–64), low-income persons with disabilities, an identifiable and significant group that is underrepresented in the workforce and one of the poorest minorities in the United States. A disability is defined by the National Institute on Disability and Rehabilitation Research, U.S. Department of Education, as "a physical, mental, or emotional impairment that requires accommodation to allow performance of functions required to carry out life activities."

For a variety of reasons, people with disabilities have a much lower chance of finding and keeping fulfilling employment. Twenty-six percent of employed people with disabilities report difficulty in getting the kind of job they wanted because of their disability. Furthermore, less than half (46%) of those employed full-time feel that their job requires their full talents and abilities. The barriers people with disabilities face in finding satisfactory employment are numerous, the most significant being that the job "didn't pay enough" (47%), that there was poor access to public facilities and transportation (27%), and that employers did not provide adequate health insurance (23%). Lack of money is considered the most serious by far of a list of potential problems: 68% of people with disabilities cite it as at least a minor problem, of which 39% feel it is the most serious problem they face. Approximately two-thirds (67%) of adults with disabilities say their disability has prevented them from "reaching their full abilities as a person" (NOD). Without question, the target population suffers economic hardship, cutting across age and sex, across type and severity of disability, and across the nation.

- Issues and trends in the employment of people with disabilities—Mary Podmostko, January 17, 2000

Despite the economic boom during the late 1990s, people with disabilities still have significantly lower employment and income rates than the general population. This paper examines some of the issues and trends in the employment of people with disabilities. The intent is to assist in the development of policy for people with disabilities that will lead to meaningful and more successful employment outcomes.

The employment and self-sufficiency levels of people with disabilities are unsatisfactory if this segment of the population is to be fully included in the workforce and the larger community. Leadership in the public sector has been cited as a major contributing factor to successful integrated employment models and outcomes (Mank, O'Neill, and Jensen, 1998), and the bottom line is that leadership is needed in all sectors, public, private, and nonprofit—and must include people with disabilities—to find more effective ways of moving people with disabilities into meaningful, financially rewarding career paths. People with disabilities currently experience significant gaps in wages, employment, and education compared with the general population; they cannot afford a leadership gap in the development of policies and practices that will include them as contributing, gainfully employed members of society.

WORK WORLD
VCU School of Business
*http://www.workworld.org/*

Work World is decision support software for personal computers designed to help people with disabilities, advocates, benefit counselors, and others explore and understand how to best use the work incentives associated with the various federal and state disability and poverty benefit programs. It automates the computation of benefits and takes into account the complex interaction of income, benefit programs, and work incentives. Initially developed by the Employment Support Institute at Virginia Commonwealth University, the software is currently being enhanced and distributed by ESI under a contract funded by the Social Security Administration.

## Vocational Rehabilitation

### Postsecondary Education as a Critical Step Toward Meaningful Employment: Vocational Rehabilitation's Role
Research to Practice Brief (4 pp, July 2001, Vol. 7 No. 4, Order #RP29)
*http://www.childrenshospital.org/ici/publications/pdf/rp29.pdf*

Postsecondary education opens up a world of opportunities for high school graduates. Research shows that access to the opportunities afforded by a postsecondary education makes an enormous difference in the employability of people with disabilities. This brief focuses on people who have received education supports from vocational rehabilitation (VR) agencies and their rehabilitation outcomes.

### Provisions in the Final Regulations Governing the State VR Program Describing the Interplay with WIA and TWWIIA
Center on State Systems and Employment (RRTC), Center on Workforce Investment and Employment Policy (RRTC)
February 2001
*http://www.childrenshospital.org/ici/publications/text/pu7text.html*

The purpose of this policy brief is to identify and describe the provisions of the final regulation describing the responsibilities of a designated state unit to design and operate the state VR program as an integral component of the statewide workforce investment system, as envisioned by WIA. The final regulations envision major systemic changes in the operation of the state VR program through the creation of a streamlined, collaborative partnership with other components of the statewide workforce investment system. This new "partnership" requires a more "activist" role for state VR agencies regarding the provision of services to persons with disabilities in the state VR program itself as well as other components of the workforce investment system.

The purpose of the policy brief is also to identify and describe the provisions in the final regulations describing the relationship between the state VR program and the designated state unit and the new Ticket to Work Program.

VOCATIONAL REHABILITATION OUTCOMES FOR PEOPLE WITH MENTAL
RETARDATION, CEREBRAL PALSY, AND EPILEPSY: AN ANALYSIS OF
TRENDS FROM 1985 TO 1998
Monograph (26 pp., 2001, $7.00, Order#MON29)
*http://www.childrenshospital.org/ici/publications/newpubs.html#rtp*
*http://www.childrenshospital.org/ici/publications/pdf/vroutcomes.pdf*

This monograph presents the results of secondary analysis of the RSA-
911 database from the Rehabilitation Services Administration. All successful
VR closures for individuals with mental retardation, cerebral palsy, and
epilepsy for six data points between 1985 and 1998 were investigated. Trends
in competitive labor market and extended employment (sheltered workshops) closures were examined. The use of supported employment in the VR
system and its outcomes were also discussed. Findings include increased
incidence of competitive labor market closures and supported employment
services, with a decrease in extended employment closures.

## WORKFORCE INVESTMENT ACT

A DESCRIPTION OF THE WORKFORCE INVESTMENT ACT LEGAL
FRAMEWORK FROM A DISABILITY POLICY PERSPECTIVE
Robert Silverstein, J.D.
January 27, 2000
*http://www.comop.org/rrtc/rrtc/Workforce.htm*

On August 7, 1998, President Clinton signed into law the Workforce Investment Act of 1998 (WIA) (Public Law 105-220). Title I of WIA
provides assistance to states interested in establishing statewide and local
workforce investment systems for all job seekers, including persons with
disabilities.

The purpose of this paper is to describe the major sections in title I of
WIA and the implementing regulations and guidance issued by the Department of Labor and to highlight key references in the statue, regulations, and
guidance of particular relevance to persons with disabilities.

This paper is intended for policy makers, researchers, individuals with
disabilities and their families, organizations representing individuals with
disabilities, state agencies serving adults with disabilities (e.g., vocational
rehabilitation, Mental Health, Mental Retardation, Developmental Disabilities, Education, Health, Welfare), community rehabilitation providers, and
other stakeholders who want to ensure that individuals with disabilities are
provided effective and meaningful opportunity to participate in the comprehensive workforce development system envisioned by WIA.

A PRELIMINARY ANALYSIS OF THE RELATIONSHIP BETWEEN
THE WORKFORCE INVESTMENT ACT AND THE FEDERAL

## DISABILITY POLICY FRAMEWORK
Robert Silverstein, J.D.
January 27, 2000
*http://www.comop.org/rrtc/rrtc/Workforce.htm*

The purpose of this paper is use the basic conceptual framework of Federal disability policy developed in a paper entitled *The Federal Disability Policy Framework: Our Nation's Goals for People with Disabilities* (Silverstein, 1999) as a lens or guidepost for:

- identifying existing DOL policies directing or encouraging states implementing WIA to address the special needs of persons with disabilities, and

- identifying issues for policy development, oversight, and implementation at the Federal, State and local levels.

This paper is targeted at four audiences. First, this paper provides policy markers with a conceptual framework for designing and assessing the extent to which WIA addresses the needs of persons with disabilities. Second, this paper provides researchers with a policy framework for studying how WIA addresses the needs of persons with disabilities. Third, this paper provides individuals with disabilities, their families, and their representatives with tools that can be used to judge the adequacy of WIA policies and procedures developed at the federal, state, and local levels from a disability policy perspective. Fourth, this paper may be used by service providers to design, implement, and evaluate the delivery of services to persons with disabilities.

## PEOPLE WITH DISABILITIES: HAVING A VOICE IN THE CREATION OF THE NEW WORKFORCE INVESTMENT SYSTEM (TOOLS FOR INCLUSION)
David Hoff
Institute for Community Inclusion/UAP Center on State Systems and Employment (RRTC)
March 2000
*http://www.childrenshospital.org/ici/publications/word/to11wordtex.doc*

Planning is currently underway that will result in major changes in the employment and training systems across the country. It is critical that people with disabilities and their advocates be a part of these planning processes, which could significantly impact services for people with disabilities.

The changes taking place are a result of the Workforce Investment Act (WIA), a federal law that states must have implemented by July 1, 2000. WIA brings together various federal job training and employment programs into one integrated system of services, which all people, including people with disabilities, can access through One-Stop Centers located in each major population area.

The purpose of this publication is to inform people with disabilities and advocates about the opportunities available for input into WIA implementation. Significant resource and service delivery decisions are being made as part of WIA. This new workforce investment system is intended to meet the needs of all job seekers. Advocacy must take place now, so that the needs of people with disabilities are not overlooked in the decisions being made about how this new system will operate. As this new workforce investment system is formed, it is important that people with disabilities and advocates be proactive in their approach, to avoid having to demand that the system be modified or "fixed" after it has been fully established.

PROVISIONS IN THE WORKFORCE INVESTMENT ACT DESCRIBING THE INTERPLAY BETWEEN WORKFORCE INVESTMENT SYSTEMS AND VOCATIONAL REHABILITATION PROGRAMS; POLICY BRIEF

Center on State Systems and Employment Outcomes (RRTC), Institute for Community Inclusion/UAP: Center on Workforce Investment and Employment Policy (RRTC), Community Options, Inc.

April 1999

*http://www.comop.org/rrtc/rrtc/Workforce.htm*

The purpose of this policy brief is to identify and describe the sections in Title I of the Workforce Investment Act (statewide and local workforce investment systems) that specifically reference the vocational rehabilitation program, individuals with disabilities, and organizations representing individuals with disabilities. The policy brief also identifies and describes specific references to statewide and local workforce investment systems in Title I of the Rehabilitation Act (the vocational rehabilitation program). This brief should provide policy makers, researchers, individuals with disabilities, organizations representing individuals with disabilities, state agencies serving adults with disabilities (e.g., Mental Health, Mental Retardation, Developmental Disabilities, Education, Health, Welfare), community rehabilitation programs, and other stakeholders a focus on some of the key areas of policy in the Workforce Investment Act, to ensure that individuals with disabilities are provided "effective and meaningful participation in workforce investment activities" [Section 100(a)(1)(G) of the Rehabilitation Act].

THE WORKFORCE INVESTMENT ACT OF 1998: A PRIMER FOR PEOPLE WITH DISABILITIES

Duke Storen and K.A. Dixon

John J. Heldrich Center for Workforce Development at Rutgers, the State University of New Jersey

November 1999

*http://www.comop.org/rrtc/rrtc/Workforce.htm*

On August 7, 1998, President Clinton signed into law the Workforce Investment Act of 1998 (WIA). The purpose of WIA is to create a national workforce preparation and employment system that meets the needs of job seekers and those seeking to advance their careers, as well as the employment needs of the nation's employers. The goal is to create an integrated workforce investment system that improves the quality of our workforce, sustains economic growth and productivity, and reduces dependency on welfare.

This primer describes the major components of the Workforce Investment Act and suggests ways to participate that ensure that individuals with disabilities have universal access to the new workforce system.

This primer is intended primarily for people with disabilities—and the parents of children with disabilities—who are looking for a job or want to advance their careers. The new law means that new services are now available to job seekers. This primer is intended to help people with disabilities make the most of the workforce system. It is also useful for teachers, advocates, and service providers who work with people with disabilities. Finally, this primer is intended for people who want to learn how they can participate in the development and implementation of this new system.

## Workforce Investment Act Fact Sheets
*http://usworkforce.org/factsheets/default.asp*

It includes a list of Department of Labor-supported activities and services that are part of America's Workforce Network that may be of particular interest to workers, employers, and workforce development professionals. All documents are in pdf format. Fact sheets with specific information on various topics are available.

## WIA One-Stop Centers

### Access for All: A Resource Manual for Meeting the Needs of One-Stop Customers with Disabilities
Resource Manual (335 pp., 2001, $25.00, Order #RES6)
*http://www.childrenshospital.org/ici/onestop/onestopmanualcomplete.pdf*

This comprehensive, 300+-page manual is designed to assist One-Stop systems in meeting the needs of individuals with disabilities. The manual contains 14 sections; each section is available as a separate pdf file. Paper copies of the manual, in three-ring binders with tab dividers, can be also be ordered from the Institute for $25.00. For ordering information, please contact the ICI Publications Office at (617) 335-6506 or *ici@tch.harvard.edu.*

### Innovative and Interesting Practices in the Provision of Quality Services to One-Stop Customers with Disabilities

One-Stop Disability Team
Washington, DC
*http://wdsc.doleta.gov/disability/htmldocs/innovative.html*

This represents a draft document based on report-outs from state and local One-Stops on innovative and interesting practices in the provision of quality services to One-Stop customers with disabilities. Each summary is followed by contact information to facilitate more detailed discussions between One-Stop practitioners.

ONE-STOP CENTERS: A GUIDE FOR JOB SEEKERS WITH
DISABILITIES (TOOLS FOR INCLUSION)

Sheila Fesko, David Hoff, Melanie Jordan, Kristin Fichera, and Cynthia
    Thomas
Institute for Community Inclusion/UAP · Center on State Systems and
    Employment (RRTC)
February 2000 (Updated November 2000)
*http://www.childrenshospital.org/ici/publications/text/onestop.html*

The One-Stop system is designed and required to meet the needs of all job seekers who want to use the system. This includes people with disabilities. The establishment of the One-Stop system across the country provides a wonderful opportunity for people with disabilities to receive services in new and different ways, right alongside everyone else. This brief is designed to help you use the One-Stop system. It includes information on what services are available, how to make the best use of those services, and how to advocate to get the services you want and need. The brief describes general information about the One-Stop system and then answers specific questions that individuals with disabilities may have about these services.

REPORT-OUT ON DISCUSSIONS WITH STATES ABOUT FACILITATED
SELF-SERVICE TO SPECIAL APPLICANT GROUPS

One-Stop Disability Team
Washington, DC
*http://wdsc.doleta.gov/disability/htmldocs/fss.html*

The information is based on report-outs from states on the innovative use of advanced technology to ensure that self-service tools are accessible to all job seekers, including—but not limited to—persons with disabilities, farmworkers, welfare-to-work enrollees, and older workers. The states included in these report-outs represent varying stages of One-Stop system development. The assistive technology described in this report is often the result of collaborative efforts between the One-Stops and other partners, such as state and local vocational rehabilitation agencies, nonprofits, for-profit companies, and universities.

## WIA and One-Stop Centers: Opportunities and Issues for the Disability Community
David Hoff
The Institute Brief
December 2000
*http://www.childrenshospital.org/ici/publications/text/wiaonestop.html*

Major changes in employment and training systems across the country are currently taking place, changes that could have a significant impact on services for people with disabilities. These changes are a result of the Workforce Investment Act (WIA), a federal law effective July 1, 2000, which governs how publicly funded workforce investment and training services operate. The new federally sponsored nationwide employment and training system established under WIA is called "America's Workforce Network." This publication provides a basic overview of WIA and examines the impact of this law on the lives of people with disabilities as well as the systems and organizations that assist them.

## Youth with Disabilities

### A Collaborative Model Promotes Career Success for Students with Disabilities: How DO-IT Does It
Sheryl Burgstahler
2000
*http://www.rrtc.hawaii.edu/products/published/MS032-H01.htm*

Many young people entering the workforce are not well prepared to meet the demands of a dynamic work environment. Students with disabilities benefit from work-based learning activities as much as, if not more than, their nondisabled peers. Unfortunately, many school-to-work programs in high school and cooperative education and internship programs in college do not fully include students with disabilities, a group that represents an increasing portion of today's school population. The University of Washington ran a three-year project to help students with disabilities head toward successful careers with a holistic and collaborative approach. Besides the students served, the team includes staff of precollege and postsecondary educational institutions, parents, mentors, employers, and community service providers. A post work experience survey was developed to answer the question, "What impact do work-based learning experiences have on career-related attitudes, knowledge, and skills for students with disabilities?" Participants reported considerable benefit from their work-based learning experiences. They gained motivation to work toward a career, learned about careers and the workplace, gaining job-related skills, learned to work with supervisors and coworkers, and developed accommodation strategies. Aspects of this model can be used by others to promote the success of people with disabilities.

A REVIEW OF SECONDARY SCHOOL FACTORS INFLUENCING
POSTSCHOOL OUTCOMES FOR YOUTH WITH DISABILITIES
R.A. Stodden, P.W. Dowrick, N.J. Stodden, and S. Gilmore
2000
*http://www.rrtc.hawaii.edu/products/published/MS043-H01.htm*

For almost two decades, federal agencies have funded hundreds of
projects to develop and evaluate programs in support of better transitions
to adulthood for youth with disabilities. State and independent agencies
have recently developed hundreds more such programs. We reviewed findings in four areas: (1) helping youth to stay in high school; (2) improving
academic outcomes; (3) transition practices, especially related to employment; and (4) preparation for postsecondary education. We built on previous selective reviews and used a multivocal literature methodology. Overall
outcomes remain poor. Compared with the general population, half as many
students with disabilities graduate from high school; the majority follow
nonacademic curricula, seven times as many adults with disabilities are
unemployed, and one-third as many attend higher education. However,
promising practices have been demonstrated to improve outcomes in all
three areas, from person-centered planning, to assistive technology, to intern-
ships. The authors conclude that better analysis of results and better dissemination of findings could effectively inform policy makers, school
districts, and teaching personnel, as well as families and advocates, to make
substantial improvements in the lives of young adults with disabilities.

HANDBOOK ON SUPPLEMENTAL SECURITY INCOME (SSI) WORK
INCENTIVES AND TRANSITION STUDENTS
Jointly developed by: The Study Group, Inc., SSI Work Incentives and
    Transitioning Youth Project, and National Transition Network
October 1998
*http://ici2.coled.umn.edu/ntn/pub/hdbk/default.html*

Provides an overview of the SSI program as it applies to transition students, SSI work incentives, and the role school personnel can play in assisting students and parents in using these benefits in the transition process
to enhance postsecondary outcomes. Includes a glossary of SSA and SSI
related terms, common concerns and questions raised by students and
parents regarding the SSI program, steps involved in the SSI application
process, applicants' rights as defined by SSA, PASS application, additional
resources, and a listing of regional social security offices.

TRANSITION TO EMPLOYMENT: FOCUS GROUP
Research Findings Brief
April 2000
*http://www.rrtc.hawaii.edu/products/pdf/4b-focus/transition.pdf*

Students with disabilities feel supported in their postsecondary education environment but fear the transition to employment. They fear workplace discrimination and employer refusal to accommodate their needs. Focus groups composed of prospective, current, and former students with disabilities were conducted at 10 sites nationally. The groups were designed, with participant input, to elicit student-consumer perspectives regarding the issues of supports and barriers in the postsecondary setting and the workplace.

## Transition to Postsecondary Education for Students with Disabilities

D.R. Johnson, M.N. Sharpe, and R.A. Stodden
2000
*http://www.rrtc.hawaii.edu/products/published/MS044-H01.htm*

The completion of high school signals the beginning of adult life. Today, more and more young people are exiting their high school programs and going on to attend public and private postsecondary vocational training programs, community colleges, and universities. Along with this have come new opportunities for young people with disabilities to participate in these postsecondary education options. Since 1990, for example, there has been a 90% increase in the number of colleges and universities, technical institutions, community colleges, and vocational and technical centers offering opportunities for persons with disabilities to continue their education (Pierangelo and Crane, 1997). Advances in assessment, instructional strategies, and the use of accommodations have made it possible for many more young people with disabilities, including individuals with severe disabilities, to access and participate in these programs. Despite this encouraging trend, enrollment of youth and young adults with disabilities in postsecondary programs is still 50% lower than enrollment among the general population.

Interfering with an individual's participation and actual completion of postsecondary education programs are a host of barriers and concerns that must be addressed and ultimately overcome to ensure a student's success. The goals of access and reasonable accommodations, outlined in Section 504 of the Rehabilitation Act of 1973, the Americans with Disabilities Education Act of 1990, and the Individuals with Disabilities Education Act (IDEA) amendments of 1997, do not guarantee students' success in postsecondary settings. Educators, parents, and students must carefully think through the decisions regarding postsecondary education participation, and such thinking should begin as early as possible in a student's educational career. This article provides an overview of several of the major issues and needs of students that must be addressed to ensure a successful transition from high school to postsecondary education.

## APPENDIX II

This document includes resources on public and private programs and services related to employment and related support services for youth and working-age adults with disabilities that is available on the Internet. The list of websites is not meant to be all-inclusive. However, the references will help to provide more detailed information on topics of relevance to the employment and support of persons with disabilities.

## DISABILITY AND BUSINESS TECHNICAL ASSISTANCE CENTERS (DBTACS)

The National Institute on Disability and Rehabilitation Research (NIDRR) has established 10 regional centers to provide information, training, and technical assistance to employers, people with disabilities, and other entities with responsibilities under the ADA. The centers act as a "one-stop" central, comprehensive resource on ADA issues in employment, public services, public accommodations, and communications. Each center works closely with local business, disability, governmental, rehabilitation, and other professional networks to provide ADA information and assistance, placing special emphasis on meeting the needs of small businesses. Programs vary in each region, but all centers provide the following:

- Technical assistance
- Education and training
- Materials dissemination
- Information and referral
- Public awareness
- Local capacity building
- *http://www.ed.gov/offices/OSERS/NIDRR/index.html*

## EMPLOYMENT RESOURCES

ASSOCIATION FOR PERSONS IN SUPPORTED EMPLOYMENT
1627 Monument Ave.
Richmond, VA 23220
804-278-9187
*apse@apse.org*
*http://www.apse.org/*

The Association for Persons in Supported Employment is a membership organization formed in 1988 to improve and expand integrated employment opportunities, services, and outcomes for persons experiencing disabilities. To accomplish this mission, APSE:

- Provides advocacy and education to customers of supported employment (SE), that is, supported employment professionals, consumers and their family members, and supported employers.
- Addresses issues and barriers that impede the growth and implementation of integrated employment services.
- Improves supported employment (SE) practice so that individuals and communities experience SE as a quality service with meaningful outcomes.
- Promotes national, state, and local policy development that enhances the social and economic inclusion and empowerment of all persons experiencing severe disabilities.
- Educates the public and the business community on the value of including persons experiencing severe disabilities as fully participating community members.

CHILDREN'S HOSPITAL
Institute for Community Inclusion
200 Longwood Ave.
Boston, MA 02115
617-355-6506; 617-355-6956 (TTY)
*ici@a1.tch.harvard.edu*
*http://www.childrenshospital.org/ici/*

The Institute for Community Inclusion (ICI) is committed to developing resources and supports for people with disabilities and their families, fostering interdependence, productivity, and inclusion in school and community settings. Programs in the Institute carry out this mission through training and consultation, services, and research and dissemination. ICI has a wide variety of activities focused on enhancing employment opportunities for people with disabilities. Through a variety of services, ICI staff work directly with people with disabilities to help them find and keep employment. ICI staff also provide training and consultation on employment issues to service providers and consumers of services across the country and internationally. ICI also does extensive research on employment issues through numerous research projects.

CHOICE EMPLOYMENT INTERNET RECRUITING
Understanding Disabilities, Expanding Opportunities
UCP of Dallas
8802 Harry Hines Blvd.
Dallas, TX 75235
*http://www.choiceemployment.com/NewSite/*

The vision of Choice Employment is to be the forerunner in substantially lowering the unemployment rate among individuals with disabilities. Choice Employment is the premier recruiting resource targeted to assist people with disabilities. Choice Employment has partnered with leading Fortune 500 companies to find the best jobs for the best people. Their partner companies are committed to hiring people with disabilities into their workforce.

Choice Employment Internet Recruiting will:

- Provide corporate partners with efficient, quality service to meet their critical workforce needs, contributing to their overall success.
- Provide clients with access to employment opportunities through companies committed to hiring people with disabilities, promoting their dreams of independence.

### PROGRAMS

Assistive Technology

*http://www.choiceemployment.com/NewSite/AssistiveTechnology.asp*

Using the newest technologies, individuals with varying disabilities can discover their potential for living productive, meaningful lives. Assistive Technology is any device that allows an individual to perform activities with greater independence. The Assistive Technology (AT) Program at UCP Dallas is equipped with state-of-the-art devices so an individual can surf the web with the sound of his or her voice, send an e-mail with the nod of his or her head, or use a mouse with a tap of his or her feet.

Career Resources

*http://www.choiceemployment.com/NewSite/Resources.asp*

- Resume Writing Information and Tips—This resource is devoted to improving the way your resume looks on paper and on the computer screen as well. The information provided will help you to fine-tune your print resume and show you how to develop an electronic version for online submission.
- College and Career Information—A section of Choice Employment dedicated to providing employment information and job opportunities for college, graduate, and high school students planning ahead—and others looking to get ahead through more education.

### THE SMALL BUSINESS AND SELF-EMPLOYMENT SERVICE

Job Accommodation Network
P.O. Box 6080
Morgantown, WV 26506-6080
800-526-7234 (V/TTY)
*kcording@wvu.edu*
*http://www.jan.wvu.edu/SBSES/*

The Small Business and Self-Employment Service (SBSES) is a service of the U.S. Department of Labor's Office of Disability Employment Policy that provides comprehensive information, counseling, and referrals about self-employment and small business ownership opportunities for people with disabilities. Entrepreneurship is an exciting opportunity for people with disabilities to realize their full potential while becoming financially self-supporting. Some of the benefits of self-employment or small business include working at home, control of your work schedule, and the independence that comes from making your own decisions.

## The State Partnership Systems Change Initiative
Virginia Commonwealth University
1314 West Main St.
P.O. Box 842011
Richmond, VA 23284-2011
804-828-1851
804-828-2494 (TTY)
*http://spiconnect.org/*

Under a March 1998 Executive Order, the President created the National Task Force on Employment of Adults with Disabilities. The first initiative under this executive order was establishment of the State Partnership Systems Change Initiative (SPI). The purpose of SPI is to support project states in the development of innovative effective service delivery systems that increase employment of individuals with disabilities, such as: employer partnerships, customer-driven services, waivers and buy-in, state policy change initiatives, benefits assistance, and employment supports and programs.

The Social Security Administration (SSA) and the Rehabilitation Services Administration (RSA) funded a combined total of 18 demonstration states. The SSA awarded grants to 12 states to develop innovative projects to assist adults with disabilities in their efforts to reenter the work force. The RSA, a branch of the Department of Education, funded Systems Change Grants in six states. These awards will help states develop statewide programs of services and support for their residents with disabilities that will increase job opportunities for them and decrease their dependence on benefits, including Social Security and Supplemental Security Income (SSI). Other federal agencies such as the Department of Labor and the Department of Health and Human Services have joined the SSA in support of these projects.

- SSA states include California, Illinois, Iowa, Minnesota, New Hampshire, New Mexico, New York, North Carolina, Ohio, Oklahoma, Vermont, and Wisconsin.
- RSA states include Alaska, Arkansas, Colorado, Iowa, Oregon, and Utah.

SUPPORTED EMPLOYMENT
Office of Disability Employment Policy
US Department of Labor
1331 F Street, N.W. Suite 300
Washington DC 20004
202-376-6200, 202-376-6205 (TTD)
*infoODEP@dol.gov*
*http://www.dol.gov/pcepd/pubs/fact/supportd.htm*

Supported employment facilitates competitive work in integrated work settings for individuals with the most severe disabilities (i.e., psychiatric, mental retardation, learning disabilities, traumatic brain injury), for whom competitive employment has not traditionally occurred, and who, because of the nature and severity of their disability, need ongoing support services to perform their job. Supported employment provides assistance such as job coaches, transportation, assistive technology, specialized job training, and individually tailored supervision.

Supported employment is a way to move people from dependence on a service delivery system to independence via competitive employment. Recent studies indicate that the provision of ongoing support services for people with severe disabilities significantly increases their rates of employment retention. Supported employment encourages people to work within their communities and encourages work, social interaction, and integration.

TRAINING RESOURCE NETWORK, INC.
PO Box 439
St. Augustine, FL 32085-0439
866-823-9800
*info@trninc.com*
*http://www.trninc.com/*

Offering resources—supported employment, person-centered planning, and self-determination—on the full inclusion of persons with disabilities in their communities. Hands-on materials for advocates, human service practitioners, people with disabilities and their families, and businesses that employ workers with disabilities.

U.S. WORKFORCE
Gateway to information on the Workforce Investment Act
Office of Career Transition Assistance
Employment and Training Administration
200 Constitution Avenue, NW
Room S4231
Washington, DC 20210
202-693-3045
*AskWIA@doleta.gov*
*http://usworkforce.org/*

U.S. Workforce.org is designed to provide answers to current and emerging questions about the implementation of the Workforce Investment Act. It represents an unprecedented collaboration between public and private sector groups and individuals to provide access to workforce information and resources and to apply that information toward innovative and effective partnerships and programs.

## Federal Resources

### Americans with Disabilities Act Home Page
U.S. Department of Justice
*http://www.usdoj.gov/crt/ada/adahom1.htm*

Through lawsuits and settlement agreements, the Department of Justice has achieved greater access for individuals with disabilities in hundreds of cases. Under general rules governing lawsuits brought by the federal government, the Department of Justice may not sue a party unless negotiations to settle the dispute have failed. The Department of Justice may file lawsuits in federal court to enforce the ADA, and courts may order compensatory damages and back pay to remedy discrimination if the Department prevails. Under Title III, the Department of Justice may also obtain civil penalties of up to $50,000 for the first violation and $100,000 for any subsequent violation.

### PROGRAMS
ADA Information Line
*http://www.usdoj.gov/crt/ada/infoline.htm*

The U.S. Department of Justice provides information about the Americans with Disabilities Act (ADA) through a toll-free ADA Information Line. This service permits businesses, state and local governments, and others to call and ask questions about general or specific ADA requirements including questions about the ADA Standards for Accessible Design. ADA specialists are available Monday through Friday from 10:00 A.M. until 6:00 P.M. (eastern time), except on Thursday, when the hours are 1:00 P.M. until 6:00 P.M.. Spanish language service is also available. For general ADA information, answers to specific technical questions, free ADA materials, or information about filing a complaint, call: 800-514-0301 (voice) or 800-514-0383 (TDD).

ADA Information Services
*http://www.usdoj.gov/crt/ada/agency.htm*

This list contains the telephone numbers and Internet addresses of federal agencies and other organizations that provide information about the ADA and informal guidance in understanding and complying with different provisions of the ADA.

ADA Technical Assistance Program
*http://www.usdoj.gov/crt/ada/taprog.htm*

The Department of Justice ADA Technical Assistance Program provides free information and technical assistance directly to businesses, nonprofit service providers, state and local governments, people with disabilities, and the general public. Technical assistance services provide the most up-to-date information about the ADA and how to comply with its requirements. The program also undertakes broad and targeted outreach initiatives to increase awareness and understanding of the ADA and operates an ADA Technical Assistance Grant Program to develop and target materials to reach specific audiences at the local level, including hotels and motels, restaurants, small businesses, builders, mayors and town officials, law enforcement, people with disabilities, and others.

ADMINISTRATION ON DEVELOPMENTAL DISABILITIES
Administration for Children and Families
U.S. Department of Health and Human Services
Mail Stop: HHH 300-F
370 L'Enfant Promenade, S.W.
Washington, DC 20447
202-690-6590
*add@acf.dhhs.gov*
*http://www.acf.dhhs.gov/programs/add/*

The major goal of these programs is a partnership with state governments, local communities, and the private sector to assist people with developmental disabilities to reach maximum potential through increased independence, productivity, and community integration. The programs address all elements of the life cycle: prevention, diagnosis, early intervention, therapy, education, training, employment, and community living and leisure opportunities. The Developmental Disabilities programs comprise three state-based programs that collaborate in different mandated activity areas. A fourth program addresses issues that are of concern to residents across the nation.

PROGRAMS
State Councils on Developmental Disabilities Program
*http://www.acf.dhhs.gov/programs/add/states/ddc.htm*

Under Part B of the Act, the State Councils on Developmental Disabilities program provides financial assistance to each state to support the activities of a Developmental Disabilities Council in that state. Councils are uniquely composed of individuals with significant disabilities, parents and family members of people with developmental disabilities, and representatives of state agencies that provide services to individuals with developmental disabilities. Together, this group of individuals develops and implements a statewide plan to address the federally mandated priority of employment and, optionally, any of three other federal priorities (case management, child development, and community living) as well as one optional state priority.

The emphasis of the Councils is to increase the independence, productivity, inclusion, and integration into the community of people with developmental disabilities through a variety of systemic change, capacity building, and advocacy activities on their behalf, including development of a state plan, which lays out activities for demonstration of new approaches to enhance their lives; training activities; supporting communities to respond positively; educating the public about their abilities, preferences, and needs; providing information to policy makers to increase their opportunities; and eliminating barriers.

State Protection and Advocacy Agencies
*http://www.acf.dhhs.gov/programs/add/states/p&a.htm*

The Developmental Disabilities Assistance and Bill of Rights Act provides for each state to establish a Protection and Advocacy (P&A) System to empower, protect, and advocate on behalf of persons with developmental disabilities. This system must be independent of service-providing agencies. The P&As are authorized to provide information and referral services and to exercise legal, administrative, and other remedies to resolve problems for individuals and groups of clients. The P&As are also required to reach out to members of minority groups that historically have been underserved. In addition to the Protection and Advocacy Program for People with Developmental Disabilities (PADD), the P&A also includes components mandated by several other federal programs to serve people with disabilities and mental illness.

National Network of University Centers for Excellence in Developmental
    Disabilities Education, Research, and Service
*http://www.acf.dhhs.gov/programs/add/states/uap.htm*

University Centers engage in four broad tasks: conducting interdisciplinary training, promoting exemplary community service programs, providing technical assistance at all levels from local service delivery to community and state governments, and conducting research and dissemination activities. UAPs provide community training and technical assistance to family and individual support service organizations, working with individuals with developmental disabilities, family members of these individuals, professionals, paraprofessionals, students, and volunteers. Direct exemplary service programs and the provision of training and technical assistance may include activities in the areas of family support, individual support, personal assistance services, clinical services, prevention services, health, education, vocational, and other direct services. The University Centers continue to contribute to the development of new knowledge through research, development and field testing of models, and the evaluation of existing as well as innovative practices.

Projects of National Significance
*http://www.acf.dhhs.gov/programs/add/pns.htm*
Under Projects of National Significance (PNS), the Administration on Developmental Disabilities awards grants and contracts to:

- promote and increase the independence, productivity, inclusion, and integration into the community of persons with developmental disabilities; and
- support the development of national and state policy, which enhances the independence, productivity, inclusion, and integration of these individuals into the community.

These Projects focus on the most pressing issues affecting people with developmental disabilities and their families. Project issues transcend the borders of states and territories, and project designs are oriented to permit local implementation of practical solutions. Examples include:

- data collection and analysis;
- technical assistance to program components;
- technical assistance to develop information and referral systems;
- projects that improve supportive living and quality of life opportunities;
- projects to educate policy makers; and
- efforts to pursue federal interagency initiatives.

National Associations
*http://www.acf.dhhs.gov/programs/add/states/natl.htm*
This section includes a listing of national organizations.

Disability.gov
*http://www.disability.gov*
The Presidential Task Force on Employment of Adults with Disabilities created this site to provide one-stop online access to resources, services, and information available throughout the federal government. The New Freedom Initiative for People with Disabilities is also part of President George W. Bush's administration goals, which call for government to use information technology to deliver government services anytime, anywhere. The site supports the administration's efforts to reduce barriers to the employment of people with disabilities.

## DISABILITY ONLINE
Employment and Training Administration/Department of Labor
*http://wdsc.doleta.gov/disability/*

The mission of disAbility Employment and initiatives unit within the Department of Labor, Employment and Training Administration is:

1. To provide leadership in the development of national policy related to programs and services under the Workforce Investment Act of 1998 that impact individuals with disabilities;

2. To provide guidance on accessibility issues and accommodations in One-Stop Center systems;

3. To facilitate the integration and coordination of WIA partnering agencies, especially those designed to serve individuals with disabilities, into the new workforce development system;

4. To represent ETA in collaborative multiagency design and policy formulation on issues of employment and training for this target population, including working closely with the President's Task Force on Employment of Adults with Disabilities; and

5. To design, develop, and administer innovative grant programs that further career and competitive employment goals of individuals with disabilities and/or support integration of the One-Stop Center system.

### PROGRAMS
Grants and Contracts
*http://wdsc.doleta.gov/disability/htmldocs/grants.html*

The Department of Labor, Employment and Training Administration, provides specialized employment and training services for individuals with disabilities through grants with 16 organizations. These disability partnerships include national organizations authorized under Title IV, Part D, Section 451, and Title III of the Job Training Partnership Act (JTPA) and are administered by the Office of National Programs. Grants were awarded July 1, 1998 for 1 year, plus 2 option years.

These disability partnership programs are designed to increase the number and quality of job opportunities for individuals with disabilities and to empower them to integrate more fully into society. Many of these programs provide outreach services, training, job development, and placement services. The organizations generally operate their programs in multistate sites and have strong linkages with local rehabilitation agency services and other private providers.

One-Stop Career Center
*http://wdsc.doleta.gov/disability/htmldocs/onestop.html*
This website provides links to relative WIA One-Stop information.

Disability Library
*http://wdsc.doleta.gov/disability/htmldocs/library.html*
This website provides links to disability-related legislation and documents.

Success Stories
*http://wdsc.doleta.gov/disability/htmldocs/success.html*
This website provides "success stories" on individuals with disabilities and meaningful employment opportunities.

### EMPLOYMENT AND TRAINING ADMINISTRATION
U.S. Department of Labor
200 Constitution Ave., NW
Washington, DC 20210
202-219-6871
*http://www.doleta.gov/*
The Employment and Training Administration (ETA) seeks to build up the labor market through the training of the workforce and the placement of workers in jobs through employment services. ETA's mission is to contribute to the more efficient and effective functioning of the U.S. labor market by providing high-quality job training, employment, labor market information, and income maintenance services primarily through state and local workforce development systems. This website is designed to direct adults, youth, dislocated workers, and workforce development professionals to information on these programs and services. Employers will find information on several areas, including tax credits and other hiring incentives, how to find and train employees, assistance with plant closures and downsizing, legislation text, and ETA grants and contracts.

#### PROGRAMS
Adult Training Programs
*http://www.doleta.gov/programs/adtrain.asp*
Funded by the Workforce Investment Act, these programs teach job skills and provide job placement services for economically disadvantaged adults.

One-Stop Centers
*http://usworkforce.org/onestop/*
An integrated, high-quality delivery system for an array of employment and training services designed to enhance the effectiveness and coordination of employer and job seeker services. One-Stop Centers connecting employment, education, and training services into a coherent network of resources at the local, state, and national levels.

Youth Training Programs
*http://www.doleta.gov/youth_services/default.asp*

These programs are designed to enhance youth education, encourage school completion through alternative educational programs, and provide exposure to the world of work through apprenticeship and career exploration. Youth programs are administered by the U.S. Department of Labor and funded in state and local communities. The website provides information and assistance about various youth employment and training activities authorized under the Workforce Investment Act of 1998.

## Guide to Disability Rights Laws
U.S. Department of Justice
Civil Rights Division
Disability Rights Section
*http://www.pueblo.gsa.gov/cic_text/misc/disability/disrits.htm*

This guide includes information on the following disability rights laws: Americans with Disabilities Act, Fair Housing Act, Air Carrier Access Act, Civil Rights of Institutionalized Persons Act, Individuals with Disabilities Education Act, Rehabilitation Act, Architectural Barriers Act, along with other sources of Disability Rights Information.

## Centers for Medicare and Medicaid Services
U.S. Department of Health and Human Services
7500 Security Blvd.
Baltimore, MD 21244
410-786-3000
*http://www.hcfa.gov*

The Centers for Medicare and Medicaid Services (CMS) is a federal agency within the U.S. Department of Health and Human Services. CMS runs the Medicare and Medicaid programs—two national health care programs that benefit about 75 million Americans. And with the Health Resources and Services Administration, CMS runs the Children's Health Insurance Program, a program that is expected to cover many of the approximately 10 million uninsured children in the United States. CMS spends over $360 billion a year buying health care services for beneficiaries of Medicare, Medicaid, and the Children's Health Insurance Program. CMS:

- ensures that the Medicaid, Medicare, and Children's Health Insurance programs are properly run by its contractors and state agencies;
- establishes policies for paying health care providers;
- conducts research on the effectiveness of various methods of health care management, treatment, and financing; and
- assesses the quality of health care facilities and services and takes enforcement actions as appropriate.

PROGRAMS

Ticket to Work and Work Incentives Improvement Act of 1999
*http://www.hcfa.gov/medicaid/twwiia/twwiiahp.htm*

Passage of this law marks the most significant advancement for people with disabilities since enactment of the Americans with Disabilities Act. This landmark legislation modernizes the employment services system for people with disabilities and makes it possible for millions of Americans with disabilities to join the workforce without fear of losing their Medicare and Medicaid coverage. States, advocacy groups, and consumers should be aware of the following:

The TWWIIA provides:

- Increased opportunities for states to limit barriers to employment for people with disabilities by improving access to health care coverage available under Medicare and Medicaid, administered by CMS. Beginning October 1, 2000, qualifying States were eligible to receive monies under two grant programs designed to support working individuals with disabilities.

  Medicaid Infrastructure Grant Program
  - $150 million available over the first 5 years for states to design, establish, and operate health care delivery systems that support the employment of individuals with disabilities.
  - States cannot use infrastructure grant funds to provide direct services to individuals with disabilities. To be eligible, states must provide personal assistance services under the Medicaid program sufficient to support the competitive employment of disabled individuals.

  Medicaid Demonstration to Increase Independence and Employment
  - Funded at $250 million over 6 years. Under the demonstration, states can provide Medicaid services to workers with potentially severe impairments that are likely to lead to blindness or disability. This demonstration gives states the opportunity to evaluate whether providing these workers with early access to Medicaid services delays the progression to actual disability.
  - States define the number of individuals with potentially severe disabilities that they decide to cover and which potentially severe impairments they will target.

- Improved access to employment training and placement services for people with disabilities who want to work administered by the Social Security Administration: *http://www.ssa.gov/work.* (For more information on the SSA portion of TWWIIA, see the Social Security Administration resource link listed below.)

Medicaid
*http://www.hcfa.gov/medicaid/medicaid.htm*

Medicaid is a jointly funded, federal-state health insurance program for certain low-income and needy people. It covers approximately 36 million individuals including children, the aged, blind, and/or disabled, and people who are eligible to receive federally assisted income maintenance payments. Although there are broad federal requirements for Medicaid, states have a wide degree of flexibility to design their program. States have authority to:

- establish eligibility standards;
- determine what benefits and services to cover; and
- set payment rates.

### PROGRAMS

Home and Community-Based Services 1915(c) Waivers
*http://www.hcfa.gov/medicaid/hpg4.htm*

Medicaid home and community-based service (HCBS) waivers afford states the flexibility to develop and implement creative alternatives to placing Medicaid-eligible individuals in hospitals, nursing facilities, or inter-mediate care facilities for persons with mental retardation. The HCBS waiver program recognizes that many individuals at risk of being placed in these facilities can be cared for in their homes and communities, preserving their independence and ties to family and friends at a cost no higher than that of institutional care.

Americans with Disabilities Act/Olmstead Decision
*http://www.hcfa.gov/medicaid/olmstead/olmshome.htm*

In July 1999, the Supreme Court issued the *Olmstead v. L. C.* decision. The Court's decision in that case clearly challenges federal, state, and local governments to develop more opportunities for individuals with disabilities through more accessible systems of cost-effective community-based services. The *Olmstead* decision interpreted Title II of the ADA and its implementing regulation, requiring states to administer their services, programs, and activities "in the most integrated setting appropriate to the needs of qualified individuals with disabilities."

Medicaid can be an important resource to assist States in meeting these goals. However, the scope of the ADA and the *Olmstead* decision are not limited to Medicaid beneficiaries or to services financed by the Medicaid program. The ADA and the *Olmstead* decision apply to all qualified individuals with disabilities regardless of age. CMS has begun consultation with states and with people with disabilities. CMS plans to review relevant federal Medicaid regulations, policies, and previous guidance to ensure that they are compatible with the requirements of the ADA and the *Olmstead* decision and to facilitate states' efforts to comply with the law. CMS is working closely with other involved Federal agencies to ensure that these reviews are consistent with the requirements of the statute and are focused on the needs of persons with disabilities.

ADA/Olmstead Decision Questions and Answers
*http://www.hcfa.gov/medicaid/olmstead/olmsfaq.htm*
This page contains ADA/Olmstead information generated by questions CMS has received from states, stakeholders and other interested entities.

Guidance on Olmstead Decision and Fact Sheet (Letter to State Medicaid Directors)
*http://www.hcfa.gov/medicaid/smd1140a.htm*

THE OFFICE OF DISABILITY, AGING, AND LONG-TERM CARE POLICY
U.S. Department of Health and Human Services
Room 424E, H.H. Humphrey Building
200 Independence Avenue, S.W.
Washington, DC 20201
202-690-6443
*DALTCP2@OSASPE.DHHS.GOV*
*http://aspe.os.dhhs.gov/daltcp/home.htm*
The Office of Disability, Aging, and Long-Term Care Policy (DALTCP) is in the Office of the Assistant Secretary for Planning and Evaluation (*http://aspe.os.dhhs.gov/*) within the U.S. Department of Health and Human Services (HHS). DALTCP is charged with developing, analyzing, evaluating, and coordinating HHS policies and programs that support the independence, productivity, health, and long-term care needs of children, working-age adults, and older persons with disabilities. The office works closely with the Administration on Aging, the Administration on Developmental Disabilities, the Health Care Financing Administration and others.

The Assistant Secretary for Planning and Evaluation (ASPE) advises the Secretary of the Department of Health and Human Services on policy development in health, disability, human services, and science and provides advice and analysis on economic policy. ASPE leads special initiatives, coordinates the Department's evaluation, research, and demonstration activities, and manages cross-Department planning activities such as strategic planning, legislative planning, and review of regulations. Integral to this role, ASPE conducts research and evaluation studies, develops policy analyses, and estimates the cost and benefits of policy alternatives under consideration by the Department or Congress. The DALTCP site includes information on topics such as:

- Disability issues
- Employment
- Home and community-based services
- Insurance issues
- Long-term care issues
- Medicaid issues
- Medicare issues

## OFFICE OF DISABILITY EMPLOYMENT POLICY
1331 F Street, N.W. Suite 300
Washington, DC 20004
202-376-6200; 202-376-6205 (TTD)
*http://www.dol.gov/dol/odep/*

In the FY 2001 budget, Congress approved a new Office of Disability Employment Policy (ODEP) for the Department of Labor. Programs and staff of the former President's Committee on Employment of People with Disabilities have been integrated in this new office. The mission of ODEP, under the leadership of an Assistant Secretary, will be to bring a heightened and permanent long-term focus to the goal of increasing employment of persons with disabilities. This will be achieved through policy analysis, technical assistance, and development of best practices, as well as outreach, education, constituent services, and promoting ODEP's mission among employers.

To support the President's New Freedom Initiative, ODEP will provide competitive grants to One-Stop Career Centers to make the centers more accessible to people with significant disabilities in a variety of ways. The centers will be expected to utilize assistive technology, provide appropriate staff training, and use best practices to provide greater access to people with significant disabilities and to provide them the services they need to get into the economic mainstream.

### PROGRAMS
Job Accommodation Network (JAN)
*http://www.dol.gov/dol/odep/public/jan.htm*

The Job Accommodation Network (JAN) is a toll-free consulting service of the U. S. Department of Labor's ODEP. JAN provides information on workplace accommodations and on the employment provisions of the Americans with Disabilities Act (ADA). Service is available via a toll-free number: 1-800-ADA-WORK (1-800-232-9675 ) or 1-800-526-7234. In addition, a Searchable Online Accommodation Resource (SOAR) is available on JAN's website.

OFFICE OF SPECIAL EDUCATION AND REHABILITATIVE SERVICES
U.S. Department of Education
400 Maryland Avenue, SW
Washington, DC 20202-0498
800-872-5327
*http://www.ed.gov/offices/OSERS/*

The Office of Special Education and Rehabilitative Services (OSERS) supports programs that assist in educating children with special needs, provides for the rehabilitation of youth and adults with disabilities, and supports research to improve the lives of individuals with disabilities.

### PROGRAMS

The Individuals with Disabilities Education Act Amendments of 1997
*http://www.ed.gov/offices/OSERS/IDEA/*

The U.S. Department of Education helps states and school districts meet their responsibility to provide a free appropriate public education for children with disabilities. Two landmark federal court decisions in the early 1970s established the constitutional right of children with disabilities to equal educational opportunity. In 1975 a federal law, now known as the Individuals with Disabilities Education Act (IDEA), P.L. 94-142, was enacted to provide a framework for appropriately serving these children as well as federal financial assistance to help pay for their education.

The Individuals with Disabilities Education Act Amendments of 1997 (IDEA '97) were signed into law on June 4, 1997. This Act strengthens academic expectations and accountability for the nation's 5.8 million children with disabilities and bridges the gap that has too often existed between what children with disabilities learn and what is required in regular curriculum.

Rehabilitation Services Administration
*http://www.ed.gov/offices/OSERS/RSA/*

The Rehabilitation Services Administration (RSA) oversees programs that help individuals with physical or mental disabilities to obtain employment through the provision of such supports as counseling, medical and psychological services, job training, and other individualized services. RSA's major formula grant program provides funds to state vocational rehabilitation agencies to provide employment-related services for individuals with disabilities, giving priority to individuals who are severely disabled. RSA maintains close liaison with federal counterpart agencies such as the Social Security Administration, the Department of Labor, the National Institute of Mental Health, the President's Committee on the Employment of Persons with Disabilities, the Office of Special Education Programs, the Office of Adult and Vocational Education, and the National Institute on Disability and Rehabilitation Research.

PRESIDENTIAL TASK FORCE ON EMPLOYMENT OF ADULTS
WITH DISABILITIES
U.S. Department of Labor
200 Constitution Avenue, NW, Suite S-2220
Washington, DC 20210
202-693-4939; 202-693-4920 (TTY)
*ptfead@dol.gov.*
*http://www.dol.gov/dol/_sec/public/programs/ptfead/main.htm*

The mission of the Presidential Task Force on Employment of Adults with Disabilities is to create a coordinated and aggressive national policy to bring adults with disabilities into gainful employment at a rate that is as close as possible to that of the general adult population. The mandate of the Task Force is to evaluate existing federal programs to determine what changes, modifications, and innovations may be necessary to remove barriers to employment opportunities faced by adults with disabilities. Some of the areas the Task Force will review include reasonable accommodations, inadequate access to health care, lack of consumer-driven, long-term supports and services, transportation, accessible and integrated housing, telecommunications, assistive technology, community services, child care, education, vocational rehabilitation, training services, employment retention, promotion and discrimination, on-the-job supports, and economic incentives to work.

SOCIAL SECURITY ADMINISTRATION
6401 Security Blvd.
Baltimore, MD 21235-0001
800-772-1213
*http://www.ssa.gov*

The Social Security Administration (SSA) manages the nation's social insurance program, consisting of retirement, survivors, and disability insurance programs, commonly known as Social Security. It also administers the Supplemental Security Income program for the aged, blind, and disabled. The Administration is responsible for studying the problems of poverty and economic insecurity among Americans and making recommendations on effective methods for solving these problems through social insurance. The Administration also assigns Social Security numbers to U.S. citizens and maintains earnings records for workers under their Social Security numbers.

*PROGRAMS*
Supplemental Security Income
*http://www.ssa.gov/notices/supplemental-security-income/*

SSI is an acronym for the Supplemental Security Income program that was established in 1974 under Title XVI of the Social Security Act and administered by the Social Security Administration. SSI is a federally administered cash assistance program for individuals who are aged, blind, or disabled and meet a financial needs test (income and resource limitations).

The SSI program operates in the 50 states, the District of Columbia, and the Northern Mariana Islands. The program also covers blind or disabled children of military parents stationed abroad and certain students studying outside the U.S. for a period of not more than 1 year. The federal government funds SSI from general tax revenues. The basic SSI amount is the same nationwide. However, many states add money to the basic benefit. Some states pay benefits to some individuals to supplement their federal benefits. Some of these states have arranged with SSA to combine their supplementary payment with the federal payment into one monthly check. Other states manage their own programs and make their payments separately.

Unlike the Social Security Disability Insurance (SSDI) program, SSI has no prior work requirements and no waiting period for cash or medical benefits. Eligible SSI applicants generally begin receiving cash benefits immediately on entitlement and, in most cases, receipt of cash benefits makes them eligible for Medicaid benefits.

### Social Security Disability Insurance
*http://www.ssa.gov/dibplan/index.htm*

SSDI is an acronym for the Social Security Disability Insurance program, which was established in 1956 under Title II of the Social Security Act. SSDI provides federal disability insurance benefits for workers who have contributed to the Social Security Trust Fund and become disabled or blind before retirement age. These contributions are the Federal Insurance Contributions Act (FICA) social security tax paid on their earnings or those of their spouses or parents. Spouses with disabilities and dependent children of fully insured workers (often referred to as the primary beneficiary) also are eligible for disabilitybenefitsontheretirement,disability,ordeathoftheprimarybeneficiary.

After becoming disabled, individuals have a waiting period of 5 months before receiving cash benefits. In addition to cash assistance, SSDI beneficiaries receive Medicare coverage after they have received cash benefits for 24 months. Beneficiaries' SSDI benefits convert to Social Security retirement benefits when beneficiaries reach age 65.

### Office of Employment Support Programs
*http://www.ssa.gov/work/index2.html*

The Office of Employment Support Programs, formerly the Division of Employment and Rehabilitation Programs, has been established to improve SSA's service to people with disabilities who want to work. The mission of the Office of Employment Support Programs consists of:

- Planning, implementing, and evaluating SSA programs and policies related to the employment of SSDI and SSI beneficiaries with disabilities;

- Promoting innovation in the design of programs and policies that increase employment opportunities for Social Security beneficiaries;
- Educating the public about SSA and other public programs that support employment and about organizations that provide employment-related services; and
- Joining with other public and private entities to remove employment barriers for people with disabilities.

Work Incentives
*http://www.ssa.gov/work/ResourcesToolkit/workincentives.html*

Once a person with a disability has returned to work, special rules called "work incentives" will help serve as a bridge from reliance on benefits to financial independence achieved by returning to work. With these incentives, the individual can continue to receive cash payments and health insurance coverage (for a period of time) until he or she is able to work regularly. There are different work incentives for persons who receive SSDI and SSI benefits. There are also special work incentives for persons who are blind and for students with disabilities.

- SSDI and SSI Work Incentives
  - Impairment-related work expenses
  - Subsidies and special conditions
  - Unincurred business expenses
  - Unsuccessful work attempts
  - Continued payments under a vocational rehabilitation program
- SSDI Work Incentives
  - Trial work period
  - Extended period of eligibility
  - Continuation of Medicare coverage
  - Medicare for people with disabilities who work
- SSI Work Incentives
  - Blind work expenses
  - Earned income exclusion
  - Student earned income exclusion
  - Plan for achieving self-support
  - Property essential to self-support
  - Special SSI payments for people who work
  - Continued Medicaid eligibility
  - Special benefits for people eligible under Section 1619 (a) or (b) who enter a medical treatment facility
  - Reinstating eligibility without a new application

Some of the ways that these incentives help people with disabilities to work is by allowing them to:

- test the ability to work for a specified period of time without losing any benefits;
- deduct from earnings the cost of certain impairment-related work items or services needed to work in determining whether earnings are too high to continue receiving benefits;
- continue Medicare coverage if disability benefits stop because earnings are too high;
- continue to receive SSI payments until the earnings that count exceed the SSI limits; and
- continue Medicaid coverage if the person depends on Medicaid to work even if earnings exceed the SSI limits until the person's earnings are sufficient to replace lost benefits.

Ticket to Work and Work Incentives Improvement Act of 1999
*http://www.ssa.gov/work/ResourcesToolkit/legisreg2.html*
This new law: increases beneficiary choice in obtaining rehabilitation and vocational services; removes barriers that require people with disabilities to choose between health care coverage and work; and ensures that more Americans with disabilities have the opportunity to participate in the workforce and lessen their dependence on public benefits.
Ticket To Work And Self-Sufficiency Program
Starting in 2001, Social Security and Supplemental Security Income (SSI) disability beneficiaries receive a "ticket" they may use to obtain vocational rehabilitation, employment, or other support services from an approved provider of their choice. The Ticket Program is voluntary. The program will be phased in nationally over a 3-year period.


## GENERAL RESOURCES

INDEPENDENT LIVING RESEARCH UTILIZATION
2323 South Shepherd, Suite 1000
Houston, TX 77019
713-520-0232
713-520-5136 [TDD]
*http://www.ilru.org*
The Independent Living Research Utilization (ILRU) program is a national center for information, training, research, and technical assistance in independent living. Its goal is to expand the body of knowledge in independent living and to improve utilization of results of research programs and demonstration projects in this field. Since ILRU was established in 1977, it has developed a variety of strategies for collecting, synthesizing, and disseminating information related to the field of independent living. ILRU staff—a majority of whom are people with disabilities—serve independent

living centers, statewide independent living councils, state and federal rehabilitation agencies, consumer organizations, educational institutions, medical facilities, and other organizations involved in the field, both nationally and internationally. ILRU has developed a variety of resource materials on independent living subjects.

## Home and Community-Based Services Resource Network
*http://hcbs.org/index.htm*

The mission of the Home and Community-Based Services (HCBS) Resource Network is to bring the federal government, states, and persons with disabilities of all ages together to expand access to high-quality, consumer-directed services in a cost-effective manner. The Resource Network will support state efforts to engage in collaborative planning and policy development within the aging and disability communities. It will focus on identifying practical and immediate next steps that can be taken to expand access to supportive services in the most integrated, least restrictive settings in ways that are realistic, equitable and affordable. The Resource Network will serve as a model for collaborative problem solving, priority setting, and styles of working between government agencies and persons with disabilities that is fundamental to continued progress in HCBS systems development.

### Programs
State Collaboration

The Resource Network will collaborate with states on HCBS systems change. These initiatives will generally begin with a process of eliciting input from stakeholders, including state agencies, consumers, families, providers, legislators, and others. Once completed, the Network will provide resources for implementing system improvements, including consulting expertise, data analysis, technology transfer among states, direct support for consumer involvement in program development activities, and convening forums and other meetings.

State Health and Social Services Web Sites in the United States
*http://hcbs.org/state_links.htm*

HCBS links to state health and social services websites

State Data
*http://www.hcbs.org/state_data.htm*

HCBS reports on state activities.

## Human Services Research Institute
2336 Massachusetts Ave.
Cambridge, MA 02140
617-876-0426
*http://www.hsri.org/*

In the fields of developmental disabilities, physical disabilities, mental health, and child welfare the Human Services Research Institute (HSRI) works to:

- Assist human service organizations and systems to develop support systems for children, adults, and families;
- Enhance the participation of individuals and their families to shape policy and service practices;
- Improve the capacity of systems, organizations, and individuals to cope with the changes in fiscal, administrative, and political realities; and
- Expand the use of research and evaluation to guide policy and practice.

*PROGRAMS*

Workforce Development Initiatives
*http://www.hsri.org/ddworkforce/about.html*

The challenge of assisting people with disabilities to determine the course of their lives has been a transforming theme throughout the last decade. This movement toward consumer empowerment as well as the increasing decentralization of support services requires that the field must redefine the direct support role to ensure that practitioners meet the unique characteristics of the contemporary service environment. The workforce development activities at HSRI are focused on building the capacity of the human service, education, and training systems to meet this challenge and to shape a competent and vital direct service workforce with the skills, knowledge, and values that will help people lead self-determined lives. Toward this end, HSRI staff is engaged in a variety of demonstration, research, and technical activities to help government and human service employers ensure a robust workforce. These activities include the development of:

- practice guidelines for direct support professionals
- competency-based curriculum aligned with contemporary practice standards
- strategic planning for improving employee recruitment, retention, and development
- performance-based assessment of practitioner competence
- planning for systemwide workforce development strategies including education and incentive programs and credentialing systems
- multimedia instructional design
- implementing measures and indices of workforce stability

Self-Advocate Leadership Network
*http://www.hsri.org/leaders/leaders.html*
The purpose of the Leadership Network is to prepare self-advocates to play a leadership role in guiding developmental disabilities systems change in ways that promote self-determination, community integration, and participant-driven supports.

QualityMall.org
150 Pillsbury Dr. SE Rm. 204
Minneapolis MN 55455
612-624-6328
612-625-6619
*rtc@icimail.coled.umn.edu*
*http://www.qualitymall.org*
QualityMall.org, a showcase of promising practices and innovations that promote quality of life for persons with developmental disabilities, was developed by the Research and Training Center on Community Living at the University of Minnesota's Institute on Community Integration (RTC/ICI), the National Association of State Directors of Developmental Disabilities Services (NASDDDS), and Human Services Research Institute (HSRI). It receives its primary funding through a grant from the federal Administration on Developmental Disabilities. Although it is not a retailer or vendor of products or services, it uses the theme of a shopping mall to help connect visitors to the best products and services available.

Stores at QualityMall.org represent broad topic areas, whereas departments provide more specific descriptions of available products and services. Products represent efforts to enhance the quality of life for persons with disabilities and may be exemplary programs, publications, video and sound recordings, training curriculum, CD-ROMs, or websites. Product pages contain detailed descriptions, contact information, and web links. Other components of the mall include the Quality Cinema, where users can view video clips, slide shows, and interactive presentations; the News Stand, where breaking information regarding quality in services to people with disabilities will be posted; and The Coffee Shop, which features bulletin boards and live chats on issues in person-centered services.

## General Resources on Youth with Disabilities

National Information Center on Children and Youth with Disabilities
P.O. Box 1492
Washington, DC 20013
800-695-0285
*http://www.nichcy.org/*

NICHCY is a national information and referral center that provides information on disabilities and disability-related issues for families, educators and other professionals. The focus is children and youth (birth to age 22). It provides links to:

- Comprehensive database of disability organizations
- Publications/Fact Sheets on specific disabilities
- Publicaciones en Espanol
- Personal responses to specific questions via email
- State Resource Sheets to assist in locating organizations/agencies within each state

## REGIONAL RESOURCE CENTERS

*http://www.dssc.org/frc/rrfc.htm*

The Regional Resource and Federal Centers (RRFC) Network is comprised of the six Regional Resource Centers (RRCs) for Special Education and the FRC. The six RRCs are specifically funded to assist state education agencies in the systemic improvement of education programs, practices, and policies that affect children and youth with disabilities. The RRCs help states and U.S. jurisdictions find integrated solutions for systemic reform, offering consultation, information services, technical assistance, training, and product development. The beneficiaries of the RRCs' work are children and youth with disabilities and the families and professionals who are associated with them.

## REHABILITATION RESEARCH AND TRAINING CENTERS

### REHABILITATION RESEARCH AND TRAINING CENTERS

Projects of the National Institute on Disability and Rehabilitation Research
400 Maryland Avenue, S.W.
Washington, DC 20202-2572
202-205-8134
*http://www.ed.gov/offices/OSERS/NIDRR/*

The new employment-focused Rehabilitation Research and Training Centers are undertaking a variety of research projects that are consistent with the "New Paradigm of Disability" and NIDRR's purpose and focus for research on the employment of people with disabilities. Following are brief introductions to the RRTCs and their research projects.

Rehabilitation Research and Training Center on Workforce
Investment and Employment Policy for Persons with Disabilities

Community Options, Inc.
1130-17th Street NW, Suite 430
Washington, DC 20036
202-721-0124
*michael.morris@comop.org*
*http://www.comop.org*

This Center helps expand, improve, and modify disability policy and other more general policies to improve the employment status of Americans with disabilities and increase their independence and self-sufficiency. Based on research from this project and other NIDRR-funded projects, this project establishes an information and technical assistance resource to government leaders and decision makers at state and federal levels, individuals with disabilities, parents and family members, and other interested parties, offering new and revised approaches to workforce development and employment policy. Studies conducted by this project include: (1) an analysis of the relationship between select federal and state policies and the employment of people with disabilities, (2) an analysis of the policy-based implications of outcome-based reimbursement on the delivery of employment and rehabilitation services to people with disabilities, and (3) an analysis of the effect of civil rights protections and multiple environmental factors on promoting or depressing the employment status of people with disabilities.

National Center for the Study of Postsecondary Educational Supports:
    A Rehabilitation Research and Training Center
University of Hawaii at Manoa
Center on Disability Studies—University Affiliated Program
1776 University Ave./UA4-6
Honolulu, HI 96822
808-956-3975
*stodden@hawaii.edu; huap@hawaii.edu; cds@hawaii.edu*
*http://www.rrtc.Hawaii.edu*

The research this project conducts on educational supports is designed to increase access to postsecondary education programs and to improve outcomes for people with disabilities. The research includes: (1) examining and evaluating the current status of educational supports, including (a) individual academic accommodations, (b) adaptive equipment, (c) case management and coordination, (d) advocacy, and (e) personal counseling and career advising; (2) identifying effective support practices and models of delivery that contribute to successful access, performance, and retention and completion of postsecondary programs; (3) identifying specific barriers to the provision of disability-related services, including policy and funding requirements; (4) assessing the effectiveness of promising educational practices and disability-related services that are important to career mobility and success in the workplace; (5) testing the effectiveness of specific models of delivery that are believed to increase the accessibility of educational supports and innovative technologies; (6) identifying the types of educational and transitional assistance that postsecondary programs provide to improve educational and subsequent labor market success; (7) providing training, technical assistance, and information to support personnel, public and private rehabilitation personnel, career placement specialists, and students with disabilities based on the findings and implications of the research program; and (8) implementing a consumer-driven empowerment evaluation plan for assessment of the Center's progress in achieving its goals.

UIC National Research and Training Center on Psychiatric Disability
University of Illinois/Chicago
Department of Psychiatry
104 South Michigan Ave., Suite 900
Chicago, IL 60603-5902
312-422-8180; 312-422-0706 (TTY)
*http://www.psych.uic.edu/uicnrtc*
    This Center conducts a comprehensive series of research and training projects that focus on increasing self-determination for persons with psychiatric disability. The Center's current projects are composed of five core areas: (1) choices in treatment decision making; (2) economic self-sufficiency; (3) consumer advocacy under managed care; (4) career development through real jobs for real wages; and (5) strengthening self-determination skills and self-advocacy. These core areas reaffirm that people with psychiatric disabilities have the right to maximal independence, which grows out of making choices in the decisions that affect their lives. Project activities are implemented by multidisciplinary workgroups composed of consumers, families, service providers, state agency administrators, researchers, and Center staff. Outcome and measurement tools developed for each core area assess key outcomes and program policies related to self-determination.

Rehabilitation Research and Training Center on State Systems and Employment
Children's Hospital
Institute for Community Inclusion
300 Longwood Ave.
Boston, MA 02115
617-335-7074
*ici@a1.tch.harvard.edu*
*http://www.childrenshospital.org/ici/rrtc*

This Center identifies effective practices in coordinated employment efforts and facilitates such development at local, regional, and state levels. It also influences policy, practice, and perceptions on the national level. Project activities include investigations, technical assistance, and public policy reviews focused on: (1) examining state service systems, including vocational rehabilitation, mental health, mental retardation, employment and training service (including one-stop career centers and welfare-to-work programs), and education to document promising policies and practices reflecting integrated and coordinated approaches to employment of people with disabilities; (2) documenting actual employment outcomes for people with disabilities through the analysis of national, state, and local data collection systems; (3) documenting strategies state agencies use for overcoming barriers to employment at the state and local levels; (4) examining, documenting, and disseminating practices at the state level that respond to the employment and support needs of SSI and SSDI beneficiaries; and (5) reviewing and evaluating strategies and approaches to develop a more integrated employment approach at the federal and state levels, to enhance the employment of people with disabilities.

Rehabilitation Research and Training Center for Economic Research on
    Employment Policy for Persons with Disabilities
Cornell University
Program on Employment and Disability
School of Industrial and Labor Relations
Ithaca, NY 14853-3901
607-255-7727; 607-255-2891 (TTY)
*smb23@cornell.edu*
*http://www.ilr.cornell.edu/rrtc*

Using principles of economics, this project conducts policy research on how environmental factors influence the work outcomes of people with disabilities. Research also addresses critical aspects of employment outcomes, recognizing the heterogeneity of people with disabilities, and explains the importance of interactions among the multiplicity of programs intended to meet the employment needs of people with disabilities. Components include: (1) a comprehensive analysis, using existing panel data, of the current employment status of people with disabilities; (2) a longitudinal analysis of the effects of labor market change on the employment and earnings of people with disabilities; (3) a longitudinal analysis of return to work after the onset of a disability; (4) a longitudinal analysis of the impact of civil rights protections on the employment and earnings of people with disabilities; (5) identification and analysis of policies that foster or impede the participation of transitioning students in rehabilitation or employment service programs; and (6) analysis of emerging and important issues affecting the employment of people with disabilities.

Rehabilitation Research and Training Center on Workplace Supports
Virginia Commonwealth University
1314 West Main St., Box 842011
Richmond, VA 23284-2011
804-828-1851; 804-828-2494 (TTY)
*tcblanke@saturn.vcu.edu*
*http://www.worksupport.com*

This Center helps to increase the national employment rate among people with disabilities by identifying factors in the work environment that inhibit or enhance employment outcomes and by sharing the results with the business community. Researchers: (1) analyze existing or new financial incentives to find those that encourage enterprises to hire or retrain workers with disabilities; (2) measure the effectiveness of disability management and return-to-work strategies; (3) assess employers' need for information, training, and resources; (4) conduct, in business settings, interventions that respond to employer needs; (5) analyze the interventions to determine their effectiveness; and (6) determine the impact of changes in work structures such as telecommuting and self-employment on the employment outcomes of people with disabilities. Stakeholders who benefit from these research, training, technical assistance, and dissemination efforts include business personnel; rehabilitation service personnel; federal and state policy-makers; people with disabilities; their guardians, advocates, and authorized representatives; students; and the general public.

Rehabilitation Research and Training Center on Community Rehabilitation
      Programs to Improve Employment Outcomes
University of Wisconsin/Stout
Stout Vocational Rehabilitation Institute
College of Human Development
715-232-2236; 715-232-5025 (TTY)
Menomonie, WI 54751
*rtc@uwstout.edu*
*http://www.rtc.uwstout.edu*

This project engages community-based rehabilitation programs (CRPs) and state rehabilitation programs in an effort to open multiple funding sources for rehabilitation and habilitation services and employment opportunities for people with disabilities. The project includes a series of interrelated studies directed toward changing outcomes and determining CRP capacities to affect economic status of people with disabilities in their communities and develops a complementary methodology for achieving utilization and application of the new knowledge. Primary research tasks include: (1) examining how CRPs are serving people with disabilities from alternate sources of funding; (2) determining the extent to which consumers pursue and receive services, compared to the intentions of the Rehabilitation

Act; (3) exploring what funding, service, and strategy capacities exist to address those intentions more coherently at the community level; (4) devising and demonstrating practice-program alternatives that materially improve outcomes from CRPs; and (5) clarifying how CRPs as an industry can be better enjoined as a complementary resource to improve the economic and community integration status of people with disabilities.

# Playing the Housing "Game": People with Down Syndrome and Their Families Can Have More Control When It Comes to Housing

## Kathleen H. McGinley, Ph.D.

### BACKGROUND

When I began to write this chapter, I made a list of issues and resources that should be covered if there is to be more decent, safe, and affordable housing available so that people with Down syndrome and their families can make real "choices" about where they want to live. Then, of course, I realized that covering all these issues would take a book—not a chapter. Therefore, my goal here is to give the reader as much basic information and guidance as possible about how to play the "housing game" and to provide a range of information sources that can help complete the picture.

My goal is for the reader to come away realizing that the following points are true.

- Housing can be the cornerstone to independence.
- People with disabilities face a housing crisis that has been ignored by many in the disability community and by policy makers.

*Down Syndrome*, Edited by William I. Cohen, Lynn Nadel, and Myra E. Madnick.
ISBN 0-471-41815-3   Copyright © 2002 by Wiley-Liss, Inc.

- For too long there has been a reliance on a separate "disability" system.
- If people are going to have real choice in housing, there has to be affordable housing from which to choose.
- People with disabilities and their families must become players in the generic housing world.
- Advocacy at the local, state, and national levels is the key to successfully increasing decent, safe, and affordable housing options in the community.

## What Is "Real" Choice?

If the goal is to ensure that people with Down syndrome and other disabilities have the opportunity to live full lives in the community, then we need to stop and ask ourselves a few questions up front.

- Where do people *want* to live? What are the variables that guide the answer to this question?—being close to friends and family; being independent from family; being close to work, stores, or place of worship; being near a bus or train route; being near parks and places to have fun?
- Once someone knows where he/she wants to live, what are the variables that influence his/her ability to really choose to live there? One of the most influential variables, whether or not a person has a disability, is money.
- In the real world, money or the lack of it can either expand or severely limit individual choice. Although someone may want to live in an apartment in a high rise, he may not be able to pay the rent. Although someone may want to buy a nice town house, she may be unable to afford a mortgage and long-term upkeep.
- As if money is not enough of an obstacle, some people with disabilities may face a number of additional obstacles, such as the need for specific services and supports to help them live independently, the need for a place large enough for both the individual and the person who provides supports, and/or the need for a place to live that is physically adaptable or accessible.
- One other factor that still limits choice is housing discrimination. Discrimination either may be intentional or may be the result of the continuing ignorance of people, who should be neighbors, as well as those people who make policy at the local, state, and national levels.

- Another potential major obstacle is—what if no one lets the person with a disability make choices? This may happen because family members are afraid that something bad will happen to the person with a disability, or it may happen because some service providers want to "fit" the person to their services and not to match the necessary supports to the person.

- Finally, the unfortunate fact is that individual choice and self-determination continue to be limited because of poorly designed federal policies. Medicaid too often requires an individual to "fit" the system or fight for flexibility. Social Security policies limit an individual's ability to make choices because they force people to live in poverty, especially those who receive Supplemental Security Income (SSI) benefits. Federal housing policies have historically ignored the needs of people with disabilities or pigeonholed them into small disability-specific programs.

I make these points not so the reader will think that finding decent, safe, and affordable housing is an impossible task but so it is clear that self-determination and choice making in relation to housing do not operate in a vacuum. There are variables in all our lives that limit choice and control. What everyone needs to learn—not only people with disabilities and their families—is how to manipulate or change variables so that real choices are available.

There are many ways that people with Down syndrome and their families can work to change the environment so that communities are welcoming places that recognize the important role that people with disabilities play in community life. Over the past several years, more and more people with disabilities, family members, and advocates have started to be housing "activists." Because of their work, more doors are already open and continued activism will ensure that additional doors open in the future.

## SELF-DETERMINATION

The following definition of "self-determination" was the first ever included in a piece of federal legislation. It is part of the 2000 reauthorization of the Developmental Disabilities Assistance and Bill of Rights Act.[1] Although the inclusion of a definition of this concept in federal law was a positive step, it has not been without controversy. One concern voiced is that the definition combines "self-determination" with "activities." Some advocates believe that the term "self-determination activities" makes it sound as though self-determination is something that someone else does for an individual

[1] Developmental Disabilities Assistance and Bill of Rights Act of 1999, P.L. 106-402.

through pre-established—and not individualized—activities, thus missing the centrality of individual choice and control to self-determination. Even with this concern, it is obvious that this definition clearly reflects many of the important characteristics that comprise real self-determination.

> SELF-DETERMINATION ACTIVITIES—The term self-determination activities means activities that result in individuals with developmental disabilities, with appropriate assistance, having—
> (A) the ability and opportunity to communicate and make personal decisions;
> (B) the ability and opportunity to communicate choices and exercise control over the type and intensity of services, supports and other assistance the individuals receive;
> (C) the authority to control resources to obtain needed services, supports and other assistance;
> (D) opportunities to participate in, and contribute to, their communities; and
> (E) support, including financial support, to advocate for themselves and others, to develop leadership skills, through training in self-advocacy, to participate in coalitions, to educate policymakers, and to play a role in the development of public policies that affect individuals with developmental disabilities.

What is not reflected in this definition are some of the intangibles that must be considered in relation to self-determination. These intangibles play an important role in ensuring that people with disabilities are truly "part" of the community. David and Faye Wetherow, in *Supporting Self Determination with Integrity*,[2] make the important point that there are beginning to be "some indications that the bare language of Self-Determination 'autonomy, choice, freedom, and responsibility'—may fail to convey the importance of engagement, companionship, contribution, and affiliation." The importance of these and similar attributes cannot be underestimated if an individual is to really "live" in his/her community.

## PEOPLE WITH DISABILITIES FACE A HOUSING CRISIS

Independence and integration are some of the most important values and goals shared by people with disabilities, their families, and advocates. The term "integration" is used in this chapter because it is a more familiar term for many people outside of the disability community than "inclusion." Most people understand that integration is the opposite of segregation and that true integration is being a welcomed member of a community.

A home of one's own—whether rented or owned—can be the cornerstone of independence for a person with a disability. When someone has decent, safe, affordable, and—if needed—accessible housing, then he or she

---

[2] Wetherow, D. and Wetherow, F. (2001) Supporting Self-Determination with Integrity.

has the opportunity to really be part of the community. With stable housing, it is much easier to achieve other important life goals, such as having a job and spending quality time with friends and family.

Local, state, and federal housing policies that affect the lives of people with disabilities should reflect the values of people with disabilities, as well as be designed to help achieve—not thwart—their goals. Unfortunately, most current policies still do not do this, although there have been recent improvements. The negative result of the historical disconnect between the wants and needs of people with disabilities and public policy is that people with disabilities face a housing crisis—a crisis that will worsen without improved public policies.

If implemented effectively, the 1999 U.S. Supreme Court decision in *Olmstead v. L.C.*[3] could be one major step toward an improved public policy for people with disabilities. This important lawsuit against the State of Georgia questioned the state's continued confinement of two individuals with mental retardation and mental illness after the state hospital's physicians had determined that they were ready to return to the community. The Supreme Court described Georgia's action as "unjustified isolation" and determined that it violated these individuals' rights under the Americans with Disabilities Act (ADA)[4]. The impact of this decision on people with disabilities who are in institutions, or who are at risk of institutionalization, has prompted a great deal of activity by advocates, states, and the federal government. It is unfortunate that the word "housing" does not appear in the *Olmstead* decision. However, the Court did use terms such as "community placements" and "less restrictive settings." For people with disabilities, including people living in institutions, these terms should translate to affordable housing of their choice in communities of their choice—including apartments, condominiums and single-family homes. Up-to-date information on state responses to the *Olmstead* decision, including contact information, is available on the National Conference of State Legislatures website at *www.ncsl.org*.

In HUD's recent *Report on Worst Case Housing Needs in 1999: New Opportunity Amid Continuing Challenges* (2001),[5] data show that there are 4.9 million households with worst-case housing needs. Worst-case needs means that people pay more than 50% of their income for rent or live in seriously substandard housing. Between 1997 and 1999, worst-case needs went down for the elderly and for families with children, but they did not go down among nonelderly people with disabilities, 60% of whom face worst-case housing problems.

---

[3] *Olmstead v. L.C.*, United States Supreme Court, Dec. 22, 1999.
[4] Americans with Disabilities Act, P.L.101-336.
[5] U.S. Department of Housing and Urban Development (2001): A Report on Worst Case Housing Needs in 1999: New Opportunity Amid Continuing Challenges.

There are a number of reasons why almost five million people have worst-case housing needs. One side effect of the economic boom of the past decade is that rents have risen to respond to increased market demand and affordable housing has been lost to those with lower incomes. In addition, there are inadequate federal, state, and local resources to either develop new affordable housing or help individuals meet increasing housing costs. Although we often hear or read in the news that people with high-paying jobs in Silicon Valley can't find a place to live, we unfortunately don't often hear about the impact on those who are really poor.

Individuals with disabilities have fared the worst. Although many people have found better-paying jobs that could help them pay higher rents or other housing costs, this has not been true for people with disabilities— the majority of whom are unemployed or underemployed. According to *Priced Out in 2000: The Crisis Continues* (2001) [6], a person with a disability who relies on SSI faces the reality that the federal SSI payment ($512) equals only 18.5% of the national median income. In addition, increases in federal benefits, such as SSI, have not kept up with real costs. Between 1998 and 2000, rents increased almost twice as much as the income of people with disabilities. The result is that people with disabilities on SSI must pay, on a national average, 98% of their SSI to rent a modest one-bedroom apartment at the published HUD Fair Market Rent. It is apparent that, without some type of housing assistance, the choices of people with disabilities will be extremely limited. People who receive Social Security Disability Insurance (SSDI) benefits are in a somewhat—but not much—better situation than those who receive SSI. The average monthly SSDI benefit in January 2001 was $649.00[7]. One year of benefits at that monthly rate totals $7795 or a mere 22% of the one-person national median income. When you measure this against the fact that the nationwide average rent for a one-bedroom apart-ment is $552, it is clear that many of these individuals also need a rental subsidy to be able to afford to live in the community.

For the past 10 years the National Low Income Housing Coalition has published a report, *Out of Reach*[8], that is designed to indicate the gap between the cost of rental housing and what poor people can pay. The year 2000 report includes the estimated "Housing Wage"—or what an individual would need to earn per hour to afford to rent a certain-size apartment. For purposes of this article, the national median housing wage for a two-bedroom apartment is $12.47 per hour. This is more than two times the federal minimum wage of $5.15 and almost four times the average hourly SSI rate of $3.23. Obviously, people with disabilities—especially those who

[6] Technical Assistance Collaborative (Boston, MA) and Consortium for Citizens with Disabili-ties Housing Task Force (Washington, DC) (2001): Priced out in 2000: the crisis continues.
[7] U.S. Social Security Administration: (2001).
[8] National Low Income Housing Coalition (Washington, DC) (2000): Out of Reach.

rely on federal benefits—need financial help if they are going to be able to make any real housing choices.

## TACKLING THE CRISIS AND MOVING US FORWARD

What can be done to address this crisis, move public policy forward, and add to the housing resources for people with disabilities? The most important answer to this question is that people with Down syndrome and their families must be at the table when housing decisions are made at the local, state, and national levels. Trying to navigate the world of "housing" may be initially frightening. However, activism by people with disabilities, their families, and advocates has and will continue to effect positive change. The following examples demonstrate that people working together—in their towns and cities, in their states, and at the national level—can make changes that have a nationwide impact.

- Of the 21 disability organizations that took the time to learn to apply for federal HOME program and Community Development Block Grant funds, 14 of them (67%) reported success. In addition, 56% of the disability groups that sought funds for rental housing production or down payment assistance from the Federal Home Loan Bank Affordable Housing Program were successful [*Going it Alone: The Struggle to Expand Housing Opportunities for People with Disabilities* (2000)][9].

- The Arc of Anne Arundel County, Maryland forged a successful partnership with the local housing authority several years ago, and together they have helped people with disabilities find housing using Federal Section 8 tenant-based rental assistance. Other areas in Maryland are working to replicate this success.

- Last year, The Arc of the Piedmont in Charlottesville, Virginia entered into a partnership with a local housing authority and a local nonprofit affordable housing organization. This alliance pools the skills of each partner and, using Federal Section 811 Mainstream tenant-based rental assistance, is finding housing for people with disabilities. This is only one of an increasing number of successful public-private partnerships around the country.

- Home of Your Own[10] and/or Fannie Mae Home Choice[11] coalitions exist in many states. Where housing is affordable and there is a good

[9] Technical Assistance Collaborative (Boston, MA) and Consortium for Citizens with Disabilities (Washington, DC) (2000): Going It Alone: The Struggle to Expand Housing Opportunities for People with Disabilities.

[10] National Home of Your Own Alliance, Institute on Disability, University of New Hampshire.

[11] Fannie Mae, Washington, DC

working relationship with lenders, people with disabilities have become homeowners. According to *Going it Alone*, the Texas Home of Your Own Coalition has helped over 35 people buy homes since 1995 and the Home Choice Coalition has helped approximately 250 people since 1996.

- Advocacy by The Arc of the United States and other members of the Consortium for Citizens with Disabilities (CCD) Housing Task Force at the national level helped add $210 million over five years to the federal budget for Section 8 tenant-based rental assistance for people with disabilities. These funds have provided approximately 35,000 vouchers, including those used in Anne Arundel County, Maryland. CCD advocacy also helped change federal law so that nonprofit disability organizations, such as The Arc of the Piedmont, are now eligible to apply for and administer Section 811 mainstream tenant-based rental assistance.

## HOUSING OPTIONS

Like all people, individuals with disabilities have a need for decent, safe, affordable, and appropriate housing. However, just like all people, individuals with disabilities vary in abilities, interests, desires, and needs over the span of their lifetime. For many people with disabilities, the need for affordable housing may be met simply by helping them find an affordable place to live, rental assistance to help them pay the rent, down payment assistance to help them buy, or funds to help them pay for accessibility modifications. For some people with more severe disabilities the need for affordable housing, which is linked with services and supports, will last throughout their lifetime.

In the effort to find affordable housing in the community, people with disabilities, their families, and advocates increasingly have been seeking various forms of federal housing assistance. This effort to access generic housing funds—funds that are targeted to all people—is a reflection of the fact that disability policy is now community based. It also is a reflection of the fact that people are beginning to realize that a separate but unequal disability "system" has not always been in their best interests. One of the major advocacy messages of the CCD Housing Task Force at the national level has been that people with disabilities should have their "fair share" of available federal, state, and local housing funds. Because people with disabilities make up a large part of those individuals characterized as having worst-case housing needs, it makes not only good sense but good policy if funds to address these needs are allocated fairly.

Consider the housing options that—in the ideal—should be available to all people in the community. Broad-based housing options should be responsive to the needs of all community members. This includes people with very low incomes, with moderate incomes, with support needs, with accessibility requirements, or with large families. Consider how people with disabilities, families, friends, advocates, and providers can best work with the community to ensure that whatever the range of housing options to be available, it meets the needs of people with disabilities.

- Rental housing should be an option, whether apartments, condominiums or cooperative units, or houses. Rental housing should be open to a person who lives alone, as part of a couple or with roommates.

- Home ownership should be an option for an individual, a couple, friends, or others who may want to buy a house, a condominium, a cooperative, or manufactured housing.

- Some individuals may want a housing option that comes with certain services or supports attached, such as assistance with daily living skills or transportation.

- Not in my back yard (NIMBY) policies or other forms of explicit or implicit discrimination must not be permitted to limit people's housing options.

## Getting to the Table

## The Consolidated Plan

The HUD Consolidated Plan (ConPlan) could be considered the "master plan" for ensuring the availability of affordable housing in local communities and states. It is of major importance to people with disabilities for a number of reasons. The ConPlan controls how federal housing funds will be used to expand affordable housing and determines who—in the community or state—will benefit from these affordable housing efforts. States and communities that receive HOME Program, Community Development Block Grant (CDBG), Emergency Shelter Grant, and/or Housing Opportunity for People with AIDS (HOPWA) funds must develop a ConPlan. HUD approval of a plan is required before federal funds can be allocated to the community or state. Requirements for public participation are built into the ConPlan process, and Congress[12] and HUD have both taken steps recently to remind states and communities that people with disabilities and their advocates must be at the table as decisions are being made. HOME and CDBG funds

---

[12] U.S. House of Representatives Appropriations Committee, Subcommittee on HUD-VA-Independent Agencies (2000) Report 106-674.

hold great potential for expanding integrated housing options for people with disabilities.

- The Home Program is a grant of federal housing funds to states and communities. HOME funds can be used for (1) rental housing production and rehabilitation loans and grants; (2) first-time homebuyer assistance; (3) rehabilitation loans for homeowners; and (4) tenant-based rental assistance. All housing developed with HOME funds must serve people with low and very low incomes. In addition, 15% of a state or locality's HOME funds must be set aside for community-based non profit organizations (CHDOs). Disability organizations can be CHDOs.

- The Community Development Block Grant program is a federal grant provided to certain larger communities and all states. States are to use their funds in smaller towns and rural areas. At least 70% of CDBG funds are to benefit individuals with low and moderate incomes. CDBG funds can be spent on such activities as (1) housing rehabilitation loans or grants to homeowners, landlords, nonprofit organizations, and developers; (2) new housing construction by nonprofit groups; (3) buying land and buildings; (4) building public facilities, neighborhood, or community centers; (5) making buildings accessible; and (6) public services such as health and child care.

## THE PUBLIC HOUSING PLAN

The more than 2,000 public housing authorities (PHAs) across the nation play a major role in providing affordable housing to individuals with low and very low incomes. Public housing reform legislation that was enacted into law in 1998 gave PHAs more flexibility as to how to use federal public housing and Section 8 rental assistance funds. However, with this additional flexibility came the requirement for additional accountability by PHAs. Beginning in 2000, each PHA was required to complete a plan that (1) describes the agency's overall mission for serving people with low and very low incomes, including people with disabilities, and (2) what it is going to do to meet their housing needs.

PHAs control public housing and Section 8 tenant-based rental assistance; therefore, they are an invaluable resource to individuals with disabilities. Although public housing may not have the best reputation in large metropolitan areas, in many places it provides the only decent, safe, affordable, and accessible housing. Section 8 tenant-based rental assistance is a very important resource for people with disabilities. Operating within certain cost and unit quality parameters, people can have more choice over what and where they rent. In addition, Section 8 can now be applied to home ownership.

Because PHAs control access to Section 8 rental assistance and public housing, it is just as important that the needs of people with disabilities be reflected in the PHA plan as in the ConPlan. The PHA plan is required to be consistent with the area's ConPlan; therefore, it is much more likely that the needs of people with disabilities will be reflected in the PHA plan if they are included in the ConPlan.

## What You Must Bring to the Table

Being at the table when important community and state decisions are being made is one thing. However, what people with disabilities and their advocates bring to the table is even more important. This is the opportunity to show that people with disabilities are constituents. It is the opportunity to provide detailed information about their varied housing wants and needs. This is the opportunity to disabuse communities of the belief that all people with disabilities want to live in "disability" housing. This is the opportunity to remind communities that people with disabilities deserve their "fair share" of federal, state, and local housing funds. This is the opportunity to remind communities that fair housing laws protect people with disabilities and discrimination will not be tolerated.

The Technical Assistance Collaborative and the CCD Housing Task Force have developed a number of useful tools to help individuals with disabilities and advocates to actively participate in the ConPlan Process. *Piecing it all Together in Your Community: Playing the Housing Game* (1999)[13] is a guide developed specifically to help the disability community learn to use HUD's Consolidated Plan process to expand housing opportunities in the community. *Priced Out in 1998: The Housing Crisis for People with Disabilities* (1999)[14] and *Priced out in 2000: The Crisis Continues* (2001) provide SSI data for each state and metropolitan statistical area. This data helps individuals with disabilities and advocates show why their needs must be a priority as states and communities plan for affordable housing. *Going It Alone: The Struggle to Expand Housing Opportunities for People with Disabilities* (2000) evaluates current efforts to expand housing options around the country. It includes not only examples of best practices in relation to expanding both rental and home ownership options but also examples of some of the barriers that still exist.

[13] Technical Assistance Collaborative (Boston, MA) (1999): Piecing It All Together in the Community: Playing the Housing Game.
[14] Technical Assistance Collaborative (Boston, MA) and Consortium for Citizens with Disabilities Housing Task Force (Washington, DC) (1999): Priced Out in 1998: The Housing Crisis for People with Disabilities.

## Housing Resources

### Section 8 Tenant-Based Rental Assistance

Section 8 tenant-based rental assistance is an extremely effective tool to help people with mental retardation and other disabilities live integrated lives in their home communities. Although rules vary from PHA to PHA, Section 8 vouchers are "portable," meaning they can be acquired in one community but used in another. Many people with Down syndrome and other disabilities are dependent on SSI benefits or have very low paying jobs. Therefore, as demonstrated earlier in this chapter, they are unable to afford a decent place to live unless they have a rent subsidy—Section 8 is such a rent subsidy. The Section 8 program has existed since 1974 and, although it has helped hundreds of thousands of people with disabilities afford decent housing, it still remains an underutilized resource by people with disabilities.

Medicaid is the major source of funding for services and supports for people with disabilities, yet it does not pay for housing. Great attention has been placed on redirecting Medicaid funds from institutions so they can support people in the community. Very little attention was paid—until recently—to where people wanted to live in the community and how those living arrangements would be paid for. As people with Down syndrome and others face a housing crisis because of their low incomes and the high cost of housing or because of the loss of housing because of elderly-only designation, as more and more people are living at home with aging parents, and as states move to implement the Supreme Court *Olmstead* decision, innovative ways to fund housing must be an issue[15].

Currently, people with disabilities who meet certain income criteria are eligible for Section 8 tenant-based rental assistance. However, people without disabilities are also eligible, so the competition is intense. It is not unheard of to find decade-long Section 8 waiting lists. One other problem currently facing the Section 8 program is that there is not enough affordable housing in many communities so it may be difficult to use a Section 8 voucher. An additional problem for people with disabilities is the lack of affordable, accessible housing. There are a number of "set asides" in the Section 8 program for people with disabilities, and there is movement in the generic Section 8 world to target a certain percentage of new vouchers to people with disabilities each year.

For the past five years, Section 8 vouchers have been available for nonelderly people with disabilities who have been affected by the loss of public or federally assisted housing that has been designated as elderly-only.

---

[15] Technical Assistance Collaborative (Boston, MA) and Consortium for Citizens with Disabilities Housing Task Force (Washington, DC) (2000): Opening Doors: A Housing Publication for the Disability Community, Issue 12 (Dec.).

This housing, until a change in federal law in the early nineties, was available to elderly individuals as well as younger people with disabilities and sometimes was the only affordable and accessible housing in a community[16].

- In the effort to offset this loss, PHAs have access to Section 8 funds from two separate HUD programs: Rental Assistance for Nonelderly Persons with Disabilities in Support of Designated Housing Plans and Rental Assistance for Nonelderly Persons with Disabilities Related to the Loss of Certain Types of Section 8 Project-Based Developments and Section 202, 221(d)(3), and 236 Developments. For 2001, funds are available to provide 3,500 one-year vouchers in *each* of these programs.

- There is a third HUD program that funds rental assistance for people with disabilities, and both PHAs *and* nonprofit disability groups can apply to administer these vouchers. The Section 811 Mainstream Tenant-Based Rental Assistance Program will fund 1,900 five-year vouchers in 2000.

The response by most PHAs to the availability of these vouchers has been less than positive unless they are enlightened or face strong advocacy by people with disabilities and their families. In addition, because of long-standing HUD neglect of the needs of people with disabilities, it is often necessary for people with disabilities and their advocates to actually inform local and regional HUD offices and PHAs about Section 8 vouchers for people with disabilities. On the other hand, the response by nonprofit disability groups to the availability of vouchers has been strong. However, nonprofits face the challenge of having to learn to negotiate the confusing world of Section 8 rules without technical assistance from HUD. In any case, if Section 8 is to be a resource in a community, the needs of people with disabilities must be reflected in the ConPlan and the PHA Plan and people with disabilities and advocates must educate and work with a PHA.

"Fair Share" vouchers are what HUD calls its generic Section 8 vouchers. Although some PHAs may have longstanding preferences for people with disabilities in their generic voucher programs, many do not. For the past few years, HUD has tried to encourage PHAs to pay more attention to people with disabilities by awarding them 15 extra points if applications target 15% of their new vouchers to people with disabilities. An additional five extra points are awarded if PHAs also agree to target vouchers to people with disabilities who are receiving Medicaid Home and Community-Based waiver funds for services and supports. There are funds for 69,000 fair share

[16] Technical Assistance Collaborative (Boston, MA) and Consortium for Citizens with Disabilities Housing Task Force (Washington, DC) (1996) Opening Doors: recommendations for a federal policy to address the housing needs of people with disabilities.

vouchers in 2001. If PHAs agree to target people with disabilities, this will help open many more doors in the community, not only to people who have been waiting in the community but also to people who will be returning to the community because of the *Olmstead* decision. In 2000, a total of 60,000 fair share vouchers were distributed to 499 PHAs nationwide. Of these PHAs, 224 received extra points for targeting people with disabilities. These 224 received a total of 35,716 vouchers—with 5,357 for people with disabilities and 3% of these for people with disabilities receiving supports through Medicaid Home and Community-Based Waivers.

One more issue that must be addressed by people with disabilities, families, and advocates is how to monitor the effectiveness of PHA administration of all these Section 8 vouchers. If vouchers are going to be used by people with disabilities in a timely manner, PHAs will have to make changes in a number of their procedures. These could include (1) reopening waiting lists, (2) making information more accessible, (3) revising house search techniques, and (4) revising notification and rent collection methods. A formalized cooperative agreement between a PHA and a disability organization(s) would benefit both people with disabilities and the PHA. In an ideal situation, both entities would bring differing, yet equally important, skills to the relationship.

## SECTION 811 SUPPORTIVE HOUSING FOR PERSONS WITH DISABILITIES

Although Section 8 provides people with disabilities the opportunity to find their own housing in the community, many communities are facing the dilemma that there is no affordable housing to be found. This is why, currently, the focus at the national level is on the production of additional housing. For many years, the Section 811 program has been a positive example of a public-private partnership that works. Section 811 plays an important role in producing new decent, safe, affordable, and accessible housing, while at the same time ensuring a level of individualized supports required by many individuals with severe disabilities. It has proven to be one of HUD's most effective programs, successfully investing federal funding through nonprofit disability organizations. The Arc of the United States and other disability groups have worked to reshape the Section 811 program so that its funds are used less and less to build large, segregated "independent living facilities" and more and more to develop small, scattered-site housing options in the community. Although some people may choose to live with others in a group setting, Section 811 options include units scattered throughout apartment or condominium or cooperative developments. Disability groups, such as The Arc, also have expended much energy in the effort to reduce the overly bureaucratic requirements of this program.

Nonprofit disability organizations are the only eligible applicants for Section 811 funding. A Section 811 award to a nonprofit group consists of capital advance funds to buy, build, or rehabilitate housing *and* project-based rental assistance for each unit. Unfortunately, this program is severely underfunded. For 2001, there are funds for only 1,367 new units nationwide.

Additional information on HUD-funded housing initiatives, including those for people with disabilities, can be found at *www.hud.gov*.

## HOME OWNERSHIP

Home ownership rates for all Americans have been at an all time high, that is, for all Americans except those with disabilities. The National Home of Your Own Alliance (HOYO) estimates that only 1% of people with developmental disabilities and less than 5% of the six million plus people with disabilities living on SSI or SSDI are homeowners.[17] In addition, federal SSI policies that limit the assets that recipients can accumulate make it very difficult for people to save for a down payment and for families to help out a member with a disability.

The good news is that over the past several years, a number of new national home ownership initiatives have been targeted specifically to people with disabilities. The first of these was HOYO, which grew from a few locally based demonstration programs to a national effort funded through the Administration on Developmental Disabilities, an agency within the U.S. Department of Health and Human Services. A few years later, Fannie Mae, the nation's largest source of mortgage funds, developed a mortgage product, Home Choice, tailored specifically to the needs of people with disabilities. The Fannie Mae Home Choice coalitions that have developed around the country are built on the earlier HOYO coalition efforts, and in some states there are joint efforts.

The home ownership coalition model includes a lead agency that coordinates the efforts of stakeholders from a wide range of areas. Coalition members include people with disabilities, family members, disability organizations, independent living centers, housing finance agencies, lenders, realtors, home ownership counseling organizations, and others. One of the major efforts of coalitions is to get community support not only from political leaders but from the financial world. Another major effort has been to find ways to assist individuals with very low incomes in getting the financial and other supports they need not only to buy a home but also to keep it for the long term.

---

[17] Technical Assistance Collaborative (Boston, MA) and Consortium for Citizens with Disabilities Housing Task Force (Washington, DC) (1998): Opening doors: a housing publication for the disability community, Issue 6 (Dec.).

One new home ownership tool for some people with disabilities is that Section 8 vouchers can now be used toward home ownership and not only for rental housing. The use of Section 8 funds to make mortgage payments could help more people qualify for mortgages through both disability and generic mortgage programs. This Section 8 home ownership effort is administered through local PHAs.

HOYO has developed a number of very useful materials related to home ownership for people with disabilities. More information about the Alliance, existing state HOYO coalitions, current activities, and publications can be found at *http://alliance.unh.edu/*. A valuable publication on homeownership was developed in cooperation with Fannie Mae. *A Home of Your Own Guide: A Resource for Housing Educators and Counselors to Assist People with Disabilities* is available at the HOYO website, or a printed copy may be ordered from the Fannie Mae Distribution Center (1-800-471-5554). More information on a number of different Fannie Mae community-lending programs is available at *www.efanniemae.com*.

## FAIR HOUSING

An understanding of the value of fair housing protections is one additional tool that people with disabilities and their families should be able to use in their effort to ensure that there is a range of housing options in the community. The enactment of the Fair Housing Amendments Act (FHAA) of 1988[18] sent a clear message that people with disabilities were not to be discriminated against when it came to housing. The FHAA established a civil rights law that repudiated the use of stereotypes, prejudice, and ignorance to exclude people with disabilities from living in housing and communities of their choice.[19] This law applied not only to where people with disabilities could live but also to the need for additional accessible housing in the community. Unfortunately, 13 years after enactment of the law, the fair housing rights of people with disabilities remain under attack. These attacks come from neighbors and communities that do not welcome people with disabilities, and they come from some members of the "housing" community who resist the requirement for new accessible multifamily housing. It is important to remember, however, that, overall, fair housing court decisions have been favorable to people with disabilities.

People with disabilities are also protected by other civil rights laws, including Section 504 of the Rehabilitation Act of 1973[20] and the Americans with Disabilities Act. These protections should ensure that housing agencies

[18] Fair Housing Amendments Act of 1998, P.L.100-430.
[19] Technical Assistance Collaborative (Boston, MA) and Consortium for Citizens with Disabilities Housing Task Force (Washington, DC) (1998): Opening doors: a housing publication for the disability community, Issue 5 (Sept.).
[20] Rehabilitation Act of 1973, P.L. 93-112.

or programs, which receive federal, state or local funding, (1) do not discriminate against people with disabilities; (2) make reasonable accommodations in rules, policies, and procedures; and (3) make their programs accessible and usable by people with disabilities. Each state has a federally mandated Protection and Advocacy (P&A) Agency. The goal of these agencies is to ensure that the rights of people with all types of disabilities are protected. More information on the P&A network is available at *www.protectionandadvocacy.org*.

## SUMMARY

Hopefully, it is now obvious to the reader that much can be done to address the housing crisis facing people with disabilities, move public policy forward, and add to the housing resources available for them. It should be equally obvious that the only way positive change will be effected is if people with Down syndrome and their families educate themselves on housing issues and are at the table when housing decisions are being made at the local, state, and national levels. Although trying to navigate the world of "housing" may be initially frightening, activism by people with disabilities, their families, and advocates has and will continue to effect positive change and open new doors in communities.

National education and technical assistance efforts like those provided through the joint TAC/CCD Housing Task Force Opening Doors Project are available to help build a cadre of people who can make real housing choice a reality. The Opening Doors Project has developed materials that include information on issues from how to be at the table when housing decisions are being made to home ownership, Section 8 tenant-based rental assistance, housing accessibility, and housing and the role it must play in the effective implementation of the *Olmstead* decision. All Opening Doors information and materials are available free of charge at *http:// www.c-c-d.org/doors.html*. Additional housing resources are available on the CCD Housing Task Force web page at *http://www.c-c-d.org/tf-housing.htm* and on the TAC web page at *www.tacinc.org*.

## APPENDIX I: CCD HOUSING TASK FORCE FEDERAL PUBLIC POLICY RECOMMENDATIONS

### RECOMMENDATION #1. PROVIDE ACCESS FOR PEOPLE WITH DISABILITIES TO ALL HUD "MAINSTREAM" PROGRAMS AND THE CONSOLIDATED PLAN PROCESS

People with disabilities should have the opportunity to benefit from all of HUD's initiatives, including tenant-based rental assistance, housing production programs, as well as home ownership. This means ensuring that people with disabilities receive their "fair share" of federal HOME and CDBG funding and that the disability community is an active participant in the development of housing strategies within state and local Consolidated Plans. Special attention should be paid to the extremely limited incomes of people with severe disabilities to ensure that all programs are made truly "affordable" to people with incomes below 20% of the median. Legitimate HUD efforts to expand home ownership opportunities should not redirect resources away from those with the lowest incomes, who will continue to need rental housing.

## RECOMMENDATION #2. CONTINUE TO TARGET NEW SECTION 8 VOUCHERS TO PEOPLE WITH DISABILITIES AND IMPROVE MONITORING OF "ELDERLY ONLY" HOUSING DESIGNATION ACTIVITIES

The important progress made through the leadership of Republican and Democratic members of Congress since 1996 to address the loss of public and assisted housing for people with disabilities through the Section 8 voucher program should continue. At least 6,000 new Section 8 vouchers will be needed each year as Public Housing Agencies and HUD-assisted housing providers continue to designate "elderly only" housing. HUD should immediately move to complete an inventory of all assisted housing projects that have been designated as elderly only. Congress directed the HUD Secretary to do this more than three years ago. The inventory is needed to prevent housing discrimination and to direct new Section 8 vouchers to communities that have experienced the greatest loss of housing for people with disabilities. Better HUD monitoring of public housing designation activities and the administration of new Section 8 vouchers set aside for people with disabilities by PHAs is also needed to remedy serious problems created by the present lack of oversight

## RECOMMENDATION #3. MODERNIZE AND IMPROVE THE SECTION 811 SUPPORTIVE HOUSING FOR PERSONS WITH DISABILITIES PROGRAM

The Section 811 program has been poorly utilized for the past several years and needs major legislative reform as well as a substantial increase in appropriations. An appropriation of $346 million for FY 2002 would restore the program's funding level to what it was a decade ago. In addition to restoring needed funding, HUD, Congress, and disability advocates should work together to ensure that Section 811 funding can be used more flexibly to develop, rehabilitate, purchase, or rent small-scale or scattered site housing desired by people with disabilities. These legislative and regulatory reforms are essential to speed up production and eliminate years of cumulative "red tape" and bureaucracy. The primary focus of the program should continue to be production of housing for people with the most severe disabilities, with no more than 25% of the funding being targeted for tenant-based rental assistance. All Section 811 funds should be provided exclusively to nonprofit disability organizations and not to PHAs.

## RECOMMENDATION #4. STRENGTHEN THE ROLE AND HOUSING CAPACITY OF NONPROFIT DISABILITY ORGANIZATIONS

The TAC/CCD Housing Task Force's most recent policy report, *Going It Alone: The Struggle to Expand Housing Opportunities for People with Disabilities,* underscores the need to provide HUD-funded technical assistance and capacity building on housing issues to nonprofit disability organizations and to the disability community in general. Unfortunately, the housing system rarely engages the disability community in housing discussions. The disability community must take the lead to establish these partnerships. To do so effectively, the disability community needs a much better understanding of federal housing programs and policies and how they can work to assist people with disabilities.

## RECOMMENDATION #5. CONTINUE TO DIRECT McKINNEY–VENTO HOMELESS ASSISTANCE FUNDS TOWARD PERMANENT HOUSING

During the past few years, HUD's policies regarding Homeless Assistance funds have been modified virtually every year, with both positive and negative outcomes. A new Administration and Congress must bring stability and accountability to these important programs and must continue to reorient them to their original purpose, which was to expand permanent supportive housing for homeless persons with disabilities. All permanent rental assistance and operating subsidy funding should be renewed by HUD for projects in compliance with statutory and regulatory guidelines. All states and localities should be provided with a clear understanding of their obligations and responsibilities with respect to any planning requirements under the Continuum of Care model.

## RECOMMENDATION #6. FORMULATE NEW AFFORDABLE HOUSING PRODUCTION POLICIES THAT INCLUDE A FOCUS ON HUD'S RESPONSE TO THE L.C. v. OLMSTEAD DECISION

Tenant-based rental assistance programs such as Section 8 cannot be the sole foundation of federal housing policies to assist households with incomes below 30% of median income. A balanced housing policy for people with disabilities and others at the bottom of the economic ladder must also include the construction of new affordable rental housing. Federal efforts to assist states in implementing plans to downsize institutions and help adults with severe disabilities move into the community under the Supreme Court's *Olmstead* decision should not focus solely on small HUD programs that only serve people with disabilities (e.g., the Section 811 program, the Section 8 Mainstream and designated housing voucher programs). They should also focus on providing access to all of HUD's mainstream housing production programs, including HOME and CDBG. HUD guidance to communities regarding the *Olmstead* decision should also suggest revising local and state Consolidated Plan needs assessments, if necessary, to include the supportive housing needs of those individuals with disabilities living unnecessarily in "restrictive settings."

## Recommendation #7. Address and Prevent Housing Discrimination and Provide Reasonable Accommodation for People with Disabilities in All HUD Programs and Policies and in the Private Housing Market Where Applicable

HUD, as well as all recipients of HUD funding, should be held accountable for compliance with the Fair Housing Act Amendments of 1988 and Section 504 of the Rehabilitation Act of 1973, including the removal of all barriers and impediments that have a negative impact on the access of people with disabilities to affordable housing programs. Training and technical assistance should be made available to the disability community regarding the reasonable accommodation and reasonable modifications provisions of the Fair Housing Act and Section 504. Steps should also be taken by HUD to ensure that people with disabilities are not being discriminated against when public housing agencies and private owners of HUD-assisted housing seek to restrict occupancy to households aged 62 and older. HUD should also work closely with the Department of Justice and the Department of the Treasury to ensure that people with disabilities have access to the units developed in federal low-income housing tax credit developments, including ending discriminatory practices such as the refusal to accept Section 8 voucher program participants. Finally, more HUD leadership is needed to ensure the full compliance and enforcement of the accessibility provisions of the Fair Housing Act Amendments of 1988 in the private housing market. Affordable and accessible housing is critically important for people with mobility or sensory impairments.

## Appendix II: Important Individuals and Entities to Know in the Effort to Increase Housing Options in the Community

| Local Level | State Level | National Level |
|---|---|---|
| Mayor | Governor | Senators and Representatives |
| Members of City/Town Council or Commission | State Delegates, Representatives, Senators | U.S. Department of Housing and Urban Development |
| City/Town Manager | State Attorney | U.S. Department of Justice |
| City/Town Attorney | State Office of Civil Rights | National Disability Advocacy and Provider Organizations |
| Zoning Commission | State Protection and Advocacy Agency | Consortium for Citizens with Disabilities |
| Office of Code Enforcement | State Housing Finance Agency, State Office of Housing and Community Development | National Low Income Housing Coalition |
| Public Housing Authority | State Housing Finance Agency | National Association of Home Builders |
| Office of Housing and Community Development | State Housing Authority | National Mortgage Bankers Association |
| Office of Affordable Housing | State Offices on Disability | National Home of Your Own Alliance |
| Office of Planning | State Disability Advocacy and Provider Organizations | Fannie Mae |
| Office of Civil Rights | Regional HUD Office | National Housing Finance Agency Organizations |
| Fair Housing Enforcement Agency | Regional Office of U.S. Department of Justice | Freddie Mac |
| Office of Disability | State Low-Income Housing Coalition | |
| Mortgage Bankers | | |
| Local Housing Finance Agency | | |
| Board of Realtors | | |
| Chamber of Commerce | | |
| Local Home Builders Association | | |
| Local Association of Multifamily Housing Managers | | |
| Local Disability Advocacy and Provider Organizations | | |

# SELF-ADVOCACY

# Having A Life

## John Peter Illarramendi, Jeffery Mattson, and Mia Peterson

### John Peter Illarramendi

#### Relationships

My name is John Peter Illarramendi, but for some others I go by my initial name, which is J. P. I belong to a bilingual Hispanic family, with some French to add to that. I have two brothers and also one sister and, of course, my parents and many others that make up my whole family. I even communicate with some of them by e-mail. I once had a relationship with my former girlfriend, and now we are just friends. We broke it off because of some complications.

#### Goals

When I was 18 years old, I learned how to vote for the first time. I have voted for all three elections, primary, local, and national. I even learned how to be an artist by making some drawings and paintings, and I even received some awards and recognitions for my body of work when I was still in high school. I was accepted to an art school in New York, Pratt Institute College of Art. But it did not go well because it was too far away from where I live.

Besides being a visual artist, I am also an actor. I have been in so many plays, and I am now starting one that is funded by the National Endowment for the Arts. I have also been active with my church activities: being an altar

*Down Syndrome,* Edited by William I. Cohen, Lynn Nadel, and Myra E. Madnick. ISBN 0-471-41815-3 Copyright © 2002 by Wiley-Liss, Inc.

server at the Church of the Little Flower Parish, as well as attending a group church meetings in another parish which I do not belong to, Our Lady of Mercy.

I have also been very active with the hobbies that I do, and some of them are three sports that I enjoy most (basketball, bowling, and swimming). Some others also include writing, which is what I am doing now for this book, and also public speaking, which I have done well, but not too often.

## Dreams

What would I like to do in the near future? Well, to be with someone who really understands me and maybe one day become husband and wife. I would even like to keep up with my writing, art, and/or acting, as well as being a speaker. And to top all that, to keep up with sports as well. Even though I am out of order, I would like to also be involved with my faith with the Church activities that I have mentioned earlier except for one, being an altar server. All in all, I would just like to be my normal self, even if I am a person with Down syndrome, but what is more difficult is also being a diabetic, which of course is more complicated!

## Jeffery Mattson

I have a great life, and volunteering has made my life even better. I work. I go to school. Next fall I will live on campus and attend Taft College near Bakersfield, California. I have great friends. I exercise and try to eat healthy. I go to church. I have a hobby and I volunteer. To have a balanced life everyone needs a chance to work, to learn, to have relationships, to stay fit, to follow their faith, and to enjoy leisure (I call it "free time"). For me, volunteering has been very important because I volunteer in a way that also lets me express my faith.

I come from a family of volunteer Young Life leaders. My Dad was a volunteer Young Life leader when he was a student at Stanford. My mother is a volunteer Young Life leader. Even my grandparents were volunteer Young Life leaders in the sixties. My brother just graduated from the University of Michigan where he was a volunteer Young Life leader, and now that I am in junior college I am a volunteer Young Life leader, too.

I went to Young Life Club when I was in high school. I was the only one there with Down syndrome. Lots of girls that go to Young Life are cute. I got to know a lot of them. I got to date some of them. That is an extra bonus of being in Young Life, going out with cute girls.

God's love is important to me and I wanted to tell my friends about Him. I wanted them to have a chance to hear about His love. Young Life clubs are inclusive and open to everyone, but many of my friends were not getting to typical Young Life clubs. Some were in wheelchairs and some had other special needs. I talked with my Young Life leader about starting a club for kids with special needs. He liked the idea and we started the club two years ago. We decided to call it High Rollers. We didn't want anything with the word "special" in the title.

I have been on the leadership team for two years now. It has been so cool. I like that Young Life has people with disabilities on their leadership teams in other parts of the country. People with disabilities can serve too! In my area I am the only Young Life leader who has Down syndrome.

During the school year one day a week, every other week, the leaders meet with club kids for dinner out. It is just a time to hang out and build relationships. One day each week I meet with my fellow Young Life leader and staff person. We play guitar and practice for club and then we meet with a small group of guys for Campaigners. Campaigners is for kids that want to know more about the Bible and Jesus Christ. Wednesday is club night, and one Sunday evening a month we meet with Young Life leaders from other high schools and junior high schools here in South Orange County for a leadership meeting. In the summer we go to a week of camp. Last summer we went to Woodleaf Camp in Northern California. Being a leader takes a lot of my time, but I don't mind. I love it.

Young Life club is so much fun. I love being in the skits. Once I was super hero "Rubber Band Man" with my sidekick "Duct Tape Mama." My favorite line in that skit was to say, "I hold things together, and I am cute too!" Once I was Skippy Claus, Santa's little brother, and on Valentine's Day I was Cupid with pantyhose wings. At Young Life club we do crazy things like bobbing for goldfish or eating an eight foot ice cream sundae without any spoons. Club is a hoot. We have a blast.

I like being part of the leadership team. I have ideas to contribute. There are a lot of things I can do, and I do everything all the other Young Life leaders do. I go to all the leadership meetings and seminars. I play the guitar and lead singing every Wednesday night. I speak at fundraising events. I pray for all the kids and other leaders. Most of all, I share how much God loves us.

This is why it is important for me as a self-advocate to be a Young Life leader: I want to continue my family's tradition of volunteering in Young Life. Why should I be any different? I like being part of the team. I like the responsibility. I like the respect I have as a leader. I like spending time with other Young Life leaders. I like spending time with the kids that come to club and camp. I want to follow Him and serve Him. I want to give back to my community. I want a chance to serve, too.

Young Life has been around since 1940. Today there are over 1900 people on staff and 9000 volunteers. Young Life has National camps, Regional camps, and Wilderness programs. Over 450,000 kids are involved in Young Life each year. Young Life is headquartered in Colorado Springs.

I think the best part about being a volunteer leader in Young Life is the friendships I have with other Young Life leaders. This fall I will be part of the wedding party for a fellow Young Life leader. I was with him when he first met his fiancée. I was there when he proposed in a skit at Young Life club. Most of all, I am excited that I will be standing in a tux watching as they get married. And if and when I get married, you can bet he will be standing with me, too.

My favorite Bible verse has always been Jeremiah 29:11: "For I know the plans I have for you . . . plans to prosper you and not to harm you, plans to give you a hope and a future." My future is better because I have had an opportunity to give back, to learn leadership skills, and to share my faith by volunteering.

## MIA PETERSON

My name is Mia Peterson and I would like to talk about "Having A Life." What I would like to do is just have a conversation with you about me.

I am 27 years old and I live in Cincinnati, Ohio. I have been a resident of Ohio for four years. I am originally from Iowa. Iowa is where my family is. Right now I am employed at the Down Syndrome Association of Greater Cincinnati, where I am the self-advocacy coordinator.

Some things that I will be doing here at the Association include working on all issues related to self-advocates, their families, and their parents. I am helping with the newsletter, the *DS News*, talking about what things self-advocates with Down syndrome want to hear that are important to them, and not just what is important for everyone else to hear. I have a column in the *DS News* about my thoughts or if anyone else has a thought they want me to add. In order for me to get their help, I need them to write me a letter about what they want to hear about or what the Down Syndrome Association of Cincinnati does. If there is something that they can't understand or if they have any questions, they ask me so we all work together and are a part of the team. The whole point of this is for me to get connected to them and for them to reach out to me. I have to be able to understand what is going on for persons with Down syndrome. I can't read their minds.

I am the first self-advocate who has Down syndrome to be working for the Down Syndrome Association of Greater Cincinnati. I have just done a survey asking questions of the self-advocates with Down syndrome what they know about having a life with Down syndrome. They are to tell me about themselves and about what they always wanted to learn and do. A part of my job is to support most of the programs for the Association. The program I am supporting is the Outreach Program. What they have is a Speakers Bureau. These are trained speakers who make presentations to medical professionals and community groups. I like this program because I get to watch the professionals make presentations. I have also learned how I can make better presentations myself. I already have a lot of skills in public speaking. I was previously employed as a self-advocacy coordinator for Capabilities Unlimited in Cincinnati.

Some other things I am involved with include being a cofacilitator for Franklin Covey in teaching using *The 7 Habits Of Highly Effective People*. I am president for the statewide chapter "People First Of Ohio." Finally, I have the opportunity to be liaison for the self-advocates to the board of NDSS. I am very proud to help NDSS with their National Conference!

One thing that I'm really excited about in my life is that I have my own apartment now and have been living there for two years. I like having my own place, because I can have a life of my own and make my own rules. I do know that it is ok to get advice when you need it the most.

I have also been taking college classes at Xavier University. I took a position as a coresearcher for a project called Healthy Lifestyles for Adults with Down syndrome: What I wanted to do was to go to college. A grant helped me to accomplish this goal. Some of the classes I have taken include Interpersonal Relationships and Presentational Speaking. I also just graduated from Ohio's Partners and Policy Making Class of 2000. I have just started taking a new class called Project Leadership. This class takes place in Washington, DC and is sponsored by Community Options, Inc. This is a national event that involves leadership, government, policymaking, and politics. The Ohio Governor's Developmental Disabilities Planning Council is sponsoring me. I am the first self-advocate from Ohio to participate in this class.

Let me tell you some fun things I have been doing in my life. I have been working on a book I am trying to write. I call it *Take The Challenge, Take The Risk*. This is based on my journal of thoughts that I have in my head. I am learning in life to face my problems instead of keeping them to myself. I have been going to my local YMCA and running, cycling, and lifting weights. Sometimes I go swimming. I also like to take dance classes. I like to go out and do things with my friends and party with them. I do have a goal I want to accomplish in my life. I would like to take acting classes. I want to learn and be an example for all people with disabilities. I want them to see that I can act and that I do have a voice.

You know, there are a lot of things that are happening to me in my life. It's a great feeling in having my own life the way I want it to be, not the way anyone else wants it to be. Please remember we, the self-advocates, can speak for ourselves and don't let anyone else speak for us.

# FOLLOW YOUR DREAMS

## CHRIS BURKE

"Obstacles are what you see when you take your eyes off the goal."

This has been a motto of mine for several years now. It means: If you have a dream you want to come true you must not let anyone or anything keep you from reaching that goal. We must work hard, never give up, and above all, believe in ourselves. It takes a lot of determination, and all of us have to face that. The harder we work, the more we will accomplish. So, don't let anyone stand in your way and who knows, you might wind up doing what you set your mind to.

From the time I was very young I wanted to be an actor in Hollywood. I didn't know how I would get there, but I knew I was going to keep trying to make it come true.

I guess the first step in the right direction was writing a letter of congratulations to Jason Kingsley after I saw him on an episode of *The Fall Guy*. What I didn't know was that his mom, Emily, was a writer and producer for *Sesame Street*. Emily wrote a letter back to me and we eventually all became friends. They are a great family.

When Emily received a call from Warner Bros. requesting names of young men who could play a role in a pilot they were shooting for a possible television series, my name was one of those she gave them. That's how my mom received the call from Warner Bros. I went on the audition and then several months later, heard from them again asking me to go out to Hollywood for a screen test. My dream was about to come true. You can imagine how excited I was! That pilot was not picked up as a series, but

*Down Syndrome*, Edited by William I. Cohen, Lynn Nadel, and Myra E. Madnick.
ISBN 0-471-41815-3   Copyright © 2002 by Wiley-Liss, Inc.

Warner Bros. thought they should give me another chance and asked Michael Braverman to write another pilot with me in it. *Life Goes On* was the result.

It was the greatest experience being on that show! I was also thrilled to know that *Life Goes On* showed the world that people with disabilities have ability, too. I was happy to be a part of that because I always wanted to help other people with disabilities.

When I was at Don Guanella School in Springfield, Pennsylvania, my second ambition was to become a reporter. So, I worked on the school newspaper, writing articles each month. Once I even wrote to President Reagan, and he took the time to write back and encourage me and all the other students to work to reach our goals in life. We printed that letter in the paper, and everybody was thrilled. My English teacher helped me a lot and that prepared me, I think, for my job as editor of *News & Views* at the National Down Syndrome Society. It is a great job and I work with super people.

I am really working hard at both of these careers, as well as going on the road with my friends, Joe and John De Masi. We entertain and speak at many schools, conferences, and performing arts camps. It is our way of making people aware!

The next thing I would like to accomplish is to become a consultant and advocate for the entertainment business. I firmly believe that people with disabilities should be portrayed by people who have that disability. I think I could also come up with some ideas for scripts—at least I would like to try.

Finally, the National Down Syndrome Society is very important to me so I would like to advocate and become a consultant for Education, Research, and Advocacy to show people it is not about our disability but our ABILITY.

The sky's the limit! Remember that!

So please: Follow your dreams

Believe in yourself

    And

Never give up.

I'm trying my best and hardest to do everything I set out to do and you should, too.

Thank you for reading this chapter.

Chris

# LIFE AFTER HIGH SCHOOL

## JOSHUA G. O'NEILL

My name is Josh O'Neill. I go to school at Chapel Haven in New Haven, Connecticut. I am learning to live independently. I would like to tell you about why I decided to go there and what I am learning.

I am from Fort Wayne, Indiana, and I went to Homestead High School. When I was in the tenth grade, my mom and dad and I started to talk about what I was going to do after high school. We talked about whether or not I would like going to school where I could learn to live on my own. This was confusing to me, and I didn't know if I wanted to do that.

My parents and I visited some programs that are for people with disabilities to attend after high school. Some of them were too hard for me. One was too far away from home. I liked Chapel Haven. I had to go there for a week to visit. That means that I had to stay there and be in the program for one week. This was so that I could see if I liked it and we could decide if the program was right for me. A few weeks after that I got a letter telling me that I was accepted. I was so happy because I was very nervous when I didn't know what I would be doing after graduation. I used to tell my mom and dad that I wanted to "wrap things up."

A few weeks later I was excited again when I found out that my friend Pat, who went to camp with me, was accepted at Chapel Haven. I graduated from high school in June, 1998 and went to Chapel Haven in July. My good friend Pat came in August.

When I started at Chapel Haven, I moved into an apartment with three other guys. All of the apartments in the building have Chapel Haven students in them, and the staff has their offices in there. My time was spent

*Down Syndrome*, Edited by William I. Cohen, Lynn Nadel, and Myra E. Madnick.
ISBN 0-471-41815-3   Copyright © 2002 by Wiley-Liss, Inc.

taking classes and also learning more about day-to-day living—cooking, cleaning, doing laundry, going to the bank, and just living with people who are not my family. My classes teach me how to live independently. A big part of what I am learning is about making choices and decisions for myself.

At first it was very hard to be away from my family. I miss them very much, but they come to visit me and I go home on vacations. It was also hard to learn how to do things like grocery shopping and making meals. I wanted to watch TV and hang out instead. Now I am used to it and it is easier.

Something that is real important to me at Chapel Haven is having friends to hang out with. It is really special having my best friend Pat there. We really care about each other. I have other friends, too and we all hang out together. It is fun to just have someone around to walk to McDonalds with, to go to CVS, or to rent a movie. On the weekends we have activities. You sign up for the things that you want to attend. If I want to go on an activity, I have to budget the money for it. Chapel Haven also has a travel club. For the last two years I have gone with the travel club to Disney World. Those trips were a lot of fun.

Since I have been at Chapel Haven, I have had some different job experiences. Some have been paid and some have been volunteer. I have worked at Goodwill, at an office, at the Yale Hospital, and at a store called McCroy's. Now I am working at the Jewish Federation. I have a job coach at my jobs. I also learned to take the bus, and now I do it myself. When I am not working I take classes, exercise, do laundry, and have free time.

The program that I am in at Chapel Haven will be over for me this summer. I have been thinking a lot about what I do next. I might stay in New Haven and live in an apartment and still be a part of Chapel Haven. There are a lot of things to figure out.

# ADVOCACY

# A Vision for the Twenty-First Century: A Blueprint for Change

## Stephanie Smith Lee

### Introduction

An essential part of the mission of the National Down Syndrome Society (NDSS) is advocating on behalf of individuals with Down syndrome and their families. With hundreds of potential policy areas to address, identifying the key priorities is an important element of a successful advocacy program. Ensuring the broad-based participation of self-advocates, families, and professionals across the country in identifying priorities and positions is critical. This chapter will outline a unique process undertaken at the NDSS conference in July 2000 to shape a vision of the future for people with Down syndrome and to identify the top priorities for research, best practice, and advocacy to achieve that vision. The chapter will also describe subsequent actions to involve additional stakeholders, expansion of the effort to include medical research, and planning for a new state-of-the-art conference on Down syndrome based on the results of this effort.

### The Twentieth Century Context

At the beginning of the twentieth century, there were close to 100,000 children in institutions. Many of those were children with Down syndrome.

*Down Syndrome,* Edited by William I. Cohen, Lynn Nadel, and Myra E. Madnick.
ISBN 0-471-41815-3   Copyright © 2002 by Wiley-Liss, Inc.

Their expected life span was about 22 years of age. For the relatively small number who resided with their families, the possibility of receiving an education did not exist. Those who were not institutionalized spent most of their adult lives at home with their families, unemployed and with no possibility for living independently with supports.

## LANDMARK EDUCATION AND CIVIL RIGHTS LEGISLATION

Until the mid-1970s, when many families had made the decision not to institutionalize their children, there were still a million children who were not allowed in the public schools. That changed in 1975 with the passage of the landmark federal special education law, PL 94-142, The Education of All Handicapped Children Act—now called the Individuals with Disabilities Education Act (IDEA)[1]. This landmark civil rights law established that *all* individuals with disabilities have the right to an individualized, free, and appropriate public education in the least restrictive environment.

The other major cornerstone of civil rights for people with disabilities is the Americans with Disabilities Act (ADA)[2], which was signed into law in 1990. According to a U.S. Department of Justice publication,[3] "The Americans with Disabilities Act gives civil rights protections to individuals with disabilities similar to those provided to individuals on the basis of race, color, sex, national origin, age and religion. It guarantees equal opportunity for individuals with disabilities in public accommodations, employment, transportation, State and local government services and telecommunications."

## A SHIFT IN FOCUS

During these past 30 years, the focus of disability public policy advocacy has been on creating legislation and policy that would allow people with disbilities to have *access* to the many domains of ordinary life—education, employment, housing, and community living. The advocacy focus is now evolving to an emphasis on quality and accountability, self-determination, opportunities for individuals with disabilities and their families to have real choices and control over services and supports, and the achievement of a level of self-sufficiency and life in the community unheard of 30 years ago.

[1] *See* Education for All Handicapped Children Act of 1975, Pub. L. No. 94-142.
[2] Americans with Disabilities Act of 1990, Pub. L. No. 101-336.
[3] *U.S. Equal Employment Opportunity Commission, U.S. Department of Justice Civil Rights Division, "Americans with Disabilities Act, "Questions and Answers"*
*http://www.usdoj.gov/crt/ada/qandaeng.htm*

## Background on NDSS Advocacy

NDSS public policy advocacy concentrates on 1) improving the lives of individuals with Down syndrome and their families through legislation, implementation of laws, and appropriations; 2) promoting best practice based on solid research; 3) encouraging public support for positive public policy through public relations efforts; and 4) involving, building, training, and mobilizing an effective grass roots. Issues affecting both children and adults are addressed with an emphasis on positive, bipartisan advocacy that promotes collaboration among self-advocates, family members, professionals, and policy makers.

During the last five years, NDSS public policy advocacy efforts—and successes—have increased substantially. A growing NDSS membership, a dramatic increase in local parent group affiliation and advocacy involvement, Board and staff support, and the establishment of an NDSS Washington office have contributed to this expansion. Notable accomplishments include playing a key role in the reauthorization of the Individuals with Disabilities Act (IDEA) Amendments of 1997 and leading a successful effort in 1999 to require the Social Security Administration to address the unique needs of individuals with more significant disabilities in the Ticket to Work and Work Incentives Improvement Act.

The NDSS Affiliate Advisory Board is helping to build an effective grass roots that assists in identifying issues and responds quickly to action alerts through the advocacy E-mail list and posts on the website. Training for parents, self-advocates, and professionals is provided at national and regional conferences and through special projects such as the Institute for Special Education Leadership (ISEL). This model project is currently assisting parent leaders in Florida in building an effective statewide coalition to ensure optimal educational opportunities for all individuals with developmental disabilities. Buddy Walks across the country are raising public awareness of the importance of including people with Down syndrome. Finally, positive media coverage of the Buddy Walks, NDSS events, and conferences; media interviews; and articles in the NDSS *Update* and other publications are promoting public acceptance and support for positive public policy.

## Developing Goals, Positions, and Priorities

The NDSS Governmental Affairs (GA) Committee consists of NDSS officers, other board members, the Executive Director, Myra Madnick, and several additional policy experts who are also parents of children with Down syndrome. It is chaired by Board Member Madeleine C. Will, Vice President for Strategic Planning and Advocacy, Community Options, Inc., and former Assistant Secretary, Office of Special Education and Rehabilitation Services (OSERS). Among other responsibilities, the GA Committee recommends strategic planning advocacy goals, policy positions, and advocacy priorities to the Board for consideration. A critical component of developing these recommendations is coming up with strategies to encourage individuals with Down syndrome, family members, and professionals to give input. Opinions are solicited through surveys, focus groups, conference sessions, contacts with affiliate leaders, recommendations from the NDSS Affiliate, Clinical, Scientific, and Self-Advocate Advisory Boards, and comments received through the NDSS information and referral service.

## SHAPING A VISION FOR THE FUTURE

## THE 2000 CONFERENCE VISION PROCESS

Given the dawning of a new century, the theme of a new vision for the twenty-first century seemed not only appropriate, but also necessary, for the NDSS annual conference in Washington, DC in the year 2000. The idea underpinning the conference was to involve a wide spectrum of stakeholders in an organized effort to shape a clear vision for the future. The challenge for conference organizers, then, was to develop an open and effective process for gathering broad input from the self-advocates, parents, other family members, affiliate leaders, and professionals about where we are now, where we need to go, and how we will get there. A variety of methods were utilized to involve participants in sharing their views about the most important priorities for achieving the goal of people with Down syndrome having the opportunity to live a full and productive life in the community. The results of this effort are helping the NDSS set priorities for research and public policy initiatives, plan future programs, determine policy recommendations, and advocate effectively on behalf of individuals with Down syndrome and their families. It is also hoped that the conference vision results will set the stage for a new state-of-the-art conference on Down syndrome.

The GA Committee played an active role in developing the vision process, planning and participating in the conference, analyzing the results, and developing recommendations to the Board based on the results. The NDSS Scientific and Clinical Advisory Boards, consisting of distinguished experts in a variety of fields, assisted in this process as well. David Patterson, Ph.D. chairs the Scientific Advisory Board, and William I. Cohen, M.D. chairs the Clinical Advisory Board. Both chairs and their respective committees were actively involved in the vision process, analyzing the results and ongoing efforts in this area. Recommendations in the medical, genetics, health, or other clinical or scientific areas are directed to these Boards for consideration.

The conference provided an opportunity for participants to reflect on accomplishments in the twentieth century, learn from top experts about best practice, and work together to identify top priorities for the identification and replication of best practice and new research initiatives. Experts in the areas of education, research, advocacy, self-determination, family support, employment, supported living, and life in the community were identified and invited to speak at plenary sessions and workshops. Each plenary session was followed by workshops that provided an opportunity for participants to speak directly with the experts. Networking sessions and focus groups on education, adult issues, and research provided further opportunities for participants, experts, NDSS Board, staff, and volunteers to discuss key issues and recommend priorities for future research, implementing best practice, and public policy advocacy. The self-advocates sessions included opportunities for individuals with Down syndrome to discuss what is most important to them and what improvements are necessary.

Before the conference, NDSS Board members, affiliate leaders, advisory board, and GA Committee members, along with the speakers, were all invited to participate in this effort. Conference attendees were encouraged to share their views directly with any of these individuals, who were identified with ribbons. Recommendations were then forwarded to the GA Committee and Scientific and Clinical Advisory Boards, either orally or on written forms. Surveys on education, adult issues, and research were developed and distributed at the conference. Cards were also provided so that participants could further comment on specific issues of concern to them. After the conference, the survey was posted on the NDSS website to obtain additional responses. Participants were enthusiastic about the opportunity to be involved in this effort and to share in shaping a vision for the future.

## THE 2001 CONFERENCE AND FOLLOW-UP

At the NDSS national conference in San Diego in July 2001, the same education and adult issues survey was distributed and responses were tabulated with the previous surveys. Researchers requested that a new survey be distributed to provide them with valuable information about the prevalence of various medical and psychological problems and to identify research and service gaps. The new research survey has been widely distributed, and survey responses continue to arrive as this book goes to print. Each year, NDSS will review and consider additional or revised surveys to further identify and document needed research, identification and replication of best practice, and policy priorities.

The next sections outline policy issues and vision survey results in the areas of education, adult issues, and research and provide a description of a new state-of-the-art conference.

## Education

## The Individuals with Disabilities Education Act (IDEA) Amendments of 1997

Disability policy has traditionally been bipartisan, with broad support for the passage of key legislation such as PL 94-142, the initial version of the federal special education act first passed in 1975. Although the Individuals with Disabilities Act (IDEA) Part B, the state grant program, is permanently authorized, various discretionary programs must be reauthorized periodically. Strong bipartisan support continued for IDEA, and improvements were made over the years, such as the additions of early intervention and preschool services, transition from school to work requirements, and increased parental involvement. However, in recent years growing concern about special education has led to a contentious debate among stakeholders that produced a stalemate over the last reauthorization of IDEA. This stalemate was finally broken by a unique bipartisan consensus process in 1995 through 1997 that involved all the interested stakeholders and key Congressional leaders and staff and resulted in the passage of IDEA 97 with widespread support.

Although the basic concepts of the law remained intact, IDEA 97 constituted a major overhaul of special education. The biggest change in IDEA 97 was the programmatic shift from access to outcomes, accountability, including students with disabilities in assessments, and tying their education to the general curriculum. IDEA 97 also addressed concerns about cost, paperwork, providing schools more flexibility in disciplining students to maintain safe schools, and the misidentification of some students and over-identification of minority students. Improvements were made in parental involvement; utilizing best practices in addressing behavioral concerns through positive interventions, strategies and supports; reducing costly litigation and due process proceedings through mediation; and school-to-work transition planning. The federal regulations implementing IDEA 97 were finally published in 1999.

## The 2002 IDEA Reauthorization

The reauthorization of IDEA in 1997 encompassed a fundamental and far-reaching reform of IDEA. The states are still in various stages of completing revisions to their own statutes and regulations to implement IDEA 97. States and local schools are still grappling with how to implement the important reforms encompassed in the last revision. Current research is not yet adequately reaching the classrooms, and a number of important research initiatives based on IDEA 97 reforms are under way and not yet complete.

Although implementation of the last reauthorization is still spotty, the next reauthorization of IDEA is scheduled to take place in 2002. This comes at a time when both general and special education are attempting to move educational reform down to the school district level and the divide between the two systems should be narrowing. Unfortunately, in many areas the gap seems just as wide and the spirit of consensus appears to have gone astray. Funding concerns complicate the policy debate and add to a growing backlash against special education.

During the policy debate on reauthorization it will be critical to directly involve families and to find ways to share their views and experiences with policymakers. Following are several areas identified by families as top priorities through the vision process. Results from the process have already been shared with top Administration officials and will be shared widely with Members of Congress.

READING INSTRUCTION.   Only 26% agreed or strongly agreed that schools provide systematic, phonics-based reading instruction with appropriate textbooks and curricular materials. Ninety-two percent agreed or strongly agreed that improved reading instruction should be a priority for research, staff training, and replication of best practice. Results indicate that both special and regular educators need training in how to integrate the National Institute of Child Health and Human Development (NICHD) research on effective reading instruction into their classroom instruction. Some students with disabilities need extended, systematic reading instruction throughout their school years. A new research initiative is needed to identify effective reading strategies for children with Down syndrome and other developmental disabilities.

INVOLVEMENT AND PROGRESS IN THE GENERAL CURRICULUM.   IDEA requires that special education and related services be designed to enable the student to be involved in and to progress in the general curriculum. Only 22% agreed/strongly agreed that educators on Individualized Education Program (I.E.P.) teams have a clear understanding of the general curriculum and enable students to be involved in and to progress in the general curriculum. Ninety-one percent agreed/strongly agreed that research in this area for students with developmental disabilities, replication of best practice, and staff training should be a top priority.

ADAPTING CURRICULUM.   Only 21% agreed/strongly agreed that teachers know how to effectively adapt the standard curriculum. Ninety-five percent agreed/strongly agreed that that this should be a top priority for research, identification, and replication of best practice. Results demonstrate the need for teacher and staff preservice and in-service training in this critical area.

POSITIVE BEHAVIOR SUPPORTS.   The Individuals with Disabilities Act (IDEA) requires the IEP team to consider positive behavioral supports, strategies, interventions to address the child's behavior if that behavior interferes with his/her learning or the learning of others. Only 30% agreed/strongly agreed that educators conduct functional behavioral assessments when necessary, including an evaluation of the instructional environment. Forty-five percent agreed/strongly agreed that educators involve parents in IEP planning to address behavioral issues with positive supports, strategies, and interventions. Eighty-nine percent agreed/strongly agreed that improving the understanding of school staff about positive behavioral supports should be a top priority for replication of best practice and teacher training. Comments indicated a real need for training and implementation in this area.

INCLUSIVE EDUCATIONAL PLACEMENTS.   IDEA requires that students with disabilities be educated in the least restrictive environment (LRE) with supports and services. Forty-three percent agreed/strongly agreed that students with Down syndrome have the opportunity to attend regular classes in their neighborhood schools with appropriate services and supports. Ninety-three percent felt promoting inclusive placements with appropriate services and supports should be a top priority. Comments indicated that inclusive placements are "rare" in many schools and school districts.

WELCOMING ENVIRONMENT.   Only 37% agreed/strongly agreed that principals and administrators create a welcoming environment. Only 36% agreed/strongly agreed that students with Down syndrome have the opportunity to be a real part of the school, with inclusive educational opportunities, social integration, peer mentors, involvement in extracurricular activities, and involvement in volunteer and community service projects. Eighty-seven percent agreed/strongly agreed that training and advocacy efforts to encourage principals and administrators to create a welcoming environment should be a top priority. Comments stressed the importance of the school boards' and superintendents' leadership, how fragmentation in special education and regular education contributes to this problem, the need for accountability for students with disabilities, the need for principals to be held responsible through their evaluations for the school environment, and the need for accountability for improved educational outcomes for students with disabilities.

POSTSECONDARY EDUCATION.   Only 17% agreed/strongly agreed that students with Down syndrome have the opportunity to attend community college with supports, and 12% agreed/strongly agreed that there are opportunities to attend college with appropriate classes and residential and special education support. Eighty-seven percent feel that this should be a priority. Despite several promising models, no more than a handful of colleges or community colleges will accept students with cognitive/developmental disabilities in nondegree or certificate programs. Results indicate that professional development for postsecondary educational faculty and administrators to increase their understanding of disabilities and educational strategies to assist diverse learners is needed. A research initiative to develop various models of nondegree postsecondary education for students with developmental disabilities would expand horizons and options for students with Down syndrome and other developmental disabilities.

TRANSITION TO WORK. Fewer than 30% agreed/strongly agreed that schools and community agencies are meeting the needs of young people with Down syndrome by providing necessary vocational and/or transition services. Top priorities for improvements in various transition services and outcomes are as follows:

- 88%—volunteer opportunities with nondisabled peers in school
- 95%—opportunities to experience real work at real jobs before leaving school at age 22
- 95%—educating the student and family about transition planning and a variety of employment options
- 90%—better collaboration with community resources
- 95%—quality education, including more individualized, appropriate instruction
- 92%—support for the student and his/her family to develop an individual budget and to choose and control employment services and supports

## ADULT ISSUES

Although the Supreme Court established that students with disabilities have a constitutional right to a free appropriate public education, there is no universal right to assistance or support after age 21. Students leaving school and their families face a confusing, complex—and often contradictory—morass of federal and state laws and regulations. Most housing, employment, and medical assistance programs require the individual to stay poor to benefit—with little support for becoming as self-sufficient as possible. Individuals with developmental disabilities are often funneled into day programs or below-minimum-wage jobs in sheltered workshops where the demands of the program—not the individuals' interests and choices—dictate employment activities. Waiting lists for housing in many areas are so long that a parent must die or the individual with a disability must become homeless before housing assistance can be obtained. Segregated sheltered work and housing make involvement in the community difficult.

However, there is hope for change. As Chapter 1 by Thomas Nerney so eloquently points out, a paradigm shift to self-determination and control of decisions, supports, and individual budgets by individuals and their families is not only possible, it is beginning to take place in some areas of the country. Chapter 2 by Michael Morris describes the policy framework, values, and systemic change necessary for a paradigm shift to economic independence and inclusion.

Moving from a system where the bureaucracy and programs determine possibilities and options to a system empowering self-determination, economic independence, and inclusion is a bit like moving a glacier ice chip by ice chip. However, it is possible, and recent actions at the federal level support the shift. The President's Task Force on the Employment of Adults with Disabilities has undertaken a wide-ranging analysis of the policy changes necessary to support "real choice, real jobs, and real wages" for individuals with significant disabilities. Research by Research, Rehabilitation, and Training Centers has helped to provide the underpinning for these policy options. *Choose Work* (2001), a publication of the Association for Persons in Supported Employment, describes the possibilities and outcomes for people with significant disabilities to work at real jobs in the community given proper support. The Ticket to Work and Work Incentives Act of 1999 will provide individuals with disabilities with a "ticket" to choose and obtain services to obtain and keep a job while retaining medical benefits. This new "outcome-based" method should mean more choice and control and better employment outcomes—*if* the regulations are written to address the equity issues concerning individuals with more significant disabilities.

On June 22, 1999, the United States Supreme Court held in *Olmstead v. L.C.* that the unnecessary segregation of individuals with disabilities in institutions may constitute discrimination based on disability. The court ruled that the Americans with Disabilities Act requires states to provide community-based services rather than institutional placements for individuals with disabilities. The federal government is funding efforts at the state level to move from funding placements in institutions to providing community-based placements. The National Organization on Disability's Accessible Congregations program is encouraging congregations of all faiths across the country to include and welcome all individuals with disabilities in a meaningful manner.

All of these developments hold hope for the future. However, the current system is firmly entrenched. It will require ongoing, concerted advocacy to accomplish a paradigm shift toward promotion of self-determination, economic independence, and inclusion. The direct involvement of individuals with disabilities and their families in this effort is critical, as is sharing information with policy makers about what self-advocates and families experience and hope for the future. Following are results from the vision process in this area.

## SELF-DETERMINATION: EMPLOYMENT

Seventy percent agreed/strongly agreed that people with Down syndrome want to work but are unable to find jobs. Sixty percent agreed/strongly agreed that many want to work but must work part-time to maintain health benefits. Fifty-nine percent think opportunities are limited to day programs. Fifty-five percent think opportunities are limited to below-minimum-wage jobs in sheltered workshops or enclaves. Only 10% agreed, and 0% strongly agreed, that people with Down syndrome have the help, resources, and support necessary to obtain and keep employment. Only 21% agreed, and only 2% strongly agreed, that opportunities for employment, at minimum wage or better, at integrated jobs in the community are available.

Top priorities for improvements in various employment services and outcomes are as follows:

- 93%—full-time work while maintaining health and other benefits
- 90%—the help, resources, and support necessary to obtain and keep employment
- 95%—opportunities for employment, at minimum wage or better, at integrated jobs in the community
- 92%—opportunities to develop an individual budget with choice and control of employment services

## SELF-DETERMINATION: HOUSING

When asked what is typically available, 85% replied "waiting for housing services." Seventy-three percent feel that there is no opportunity for the individual and his/her family to decide with whom to live and where, and ninety-six percent agreed this should be a top priority for improvement. Only 17% agreed that the individual and his/her families have the opportunity to develop an individual budget with choice and control of support services for housing, and 98% agree this should be a top priority. An interesting note is that although only 11% agreed that support is available to a married couple to live in an apartment, group home, or home of their own, 90% agreed that this should be a priority.

## SELF-DETERMINATION: CREATING AN INDEPENDENT LIFE IN THE COMMUNITY

Many comments concerned the importance of making friends, having a well-rounded life, self-determination, including siblings in programs, training for professionals and family members, educating the community at large, and "learning to succeed in life."

## RESEARCH

Since 1983 NDSS has funded more than one million dollars to advance knowledge about Down syndrome. Support for basic and applied research in areas such as sensory motor function, aging, health care, genetics, language, cognition, and behavior has included funding for specific research projects and scientific symposiums. The Charles J. Epstein Down Syndrome Research Award provides grants to postdoctoral investigators interested in basic or applied research in clinical care, molecular biology, neurobiology, genetics, developmental biology, and psychology.

Since 1998 NDSS has provided $600,000 as part of a $3.9 million partnership with the National Institute of Child Health and Human Development and the National Institute of Neurological Disorders and Stroke of NIH to support research in cognition and behavior. The distinguished experts on the NDSS Scientific and Clinical Advisory Boards are directly involved in cutting edge research on Down syndrome, such as the sequencing of chromosome 21 and research projects involving cognition, behavior, and language.

Research in these areas is directly related to how children and adults with Down syndrome learn and function in society. The NDSS research focus has expanded to include educational interventions, new models of employment and training, and identifying and promoting best practice in a wide range of areas. A growing number of parents are keenly interested in these research areas.

## THE 2000 CONFERENCE

The research portion of the visions survey distributed at the 2000 conference in Washington, DC included a variety of questions. Results include the following:

TYPES OF RESEARCH SUPPORTED/NEEDED. A long list of suggestions of needed research included a wide variety of topics in the areas of health, cognition, basic and clinical research, education, inclusion, aging, etc.

SUFFICIENT RESEARCH? Responses to the question, "Do you think there has been sufficient research in the following areas?" included the following results: basic genetics—53% agreed; cognitive skills—12 % agreed; behavior—20% agreed; language development—19% agreed; mental health—21% agreed; health care—33% agreed; aging—16% agreed.

SEQUENCING CHROMOSOME 21. A number of people responded with excitement and hope in response to a question about the impact the recent sequencing of chromosome 21 will have on therapy for people with Down syndrome.

ETHICAL ISSUES. Quite a few comments on surveys and cards expressed concern about a perceived emphasis at NIH on prenatal research and a push for prenatal testing. Concerns were expressed about the potential impact both on individuals with Down syndrome and their families and on the underfunding of NIH research on improving the lives of individuals with Down syndrome. Comments included: "I hope it won't eliminate trisomy 21 from the world. We need people with DS." "Why is NIH spending so much money on prevention and so little on children and adults with Down syndrome?"

PEDIATRICIANS. Fifty-five percent agreed that their pediatrician or other physician is knowledgeable in the area of Down syndrome; forty-five percent disagreed.

## THE 2001 CONFERENCE AND FOLLOW-UP

Important new areas of research on Down syndrome are currently being investigated. NDSS was asked to assist in gathering survey information from parents about the prevalence of various medical conditions and behavioral issues and the availability of appropriate diagnosis and care. Results will help identify research and/or service gaps and will help make a stronger case for public and private funding of research in areas identified by families. Survey questions addressed sleep difficulties, attentional difficulties, wandering, repetitive/compulsive behaviors, aggressive behavior, self-stimulating behavior, "shutting down" behavior, self-talk, depression, and the use of computers and assistive technology. Further research in these areas would identify best practice in treatment and should assist individuals with Down syndrome, their families and schools, and professionals. The research survey was widely distributed, and results are still coming in as this book goes to print.

## ACHIEVING THE VISION

## A NEW STATE-OF-THE-ART CONFERENCE ON DOWN SYNDROME

HISTORY. One of the goals of the "Shaping a Vision for the Future" effort was to set the stage for a new state-of-the-art conference on Down syndrome. The last such conference was held in April 1985 and was funded by a grant through the National Institute of Handicapped Research, now known as the National Institute on Disability and Rehabilitation Research (NIDRR). The conference brought together experts in the topics of biomedical research, education, psychosocial aspects, and community living. These experts joined individuals with Down syndrome and family members in addressing life span issues from different perspectives. Recommendations for paradigm shifts in the delivery of services and areas requiring research initiatives resulted from that conference. After the conference, the book *New Perspectives in Down Syndrome* was published in 1987 by Paul H. Brooks Publishing Co. This book is currently out of print.

CHANGES SINCE L985.   Great strides have been made in many aspects of fields relating to Down syndrome. People with Down syndrome are living longer, fuller lives and are more likely to be included in schools, the workplace, and community life. Many advances in health care have contributed to longer life spans. In genetic research, the recent sequencing of chromosome 21 will open many new avenues of discovery about Down syndrome. Other research areas—such as how children with Down syndrome best learn to read—are still woefully neglected.

ANOTHER STATE-OF-THE-ART CONFERENCE.   The need for another state-of-the-art conference on Down syndrome to explore these and other relevant issues is critical. Outcomes of such a conference would include recommendations for research; identification and replication of best practice; policy, social/ethical, and educational agendas; as well as wide distribution of the results.

ROUNDTABLE PLANNING MEETING.   The Administration on Developmental Disabilities (ADD) and NDSS cosponsored a Roundtable Meeting to plan for a new state-of-the-art conference on Down syndrome on October 11–12, 2000 in Washington, DC. The meeting brought together experts from around the country in such diverse fields as self-determination, government, biomedical research, education, employment, social insurance, psychosocial aspects, and community living. These experts worked together to strategize about how to develop the topics, organization, and funding of a future state-of-the-art conference on Down syndrome. Participants worked together to: identify major topics that should be addressed; recommend speakers and experts; recommend the structure, organization, and formation of a steering committee; plan how to involve families and self-advocates; plan how to disseminate information and results; and recommend the next steps in the planning process. Vision survey results were used to identify areas that need to be addressed and to determine priorities.

NEXT STEPS.   The Roundtable Meeting was quite a success and provided valuable guidance and assistance in planning for a new conference, as well as commitments to continue involvement with the project. Currently, NDSS is exploring possible private and/or public funding for such a conference.

Once funding is obtained, a steering committee will continue with the planning. It is probable that this effort will encompass more than one conference and a book. It may involve "teams" of experts, self-advocates, and parents addressing specific issues and then meeting together. Planning challenges will include developing strategies to involve self-advocates and parents in the process and deciding how to put knowledge gained from the project in a format that is useful and readily accessible to self-advocates, parents, and professionals. A state-of-the-art conference project will bring together public and private experts, researchers, self-advocates, and parents to identify major accomplishments and best practice and areas that need to be addressed through research and public policy advances. It will provide a unique opportunity for everyone to learn what everyone else is doing and to share ideas and knowledge. Finally, results will be communicated to self-advocates, parents, and professionals to improve the lives of individuals with Down syndrome and their families.

## CONCLUSION: THE FUTURE

The challenges to disability advocates are in some ways different now than they were 30 years ago. After many years of fighting for legislative improvements, advocates must now work to protect those gains against a rising tide of opposition and backlash. At the same time, advocates must move forward to promote implementation of the laws, research to practice effect, accountability, self-determination, and the participation and involvement of self-advocates and parents in the major challenges of the field. The efforts outlined in this chapter will assist NDSS in our positive, proactive, and collaborative advocacy work to improve the future for individuals with Down syndrome and their families. With all of us working together, we *can* achieve the vision of all people with Down syndrome reaching their fullest potential in the larger community.

## REFERENCE

Geary T, Di Leo D (2001): Choose Work. Richmard, VA: Association for Persons in Supported Employment.

# ROLE OF THE FAMILY

# THE GIFTS OF DOWN SYNDROME: SOME THOUGHTS FOR NEW PARENTS

## MARTHA BECK, PH.D.

"Things will never be the same for you or your family," a grave-faced doctor told me one bleak winter day in 1988, just after my son Adam was diagnosed with Down syndrome. "You're throwing your life away."

I doubt he would have been so blunt if my baby had already been born, but Adam's diagnosis came through amniocentesis, three months before my due date. I'd decided not to end the pregnancy, and now my obstetrician was trying to change my mind. I knew he was motivated by a sincere desire to help, that he truly believed his dire predictions about my future were right. In a way, I guess, they were. It's true that things haven't been the same for me since Adam was born, and that when I refused a therapeutic abortion I "threw away" the life I'd always thought I would have. What I didn't know back in 1988 was that the life I was throwing away was far less interesting, fulfilling, and happy than the one I would get in return. Fourteen years ago, confronting my disapproving doctor, I shuddered to think about what lay ahead for me as the parent of a child with trisomy 21. Since then, many times, I have shuddered to think what I might have missed if I'd followed the doctor's advice instead of my heart.

I'm not saying it's morally wrong to end a pregnancy after a diagnosis of Down syndrome; I don't believe that. What I am saying is that, for me, having a child with this syndrome is nothing like the awful burden I once

*Down Syndrome*, Edited by William I. Cohen, Lynn Nadel and Myra E. Madnick.
ISBN 0-471-41815-3   Copyright © 2002 by Wiley-Liss, Inc.

thought it would be. The fears and disadvantages of having such a child hit like a hammer blow at the moment of diagnosis. The gifts that come with these exceptional people make themselves known more slowly and subtly, over months, years, and decades. But for me, and most other parents of children with Down syndrome, I know these gifts end up far outweighing any pain or disappointment we may suffer because of our children's disabilities.

Maybe you don't even need this kind of reassurance. Maybe you're one of those parents—I've met several—who say they never experienced a moment of concern or sadness about their child's having Down syndrome. If so, I'd like to know what kind of drugs you're on and whether you could get someone to prescribe the same thing for me. I went through months of mental anguish, both before and after my son was born, grieving for the "perfect" baby I'd lost and fearing for the baby I'd gotten instead. I think this is a normal reaction. If you have just learned that your child has Down syndrome, I urge you to let the emotions flow as intensely, and as long, as you want. Don't let anyone tell you to buck up, look on the bright side, stop feeling what you feel. The only "wrong" reaction is an inauthentic one, including any false show of resignation or cheer. If you let yourself grieve, you will find that the terrible feelings are finite, and that accepting them allows you to move on to a happier place.

## DOWN SYNDROME IN AN IQ-OBSESSED CULTURE

It took me a long time to finish my own grieving process, probably because in the entire history of the world, there has never been a person less interested than I was in having a child with mental retardation. At the time of Adam's diagnosis, my husband John and I were both halfway through Ph.D. programs at Harvard, where we'd also earned our undergraduate degrees. Both of us were "faculty brats," born and raised in the families of committed and successful academics. In short, from the time we were born, we had lived in environments where being smart was the single most highly valued characteristic in the human repertoire. From this perspective, any degree of cognitive retardation is the very definition of catastrophe.

Not everyone lives in an academic ivory tower world like the one John and I inhabited. But almost anyone reading this will have grown up in a society that glorifies what we call the "rational mind" and will have spent years participating in an educational system that constantly ranks children according to their ability to pass certain very narrowly defined tests of intelligence. This social system teaches all of us, in a thousand ways, that our ability to earn money, respect, and status all depend on how smart we are. No wonder Down syndrome is so feared in our culture! No wonder it's hard to think of any circumstances under which you would actually *want* to have a child with trisomy 21! To receive the gifts of Down syndrome, you have to let go of the way you've been taught to think about the value of human life itself—your child's life, your own life, the life of every person you encounter.

I learned this the hard way. During the final weeks of my pregnancy and the early days of Adam's life, I spent most of my time brooding, crying, reading horribly depressing books about chromosomal defects, and developing elaborate catastrophic fantasies about the terrors that awaited my family. Nowadays, I actually look back on those fears when I need comfort, for every one of them either proved to be false or led to some transformative experience that ultimately left me happier than I'd been before.

Of course, I was very lucky: Adam was born with no major health problems. He never had to cope with life-threatening heart defects, seizures, or neonatal surgery. I know hundreds of parents and children who made it through these awful eventualities and emerged on the other side strong and happy, but I don't claim to understand the depth of their trauma. Any problems I have faced are those that relate to having a child with Down syndrome who is basically healthy, and they seem almost trivial to me now. At the time of his diagnosis, however, they were utterly terrifying. Because you might have some of these fears yourself, I'd like to tell you how mine turned out.

## Unfounded Fears

### Fear #1: My child would be repugnant to me and other "normal" people

I'm not proud to admit that this was one of my biggest fears before Adam was born. Because I had months to imagine how he would look and behave before I ever actually saw him, I think my dread was more exaggerated than it would have been if I'd learned of his diagnosis after his birth. I was terrified of having a child who looked and acted (to use one of the most hated words in the Down's community) "mongoloid." This primitive fear came from my early exposure to people with trisomy 21, which consisted largely of once-a-year Christmas caroling expeditions to a "training school" near my childhood home. The residents at this "school" had been institutionalized since birth, lumped together with others who had all manner of physical and intellectual disabilities, and left to the care of overworked, underpaid state employees who didn't understand their needs.

My fear of Adam's visible differences began to fade from the time a geneticist assured me that kids with Down syndrome who are raised at home tend—like all children—to look and behave like the other members of their families. I was also enormously relieved when Adam was finally born and

I could see that far from being a monster, he was an absolutely adorable baby. Still, as he has grown up, I've been continually surprised by Adam's finely tuned social sensibilities, his ease around people, the stylish way he dresses and combs his hair. By the age of two, he was a clotheshorse with strong preferences about his attire. By three-and-a-half, he'd decided that he felt most comfortable in a dark suit, with a white shirt and a conservative tie. He dressed like this almost daily to attend preschool and elementary school. Now thirteen, he will don (stylish) casual clothes when the occasion calls for them, but he adores formal occasions when he can wear suits or— even better—black tie and tux. Adam's style sense, all by itself, eliminates most of the "strangeness" I saw in neglected, institutionalized people with Down syndrome years ago.

Adam's manners are as formal as his clothing tastes, not just acceptable but downright gracious. You may well find, as I have, that your child with Down syndrome is the only one of your offspring who never has to be reminded to say "please" and "thank you," who offers help as soon as he sees that someone needs it, who is quick with a joke to lighten a tense situation, who works carefully, subtly, and effectively to make shy children feel that they belong. I'd like to claim that Adam's enormously likable personality is due to good genes and devoted parenting, but I think the extra chromosome has something to do with it. If they aren't exposed to a normal social environment, people with Down syndrome certainly may look and act in ways others find strange. But when allowed to function in the world like any other person, these children tend to turn out as socially skilled as those without Down syndrome, if not more so.

## FEAR #2: MY CHILD WOULD HAVE A MISERABLE LIFE

The most upsetting thing my ob-gyn doctor said as he tried to talk me into a therapeutic abortion was, "You know this child will never be happy." He compared Adam to a malignant tumor, a cellular accident that, left to grow, would lead to untold misery. As I absorbed this image, it suddenly occurred to me that the doctor himself didn't seem to be a particularly happy person. I suspected that, like so many people I knew at Harvard, he was probably intensely driven, determined to prove his brilliance at any cost. I would have bet my last dime that he wasn't basing his judgment of Adam's potential happiness on any experience with people who actually had Down syndrome. Instead, his dire predictions were based on his own belief that human value and importance were inextricably linked with IQ. In my doctor's universe, intellectual achievement was the only possible route to self-esteem and satisfaction.

I'd shared this viewpoint all my life. I was convinced that the more tests I passed, the more degrees I won, the happier I would be. But even before Adam was born, his diagnosis led me to reexamine this belief. It occurred to me that I'd already passed a great many academic tests, and none of them had ever brought me any deep or lasting happiness. I wasn't sure why this was true, but somehow I sensed that I was about to find out.

And find out I did, almost from the moment Adam was born. His very first independent act, before his umbilical cord had been cut, was to enthusiastically pee in the face of the obstetrician who had called him a malignant tumor. He followed up this literal in-your-face performance by proceeding to live one of the happiest lives I've ever witnessed. This is not because people with Down syndrome are "always content"—that's just one of the many saccharine myths you might hear from people who are trying to deal with their own uneasiness about mental retardation. In truth, people with Down syndrome have a full and normal emotional range and can become clinically depressed just like the rest of us if they're badly treated or isolated. Furthermore, their personalities are unique; they are as different from each other as so-called "normal" human beings. But at the risk of overgeneralizing, I'd say that individuals with Down syndrome tend to be more clear-sighted than the rest of us in one crucial way: Instead of being diverted into chasing self-esteem in the form of honors, power, wealth, and competition, they tend to remain focused on one primary criterion—love.

When people have near-death experiences, they tend to react by putting love at the center of their lives. The years they may have spent chasing happiness through conquest or acquisitiveness come to seem meaningless in comparison to the time they spent with the people and activities they most love. Adam, like other people with Down syndrome I know, never loses this perspective. He refuses to spend time on things he doesn't love (fortunately, he loves doing his homework, keeping things orderly, doing kind things for others, and challenging himself mentally and physically). On the other hand, he zeroes in on anything there is to love about anyone and anything that crosses his path. He is a natural optimist, constantly finding things about which to feel enthusiastically pleased.

I can't express how wonderfully it changes your daily life to spend it with someone who thinks this way. For fourteen years, Adam has been turning my attention to the happiness available in almost any situation: the appreciation of a good hamburger, the hilarity of playing with our dog, the fabulous feel of clean sheets. Every day, his ready grin and easy gratitude teach me more about how to enjoy life than I learned during the twenty-plus years of my formal education. As Adam's younger sister put it one day when he was delightedly exploring the way his new electric toothbrush worked, "Well, Adam's overwhelmed by joy again." The miserable, half-human being my doctor told me to expect never did show up in Adam's skin; instead, I got a son who seems to have come equipped with an enlightened perspective that intelligently and patiently reaches out to teach me how to be happy. I can only hope that my former obstetrician ever receives such a miraculous gift.

## FEAR #3: MY CHILD AND I WOULD BE ISOLATED IN AN UNFRIENDLY WORLD

Several weeks before Adam was born, I read an awful book, written in the 1940s (or was it the 1490s?) about how to manage children with Down syndrome so that they would act marginally human. The author mentioned that it was important for these children to receive a lot of positive reinforcement from people who loved them—which, in most cases, would mean only the mother. This book was another little treasure (and I say that with heavy irony) from the era of institutionalization, but I didn't know how outdated and unfounded it was. I really believed that my life with Adam would isolate me from the company of others, that people would avoid us both, leaving us locked in a prison caused by genetic accident. I couldn't have been more wrong.

In the past few decades, most societies in the developed world have made enormous strides toward accepting, including, and socializing children with all disabilities. There's a long way still to go, but for those of us lucky enough to have access to forward-thinking communities, the horror stories of just a few years ago are rapidly fading into history. The reason for this change is that a large group of people, perhaps even a bona fide social movement, is committed to upholding the basic value and dignity of those with developmental disabilities. You may already have met some of these people through your hospital or pediatrician, and you will meet many more as your child grows up. Moreover, you will benefit from the changes they are continuing to create in social norms and values. This will be a terrific experience for your child, and I predict it will be an even better one for you.

It's true that that since Adam was born, I have encountered people who were horrified and repelled by the very thought of his disability. When he was three days old, I strapped him into his little front-pack and walked to Harvard campus, where I talked to several of my classmates, friends, and professors. Not one person either looked directly at Adam or acknowledged in any way that he had been born. He might as well have been invisible. I was cut to the quick by this reaction, not experienced enough to know that if I simply acted as though Adam was a normal baby—which in almost every way, he was—others would relax and respond more appropriately.

Fortunately, the many specialists and therapists who began doing Adam's "early intervention" quickly helped me realize that there are few people as badly educated as Harvard folks when it comes to social inclusion. Through my son, I began to meet more and more people who taught me how accepting human beings can truly be. In the parents of other special-needs kids, the educators who assisted in Adam's schooling, the good people who run Special Olympics, and countless others, I found new friends who are down-to-earth, wise, funny, kind, and giving. As Adam grew up, I noticed that my view of humanity became steadily less cynical than that of the Ivy League scholars and high-achieving professionals with whom I worked. Completely absorbed in the proverbial rat race, my colleagues tend to see people in general as rats. But because of Adam's presence in my life, I have come to believe that most people are enormously good at heart, willing to accept anyone who is willing to accept them.

When Adam has been singled out because of his Down syndrome, the distinction is more often positive than negative. One example: When our family was vacationing in Hawaii, we boarded a small boat with about 50 other tourists to visit a coral reef where we could snorkel. The boat was equipped with a slippery slide that dropped swimmers off about ten feet above the water. Eight-year-old Adam, who could already swim like a fish, decided he wanted to go down the slide, but when he got up there, he realized the fall was a lot further than he'd expected. Carefully, gripping the edges of the slide, he inched down toward the water, then paused for a full minute, getting up the nerve to take the plunge. Finally, he drew in a deep breath, raised his arms, and flew off the slide into the water. I'd been so absorbed in encouraging him that I hadn't noticed the other people on the boat, so I was as surprised as Adam when an enormous, spontaneous cheer went up from everyone aboard. There was nothing forced or condescending about it; these people simply wanted Adam to succeed, and their joy when he did was absolutely genuine. Perhaps it was because, at some point, each of them had been some kind of underdog and could identify both with Adam's fear and his courage. With typical insouciance, Adam climbed back into the boat, bowed to his cheering audience, and spent the rest of the voyage helping other kids overcome their fear of the water slide.

This is the kind of response I have encountered almost everywhere our family goes. There have been occasions when Adam has been taunted at school, but much more rarely and mildly than I expected—no more than I was taunted as a child for being a bookworm. He has always loved school, always had true friends, always excelled at sports, always fully and realistically anticipated a happy future surrounded by people who care. In the process, he's opened my eyes to a kinder and more accepting world, as well. I once thought living with the social repercussions of Adam's disability would be unbearable. Now, I don't think I could bear to live without them.

## Fear #4: My husband and I would never achieve our personal dreams and goals

After Adam was diagnosed, but before he was born, John and I both worried that our own dreams were fatally wounded. It didn't help that several advisors (in addition to the obstetrical staff) tried to convince us that our lives would fall apart if we kept our baby. One mentor told John that neither of us would ever finish our degree programs at Harvard and that our careers would be scuttled before they began. Again, we were hearing predictions based on fear and illusion, not fact. Because of Adam's easygoing personality, he was in many ways easier to raise than his two sisters and certainly didn't interfere with his parents' career goals any more than a "normal" baby would have.

It is true, though, that both John and I have had different professional lives than we might have if Adam had not come along when he did. This is not because he interfered with our plans, but because his birth led us to recognize that the academic world we had always lived in didn't really suit our personalities. Raising Adam helped us shift our thinking away from trying to create a "perfect" child. We began to see that every child is perfect, that each person has a unique contribution to give the world and will be happiest only when allowed to make that contribution.

Our careers took new courses when we began to apply this perspective to ourselves. Although we did finish our degrees and got good jobs as tenure-track professors, both of us eventually quit to do things we liked more. John, who loves travel above all else, became an international business consultant. I became a writer and career counselor, which I find infinitely preferable to having a real job. Not to boast, but to assure you that your professional life is not irrevocably damaged, I should mention that we've each made considerably more money by following our real dreams than we would have if we'd stayed on our previous career track. You might be interested to know that people like Charles de Gaulle, writer Pearl S. Buck, essayist George Will, football coach Gene Stallings, and a host of other successful people all have had children with Down syndrome. There are challenges combining any career with parenting, but your child's condition is by no means an insuperable obstacle to your own life goals.

One final note: Within weeks after Adam was born, several other parents in the Down syndrome community told me that I had a wonderful life ahead of me as an advocate for the mentally retarded. I was not comforted. Frankly, I'd had other plans. For several years, out of guilt, I made half-hearted attempts to join in the fund-raisers, political initiatives, and educational policy meetings attended by other parents, but I never felt any enthusiasm about them. However, when Adam was nine and I'd decided I wanted to be an author, it seemed natural to write about him, so I did—not with any noble intent, but because it was what I felt like doing. I am always surprised when people tell me that I've contributed to the cause of achieving full inclusion for "special" kids, because my actions were entirely selfish.

Because of this experience, I believe that the best way for any parent to advocate for his or her child is not to drop all previous ambitions and devote full-time attention to "the cause," but to continue following whatever dreams you cherished before your child was diagnosed. As you discover your own mission in life while simultaneously coming to adore your child, you will inevitably make contributions to people with Down syndrome, and help the world recognize how deeply it needs their extraordinary presence.

## FEAR #5: MY OTHER CHILDREN'S LIVES WOULD BE RUINED

Another cheery prediction I received from my obstetrician was that Adam's presence would destroy the life of my 18-month-old daughter, as well as any other children I might have in the future. Today, in the interests of unbiased reporting, I asked my two daughters how having a brother with Down syndrome has affected their lives. Kate is fifteen, two years older than Adam, and Lizzy is eleven, two years Adam's junior. Although I interviewed them separately, their answers to most of my questions were almost identical. They were also kind of boring. Nevertheless, I will list them here, because it would have helped me immeasurably to know them when I was first adjusting to Adam's diagnosis.

Q: How do you feel about having a brother with Down syndrome?
A (both girls): Hard to say. I can't imagine *not* having a brother with Down syndrome.
Q: Are you ever unhappy about it?
A (both girls): No.
Q: How do you think it affects your social life?
A (both girls): It doesn't.
Q: Do you worry about having to help care for Adam as you get older?
A (both girls): No. He'll do the same for me.
Q: Have you ever wished Adam didn't have Down syndrome?
A (both girls): Never really thought about it.
Q: Do you ever feel that you get less attention because of Adam's special needs?
A (both girls): No.
Q: How do you think your life might be different if Adam didn't have Down syndrome?
A (Kate): It wouldn't be any different.
A (Lizzy): I think if he didn't have Down syndrome, he might pick on me.

That's it, my daughters' own account of their terrible struggle to make peace with their brother's chromosomal abnormality. As I've said before, our family has been very lucky in that Adam has a basically healthy body and an extremely likable personality. If those conditions were different, my daughters might have experienced much more trauma because of his condition. But their answers reveal that the mere presence of a child with trisomy 21 doesn't necessarily spell disaster for "normal" siblings.

My own perception of my daughters is that they are unusually accepting children, unfazed by kids who are different from them in any way. They welcome people of other cultures, races, religions, or socioeconomic status and consider prejudice a ridiculous waste of time. Whether they would have been this way with or without Adam's Down syndrome we can never know, but my personal opinion is that my daughters' minds are broader and deeper because Adam is their brother.

## Fear #6: I would be sad forever

This is another fear that was reinforced by studies I read while I was still pregnant with Adam. You may know that all human beings go through a predictable "grieving process" when something tragic happens to them. It includes denial, "bargaining," anger, grief, and finally acceptance. While expecting Adam, I was told that according to some research, parents who have a disabled child (unlike parents whose children die) never reach acceptance. They just rattle around the grieving process, from denial to bargaining to sorrow to anger and back again, for the rest of their natural lives.

This was probably the most disheartening thing I heard during the whole scary, heartbroken time between Adam's diagnosis and his birth. The idea of feeling that way forever, or at least for as long as both Adam and I were alive, was about as much fun as heading off to serve an indefinite sentence at Alcatraz. Fortunately, the prophecies of eternal grieving turned out, like my other fears, to be false. Having a child with Down syndrome does not mean that you will be eternally miserable. On the other hand, it doesn't mean that you'll be eternally happy. No child, whatever his or her genetic profile, has the power to determine his/her parents' life experience. Our children can only create opportunities for us to make sense of our own lives and come to terms with our own difficulties. Our happiness is not in their hands, but in our own.

That said, the key to adapting when your child has Down syndrome is letting go of your ideas about what you think your child should be and enjoying what your child actually is. I often compare the experience to buying a pet, thinking you've got a puppy, then taking it home to discover that it is actually a kitten. If you spend all your time trying to force your kitten to act like a puppy, you might forget to enjoy all the innately wonderful things about kittens. People who have Down syndrome are no better or worse than people who don't, but they are different in some ways. Those differences can be a source of disappointment, but they can also be a source of unexpected delight.

Simply saying this cannot convey how true it is; you'll have to discover the joys of your situation by watching your own wonderful baby develop. All I can tell you is that for me, raising Adam has been a source of continual, small epiphanies, moments when his quirky intelligence allows me to see the world in new ways. I am writing this just days after September 11, 2001, when terrorists attacked the United States and changed the American psyche forever. As I watched news coverage of the smoking rubble that had been the Twin Towers, Adam came to ask me which tie I thought he should wear to his school's homecoming dance. After I helped him decide, I pointed to the TV. We'd spent several hours talking about the disaster as a family, and I wondered what sense Adam might be making of it.

"What do you think America should do about this terrible thing?" I asked him. Adam contemplated the televised ruins, wrinkled his brow in thought, and said, "Well, we just have to keep dancing."

This is my advice to you, if you are living through your own personal devastation, the destruction of your own hopes for you and your child. I know that it's possible to descend into eternal grief, but in a society filled with options for our kids, this is far from the only choice. If you allow yourself to simply love your child as he or she is, that love will open new ways of seeing, thinking, and experiencing life. Your emotional range will probably become wider than if your child were "normal"—you'll experience more pain in some ways, but you'll also experience more joy. Some people may think of this as a burden. To me, it feels like a privilege.

Several years after Adam was born, a friend I'd known in high school called to say that she had just given birth to a son with Down syndrome. I had to restrain myself from saying, "Wow, congratulations! That's wonderful!" I had to remind myself to respect her sorrow, her fear, the pain of her dashed dreams. I respect those things in you, as well, so for now, please accept my deepest sympathy. But I'd like to leave you a message for later, when you've seen for yourself what a remarkable little person has entered your life. Just like my old doctor said, your life will never be the same again—but in many ways it will be better than that good doctor will ever know. You have a baby with Down syndrome. Life will never be the same for you or your family. Congratulations. It's going to be wonderful.

# A Personal Account

## Siegfried M. Pueschel, M.D., Ph.D., J.D., M.P.H.

One day, some 35 years ago, while I was working as Senior Resident in the Emergency Clinic of Montreal Children's Hospital, I admitted an eight-year-old girl with Down syndrome who complained of severe abdominal pain. The initial cursory physical examination revealed that she had an acute abdomen and was in severe distress. After a few essential laboratory tests, we immediately transported the patient to the operating room. The surgeons found a ruptured ovarian cyst with significant intra-abdominal bleeding. Fortunately, the girl recovered well.

Postoperatively, we had more time to examine her thoroughly. We noted that not only did she have most of the characteristics of a person with Down syndrome, but she also had signs of hypothyroidism, verified by appropriate laboratory examinations, and precocious sexual development (Pueschel et al., 1966). The subsequent investigations of the interrelationship of Down syndrome, hypothyroidism, and sexual precocity led to my first publication on the subject of Down syndrome. And during this time period, my son Christian was born.

Like many expectant parents, my wife and I had been looking forward to the happy event of the birth of a healthy baby. Our dreams, however, soon were shattered when we found out that our son had Down syndrome. After this initial traumatic experience, our profound sadness and despair were soon transformed into joy and true happiness because Chris' smiles and his pleasant personality conquered our hearts, and thus we started to celebrate

*Down Syndrome,* Edited by William I. Cohen, Lynn Nadel, and Myra E. Madnick.
ISBN 0-471-41815-3   Copyright © 2002 by Wiley-Liss, Inc.

Chris' life. My daughter Jeanette could not have said it more precisely: Chris was the sunshine of our family.

Although I had been involved in Down syndrome research before his birth, Chris undoubtedly had a significant impact on my future existence. Foremost, Chris gave direction and meaning to my professional life and in many ways shaped my personal life as well. Moreover, during his short life, Chris touched the hearts of so many other people, directly and indirectly.

I could dwell on many fascinating stories about Chris because he was such an engaging and captivating young man; however, I would rather tell you of how his life was interwoven with my career as a physician and researcher. In the following, I shall briefly touch upon three selected investigations that somehow interrelate with my son's overall development, his medical concerns, and his specific cognitive functions.

I shall first elaborate on a comprehensive study that included 114 children with Down syndrome who were followed closely from birth to their third birthday. One of the objectives of this investigation was to study the interrelationships of biological, environmental, and competency variables of these children (Reed and Pueschel, 1980).

We found that the presence of significant congenital heart disease adversely influenced muscle tone and the parent's ability to follow through with provided guidance. Muscle tone, in turn, was a powerful predictor of other outcomes including motor and social developments, cognitive functioning, and language acquisition. The general development at six months of age was noted to influence both future language acquisition and mental development. The ability to follow through with instructions pertaining to early intervention was affected by muscle tone and by the parent's ability to cope. In turn, early intervention efforts had a significant influence on cognitive functioning.

This type of analysis signifies the importance of the study of variable interrelationships because it provides information on predictability of specific biological conditions and environmental circumstances. Such assessments also give us a better understanding of developmental and maturational processes of children with Down syndrome.

Pertaining to my son's development, his severe congenital heart disease (complete atrioventricular canal) affected negatively his muscle tone and his motor development. In addition, Chris had numerous illnesses during the first few years of life. Moreover, early intervention, as we know it today, was not available at the time. Thus his competency variables including cognitive and language developments were decreased, although Chris had other strengths; I shall elaborate on later in this chapter.

We also carried out several investigations relative to thyroid function in children with Down syndrome. Whereas only a few children in our study presented with hyperthyroidism (Pueschel and Pezzullo, 1985), among 151 children with Down syndrome, 10 children had uncompensated hypothyroidism with significantly increased thyroid stimulating hormone and sig-

TABLE 9.1. NUMBER OF PATIENTS WITH ABNORMAL AND NORMAL TSH AND/OR $T_4$ VALUES CONTRASTING ANTIBODY TITER RESULTS*

| | No. of Patients | | | | |
| | With Increase in Antibody Titers | | | | |
| Hormonal Values | ATA and AMA | ATA | AMA | Without Increase in Antibody Titers | Total Patients |
|---|---|---|---|---|---|
| Increased TSH and decreased $T_4$ | 1 | 0 | 7 | 2 | 10 |
| Increased TSH and normal $T_4$ | 2 | 0 | 4 | 15 | 21 |
| Normal TSH and increased $T_4$ | 3 | 0 | 1 | 3 | 7 |
| Normal TSH and decreased $T_4$ | 0 | 0 | 1 | 2 | 3 |
| Normal TSH and normal $T_4$ | 8 | 5 | 15 | 82 | 110 |
| Total | 14 | 5 | 28 | 104 | 151 |

*TSH indicates thyroid-stimulating hormone; $T_4$, thyroxine; ATA, antithyroglobulin antibody; and AMA, antimicrosomal antibody.

nificantly decreased thyroxine. Another 20 children had compensated hypothyroidism with significantly high thyroid stimulating hormone, but normal thyroxine levels. We also studied the relationship between thyroid autoimmunity and thyroid function (Pueschel and Pezzullo, 1985). Moreover, we observed that as individuals with Down syndrome advance in age, there is a gradual decrease of thyroxine and triiodothyronine. Also, my son Chris developed hypothyroidism during adolescence (Table 9.1).

In further investigations we found that individuals with Down syndrome and untreated hypothyroidism have a significantly lower IQ than those who have normal thyroid function (Pueschel et al., 1991) (Table 9.2). Therefore, we recommended periodic (at least annual) thyroid function testing and not waiting for clinical symptoms to occur. We also observed that after initiation of thyroxine therapy, Chris became more alert and was able to study more effectively.

I will now briefly discuss another important study that was designed to investigate the cognitive and learning processes in children with Down syndrome by using primarily the Sequential and Simultaneous Processing Scales of the Kaufman Assessment Battery for Children. Whereas other intelligence tests tend to be more content-oriented, intelligence, as measured by the Kaufman test, is defined in terms of an individual's style of solving problems and processing information.

TABLE 9.2. IQS OF PATIENTS WITH DOWN SYNDROME*

| Hormonal and Thyroid Function Values of Patients With Down Syndrome | N | IQ | |
|---|---|---|---|
| | | $\bar{X}$ | SD |
| Increased TSH and decreased $T_4$ | 10 | 41.7 | 5.4 |
| Increased TSH and normal $T_4$ | 15 | 53.8 | 6.2 |
| Normal TSH and Normal $T_4$ | 21 | 55.3 | 6.9 |

*TSH indicates thyroid-stimulating hormone; $T_4$, thyroxine.

TABLE 9.3. MEANS AND STANDARD DEVIATIONS OF STANDARD SCORES OF SEQUENTIAL AND SIMULTANEOUS PROCESSING SCALES FOR CHILDREN IN THE EXPERIMENTAL AND THE CONTROL GROUPS

| | N | Sequential Processing* | | Simultaneous Processing** | |
|---|---|---|---|---|---|
| | | X | SD | X | SD |
| Down syndrome | 20 | 53.7 | 8.03 | 54.9 | 8.74 |
| Siblings | 20 | 108.3 | 12.26 | 104.9 | 12.91 |
| MA-matched | 20 | 90.3 | 10.67 | 94.0 | 13.00 |

*$F = 141.02$, $df = 57$, $p < .0001$.
**$F = 100.61$; $df = 57$, $p < .00001$.

The results of these investigations revealed that children with Down syndrome differ significantly in their sequential and simultaneous processing abilities when compared with those of their brothers and sisters and with mental age-matched a group of children without mental retardation (Table 9.3). Most importantly, we found that children with Down syndrome had more difficulties with auditory-motor and auditory-vocal processing than with visual-motor and visual-vocal processing (Pueschel et al., 1987) (Table 9.4).

An important aspect of these investigations concerns the psychoeducational implications and the educational planning. Because a child's preferred mode of processing information relates closely to his or her learning style, teaching strategies should capitalize on the child's strengths and should focus on visual-vocal and visual-motor processing modalities in the education of children with Down syndrome.

My son Chris actually had demonstrated the above strength in visual processing in a practical way some time ago. One day Chris and I were in the process of going shopping. After we had climbed into the car, I was unable to get the car started. While I was getting frustrated, Chris was smiling and said, "Why don't you put the shift into neutral." Of course, after I had done so, I was able to start the car. I then asked Chris, "Would you like to drive the car?" When he said "Yes," we switched seats and Chris started

TABLE 9.4. Means and Standard Deviations of Scaled Scores of Subtests Hand Movement, Gestalt Closure, Number Recall, and Word Order for Children in the Experimental and the Control Groups

| | Down Syndrome | | Siblings | | MA-Matched | |
|---|---|---|---|---|---|---|
| | X | SD | X | SD | X | SD |
| Hand Movement | 3.15 | 1.69 | 10.60 | 2.98 | 7.95 | 1.90 |
| Gestalt Closure | 4.55 | 2.35 | 10.25 | 2.83 | 8.05 | 2.33 |
| Number Recall | 2.35 | 1.46 | 12.25 | 1.92 | 9.00 | 2.60 |
| Word Order | 1.70 | 1.34 | 11.60 | 2.72 | 8.35 | 1.95 |

the car. Although nobody ever had taught or instructed him how to drive a car, he had been so observant in the past and he had visually memorized how to operate an automobile. And after that day he was driving, without ever having an accident. In particular, Chris enjoyed driving a golf cart during Special Olympics State Games, when he drove me from venue to venue where I had to examine injured and sick athletes. Thus he demonstrated so well what we had found in our study, namely, that visual processing skills are amplified in people with Down syndrome.

Of course, there are other studies I could discuss either to which Chris had provided an impetus or that relate to one of his medical problems. Instead, however, I would like to provide some insights about Chris as a person.

Throughout his short life, Chris was a teacher par excellence. In many ways, he made me ask probing questions about important human values such as "How do we measure human worth?" and "How do we as a just and concerned society provide the most appropriate care for those who are unable to care for themselves?"

It was Chris who made it very clear to me what our values should be and how these values should influence our behavior. Above all, Chris let me know that the basic value should be the recognition of the dignity and worth of people with Down syndrome as well as those with other developmental disabilities. He instilled in me that service to humanity must rank higher than personal gratification in professional life and private enterprise. Chris taught me that in the end, material accomplishments won't matter at all— but what will endure is the quality of life and the love that we have given to others. Chris made me aware that beyond intellectual achievement and earthly accomplishments we so highly value in our culture, there are more important human qualities we should embrace. Chris taught me not to take life for granted, but to be more aware and thankful of its simple pleasures. He taught me to use time wisely—because it is too precious to be wasted on unimportant things.

Chris taught me that individuals with Down syndrome are persons in their own right despite their limited capacity for academic achievement. Moreover, he taught me that an IQ score is a demeaning measure of human potential and human qualities. He let me know that persons with Down syndrome have an intrinsic value of humanity and that they can contribute to society and perform tasks that previously were never expected of them. Chris showed me that using quality as a measure of relationships brings a dimension that quantity just cannot match. Chris so well exemplified that there is a goodness, humanity, and magic in our children with Down syndrome that must be protected and never be betrayed.

Because many of us have chosen to spend our lives providing care for individuals with developmental disabilities including those with Down syndrome, it is fair to assume that we share a strong belief in the intrinsic value of those human beings, rich or poor, severely mentally retarded or with borderline intellectual functioning. Only human cowardice would allow us to walk away from these individuals. In this vein, the late President John F. Kennedy said some time ago, "These children may be the victim of fate, but they shall not be the victim of our neglect."

## REFERENCES

Pueschel, SM, Gallagher, PL, Zartler, AS, Pezzullo, JC (1987): Cognitive and learning processes in children with Down syndrome. Res Devel Dis 8:21–37.

Pueschel, SM, Jackson, IMD, Giesswein, P, Dean, MK, Pezzullo, JC (1991): Thyroid function in Down syndrome. Res Devel Dis 12:287–296.

Pueschel, SM, Pabst, JF, Hillman, DA (1966): Etiologic interrelationship in Down syndrome, hypothyroidism, and precocious sexual development. Canadian Paediatric Society. Halifax, Nova Scotia, July 11–13.

Pueschel, SM, Pezzullo, JC(1985): Thyroid dysfunction in Down syndrome. Am J Dis Child 139:636–639.

Reed, RB, Pueschel, SM, Schnell, RR, Cronk, CE (1980): Interrelationship of biological, environmental, and competency variables in young children with Down syndrome. Appl Res Ment Retard 1:161–174.

# Being a Dad—As I Know It

## Thomas J. O'Neill

For 31 years before I became a dad, I was a son. It was the lessons learned as a son that have heavily influenced me as I travel the journey as a dad.

This journey began on August 31, 1978. My first son, Joshua, was born that day at 12:25 in the afternoon. According to my wife Rita's obstetrician, Joshua was due to arrive on August 10th. That day, along with twenty subsequent days, came and went without any signs of labor. Finally, in the mid-evening hours of August 30th, Rita said that labor was starting. Later that night we were off to Lake Forest Hospital.

Just before leaving our house for the hospital Rita and I gently hugged, laughed, and talked about the impact that the birth of this child, a child both of us really wanted, would have on our lives. At that time, little did we know or understand the essence or the serene beauty of our naiveté. The only thing we really understood during those wee hours of darkness on that August night was that a child would soon be born. We knew that our lives would be changing; we just did not understand the total impact.

My journey as a son started on February 12, 1947. I am part of the baby boomer generation, a child of post-World War II America. My dad had been in the war, spending part of his two-year Navy career overseas. During those years my mother stayed at home, ran the family business, and cared for their other four children. I arrived two years after World War II ended, the second son and fifth and last child. My family's roots are Midwestern, working class.

If, as Kierkegaard said, "Life can only be understood backwards; but it must be lived forward," I know that the depth of my relationship with my

*Down Syndrome*, Edited by William I. Cohen, Lynn Nadel, and Myra E. Madnick.
ISBN 0-471-41815-3   Copyright © 2002 by Wiley-Liss, Inc.

dad came to light during the 12 years before his death. My dad spent those 12 years in a nursing home. Although my dad's body was limited by strokes and other cardiovascular problems, his mind remained alert until two days before he died. In watching and visiting with my dad during those years, that alertness of mind, with his ravaged body, frequently seemed like the ultimate act of nature's cruelty. My dad died at the age of eighty-six. Although his mind was alert until the end, his ability to communicate and his mobility had been seriously impaired.

From the time that I was a little boy, I knew that I had never had a real conversation with my dad, a real father-son connection. It just had not been! When my dad was older and his health problems were mounting, I knew two things. I knew that I longed for a real father-son relationship with him, and I instinctively knew that he longed for the same with me. Although that longing was there, that longing and need to connect as father and son, something existed that thwarted it. If I have a regret as a middle-aged man, it is that my dad and I were never able to connect as both of us had desired and as both of us needed.

I know that my dad loved me, as I believe he loved my mother, my sisters, and my brother. My dad was simply someone who could not express it. He had a hard time giving and receiving gifts or compliments and expressing a normal sense of love; a normal love that comes to exist in a healthy family.

My opportunity to again experience the father-son relationship issues started with the birth of my first son in 1978 and continued with the birth of my second son in 1981. Coming from a place where I had not had the relationship I knew that I desired and needed, I sometimes supplemented that need with the idealized world of the television families of the 1950s and the early 1960s. I grew up with *Father Knows Best* and *Ozzie and Harriet*. My vision of the family, and probably the perfect family, may have actually compromised my understanding of the real father figure. Who could father better than Ozzie Nelson or Robert Anderson? Was this not the way dads treated and acted with their families?

When my own opportunity to be a dad came, I started with the premise that I wanted to do it better than my dad had done and that to do so I should compensate for what had not been and I would do it perfectly. To do this would require that I be the perfect dad, and having perfect children would also aid this effort. How quickly nature taught me about reality!

When my son Joshua was born, he was not born in perfect condition. In fact, he was born in critical condition, close to death. Besides numerous health problems, he was also born with Down syndrome. I will forever remember the words and the feeling that permeated me when a neonatologist, a doctor neither Rita nor I had ever met before, told us about our son's developmental issues. This man, this complete stranger, was kind, compassionate, and understanding; but when he told us about Joshua probably having Down syndrome and his other health problems, it felt as though our world had just been pulled out from underneath us. The doctor also told us that Joshua would need to be transferred immediately to another hospital— a facility that was medically equipped to care for him.

Joshua spent the first 37 days of his life in a neonatology unit. Before Joshua's birth, I did not even know the meaning of the word neonatology. Besides learning a whole new vocabulary, a vocabulary that came to extend far beyond the word neonatology, we would also come to learn the "alphabet soup" of the doctors, the bureaucracies, and the systems that would interact with our family.

In my encounters with the medical community, as well as the community of service and care providers, I learned that as a dad I was often ignored. The dynamics of the interactions sometimes amused me, sometimes amazed me, and sometimes angered me. The interactions of which I speak were generally three-way meetings, i.e., the care provider, Rita, and me. As this triangle exists, I found that the conversation would generally flow from the care provider to Rita, with me being regarded as an outsider. The messages that I frequently received were verbal exclusion and body language that did not include me, my input, or my ideas as Joshua's dad. In a Family Support Bulletin entitled "What About Fathers" (May, 1991), James E. May talks about the dangers of excluding dads from direct involvement with their children. According to May, the research indicates that it is the dad who sets the tone for how the family deals with and handles issues related to having a child with special needs (Davis and May, 1991). Following this thinking, it is imperative that ways be found to include dads in all facets of a child's care. I found myself becoming more successful as I discovered positive ways to include my thoughts pertaining to Joshua's medical care and his various therapies. It was also easier for me to accomplish this as Rita and I shared our thoughts about Joshua, how we were feeling about what was happening with him and us, and what it was that we wanted for him and his future. Our thinking was generally complementary.

When Joshua was about 18 months old, he and I were waiting for Rita in a local shopping center; Joshua was in his stroller. A couple walked by and I heard the lady inform her companion that the child in the stroller was a "mongoloid baby." Oh, the pain of it! The baby was my son. The pain I felt that night was piercing. The only thing I could think was how dare she refer to my son in that way, using a word that is regarded as degrading and dehumanizing. My son is not a mongoloid, he is not a "Downs"; he is a person, a person who happens to have Down syndrome.

Over the course of many years I have come to have that same sense with some other people as I have seen them interact with Joshua. Some people, such as this lady, see Joshua and see a disability. Other people see Joshua and they see a person. Sometimes I have found that there are things that I can do to help ease these situations, and at other times there is virtually nothing that I can do. Some people will never look beyond the diagnosis of Down syndrome. But what I have also found is how disarming Joshua can be and what an incredible ambassador of information he is to people who leave themselves open to him.

On more than one occasion I have found myself one of Joshua's more astute students. When I have feared him trying something new, or my letting go of him, I have found myself needing to sit back and listen to what it was that he was telling me. Sometimes he has done this in a fairly orderly fashion, whereas at other times I have needed to learn through observation. Both Rita and I have found that as Joshua needs new opportunities, and as he is aware of this, he tells us. The challenge for us is learning how to listen and understanding the meaning and the need related to what he is saying.

Communication is the vital link to family life. It is the fabric that weaves a family together. In my own experience, I never really had a conversation or connection with my dad. I wanted and needed an in-depth dialogue that would bond Joshua and me as father and son. So how was I, as the dad of a child with a cognitive disability, to engage my son in full communication?

Being sensitive to this issue, and knowing that both Joshua and I needed this communication and this connection, it is interesting to me as I look back on these last 23 years. For me the communication, or maybe more appropriately the bonding, started with Joshua and me the night that he was born.

Late that evening my sister-in-law Leah and I went to Evanston Hospital, where Joshua had been transferred earlier that day. I had to officially check him into the hospital, and I also wanted to visit him. That night I found him on a ventilator in a bed that was basically a mobile medical unit. It contained the support systems necessary for the various medical emergencies that could arise. That night it was very quiet in the neonatology unit. The doctor in charge was finishing the last year of his neonatology residency. In spending time with this doctor I knew, although he never stated so exactly, that he did not expect Joshua to live until morning. However, as I spent time alone with Joshua that night I knew from some place deep inside that the morning would be his, that he would live to see another day. As Joshua and I spent time alone together that night, the bonding and the communication between us started. For me the bonding began when I "talked" with Joshua. From him I "heard" and I understood an incredible strength. Something told me how much he wanted to live, and I knew how much I wanted him as my son.

After that night and over the course of many years, I have learned that bonding is not something that sits in isolation or something that merely happens at the time of birth. Bonding is part of the lifetime journey of being a dad. The dynamics of bonding are both unique and parallel with each of my sons.

Joshua brings certain issues to our relationship merely because he has specific challenges in his life. But Joshua also brings issues to our relationship because he is the person and the personality that he is today. As Marcia Van Riper states in her research findings, "…The birth of a child with Down syndrome involves a change of plans for families, but it does not have to be a negative experience. In fact, for many families, it is a positive growth producing experience" (Van Riper, 1999). My son Noah, who is a healthy 20-year-old and a junior in college, brings issues to our relationship because he, too, is a unique individual. Although there are differences with Joshua and Noah, those differences are more related to two individual personalities than they are defined by Down syndrome.

Fifty-four years of living, blended with twenty-three years as a dad, have taught me a great deal about the daily experiences of life. I can sit back today and be very aware of the traumatic and painful situations that have been part of the experience of being the dad of a young man with Down syndrome. However, this all needs to be placed in perspective. The joys and the incredible sense of pride in Joshua far overshadow the other issues. I can remember the day of his Bar Mitzvah, the Cub Scout awards banquets, watching Joshua play YMCA basketball, the night he graduated from high school, diploma in hand, and I could go on and on, with events big and small, that have given me a total perspective on life. To use the metaphor of a mountain, to really understand what a mountain looks and feels like it cannot be embraced merely from its highest point. Rather, looking at and understanding the height from the valley adds an extra dimension.

During the fatherhood journey I have had to find ways to deal with the issues that I brought from my experiences as a son and to incorporate those experiences and to find healthy ways to be a dad to my two sons. One of the big lessons I have learned on numerous occasions is that being a good and loving dad is not about being the perfect dad. It's about making mistakes, loving my kids, being kind to them and myself, being there for them, and learning from the day-to-day issues that are part of life. I've had to find ways to deal with and sometimes forgive myself as I've made mistakes as a dad. In so doing, and because so much of who we are comes from where we came, I've discovered that I've had to find good ways to cope with the lack of communication and connectedness that I had not experienced with my own dad. This process, the knowledge and understanding of myself as both a son and dad, has also helped me forgive my dad for the mistakes he may have made. In a silver lining sense, the mistakes that my dad made may, in fact, have only served to enrich the relationships that I am experiencing with each of my sons.

If hindsight offers great vision, I would like to suggest some things that have been helpful to me in being dad to both of my sons:

- Enjoy your kids.
- Enjoy yourself as a dad.

- Remember you're a dad—not a professional, not a caretaker, not a therapist or a medical provider.
- Develop a level of comfort in responding and acting on what it is that your "gut" is telling you as a dad.
- Work on the special relationship you share with your spouse or the significant person in your life.
- Be aware of your expectations and needs.
- Be aware of the various needs of your family—you need not act on everyone's needs, but being aware of the needs is helpful.
- Be aware of the dynamics of the family of which you are a part.
- Although you cannot make Down syndrome go away, you can find healthy ways to embrace it and to deal with it.
- Get to know other dads who have family experiences similar to yours.
- You are your child's advocate; find ways to act on it.
- Be knowledgeable about your child's rights, his/her school program, health care needs, and social, athletic, and extracurricular activities.
- Don't expect other people to do the job that you need to do.
- Find time for yourself.
- Live and enjoy today while planning for tomorrow.

Some of these suggestions may be particularly germane to issues that arise because of having a child with special needs. However, most of these suggestions translate to any dad who is experiencing the joys and the trials of fatherhood.

At some point a question that dads will invariably ask is whether or not the journey of fatherhood is worth it and if there is much that would be changed, given the opportunity. For me, I can only look at where I am in this journey and know that my sons are just right, just the way they are—That my sons and I are doing fine—That there is little I would change—That the experiences we are having are just right—That being Joshua and Noah's dad is not perfect, but it is just right, just the way it is.

## REFERENCES

Davis, Phillip and May, James E. (1991): Involving fathers in early intervention programs: Issues and strategies. CHC, Spring 1991, Vol. 20 (2).

May, James E. (1991): Family Support Bulletin, What About Fathers, Spring 1991.

Van Riper, Marcia (1999): Living with Down syndrome: The family experience. Down Syndrome Q, March 1999.

## ORGANIZATIONS

National Fathers Network
Fathers Network
16120 NE 8th St.
Bellevue, WA 98008-3937
(425)747 4004, ext. 218
*www.fathersnetwork.org/*
    The National Fathers Network's mission is to celebrate and support fathers and families raising children with special health care needs and developmental disabilities. Their organization provides information and referral to fathers throughout the United States. Their website also contains articles, resources, and general information.

National Parent Network on Disabilities
1130 17th St, NW. Suite 400
Washington, DC 20036
(202)463-2299/fax (202)463-9405
*www.npnd.org/main.htm*
    NPND is a nonprofit organization dedicated to empowering parents. Located in Washington, DC, NPND has the unique capability to provide its members with the most up-to-date information on the activities of all three branches of government that affect individuals with disabilities and their families.

## PUBLICATIONS

Special Children, Challenged Parents: The Struggles and Rewards of Raising a Child with a Disability, Revised Edition. Naseef, Robert A. Ph.D. (2001) Baltimore, MD: Paul H. Brooks. Available through Paul H. Brooks Publishing Co., PO Box 10624, Baltimore, MD 21285-0624; tel.: (800) 638-3775.

Uncommon Fathers: Reflections on Raising a Child With a Disability. Meyer, Donald J. (1995) Bethesda, MD: Woodbine House. Available through Woodbine House, 6510 Bells Mill Road, Bethesda, MD 20817; tel: (800) 843-7323

Living with Down Syndrome: The Family Experience. Van Riper, Marcia. In: Down Syndrome Quarterly, Volume 4, Number 1, March, 1999. Available through Samuel J. Thios, Editor. Denison University, Granville, OH 43023; fax: (740)587-6601.

# THE SIBLING RELATIONSHIP: ATTENDING TO THE NEEDS OF THE OTHER CHILDREN IN THE FAMILY

## SUSAN P. LEVINE, M.A., C.S.W.

Everyone would agree that giving birth to a child with Down syndrome is a profound and life-changing experience. Although the struggles can be numerous (particularly struggles with schooling, adult services, and medical needs), many families feel that their child with special needs is truly a gift. However, a child with Down syndrome is born not only to parents but also to membership in the entire family. Brothers and sisters are an important part of the life of their sibling. How are they affected by growing up with a child who has Down syndrome in the family? Is the experience for siblings as profound as it is for parents? Is the overall experience viewed as a gift for them or as a struggle?

For the last 25 years, I have had the distinct privilege of running sibling groups and writing newsletters for brothers and sisters of children with Down syndrome and other disabilities who live in the central New Jersey area. These children have shared their thoughts and feelings with me, providing me with a first-hand view of the needs of siblings. In this chapter, with the help of those students, we will examine the sibling relationship in general and, more specifically, the experience related to having a child with Down syndrome in the family. We will also look at ways parents can address the needs of their children without disabilities and assist them in experiencing their sibling as more of a "gift" than a difficulty.

*Down Syndrome*, Edited by William I. Cohen, Lynn Nadel, and Myra E. Madnick.
ISBN 0-471-41815-3   Copyright © 2002 by Wiley-Liss, Inc.

## THE SIBLING RELATIONSHIP

One of my favorite children's poems provides a sweet and childlike view of the birth of a sibling. The poem reflects on the fact that the firstborn child is the star of the family. So if he is the center of their universe, why do his parents need to have another baby? Children have difficulty comprehending their parents' ability to boundlessly love each of their children differently but equally. It is hard for them to share the attention of parents under the best of circumstances.

Every sibling relationship in every family involves the experience of many conflicting emotions. Even those who maintain that their relationship with a brother or sister was without conflict certainly had, on at least a couple of occasions, felt a negative feeling or two. I like to ask parents who have concerns about their children's relationships to think back on their own sibling relationships when they were growing up. Ninety percent of the time, I find that parents will list a few negative emotions remembered from the past before they think of listing something like love! All sibling relationships contain a measure of jealousy, anger, fear, worry, embarrassment, and even hatred on the worst of days, along with love, admiration, respect, and friendship. The hope, of course, is that siblings will come into adulthood with a mainly positive view of their brothers and sisters. Most of the time, this is exactly what happens. However, many adults continue to work on issues with siblings in their adult lives, including, for some, the feeling that "Mom always loved her best!"

The point here is that, even in the most sensitive and caring family setting, sibling relationships are a challenge and a struggle. They provide the opportunity for wonderful shared memories as well as experience with some of our darker emotions. Through relationships with brothers and sisters, we learn about important things like sharing, empathy, worry, and love. It is helpful for parents of children with special needs to remember that life with a sibling is never just "a bed of roses." Challenges, fights, and struggles are the norm even in the best setting.

## WHEN A SIBLING HAS A DISABILITY

Given that sibling relationships are, by definition, intense and complex, adding a disability like Down syndrome to the mix serves to make things even more interesting! When any new baby is brought home from the hospital, there is a shift in the parents' attention from other siblings to giving the needs of the baby high priority much of the time. When the baby has Down syndrome, that shift can be even more extreme as parents struggle with their own emotions and focus on this thing called Down syndrome. As children with Down syndrome grow, parents' protectiveness and increased attention to their medical, school, and social needs may continue. Although siblings may understand the parents' concerns, they are certainly aware that the family spotlight can rest on the child with Down syndrome a disproportionate amount of the time. Children with developmental disabilities might require more help with homework, and brothers and sisters who are quite capable of doing their own work independently can perceive this as unfair. The attention of parents, after all, is the hardest thing for children to share.

In many families, the birth order of siblings actually appears to shift when there is a child with a disability. If the child with Down syndrome is older, there is a distinct point in time when it becomes apparent that the younger child is actually more capable than the older sibling. This can be frustrating for the child with Down syndrome as well as for the sibling. When Ann, who has Down syndrome, and her sister Mary, who was two years younger, were preteens and teenagers, there would be a great deal of discussion about who was in charge when their parents weren't home. Ann was frustrated that her younger sister wouldn't listen to her, and Mary was frustrated that Ann wouldn't follow her rules! Each child felt that she was the "older" one. An 8-year-old boy shared the following story with me about his sister Cathy, aged 6, and his 2-year-old brother Timmy. Cathy loved to play school and would try to teach Timmy to say certain words. The only problem was Timmy could say the words perfectly and his "teacher" couldn't. Children notice these differences in abilities and feel the subtle shift in responsibilities in the family.

As part of that responsibility, siblings are aware of the limitations of their siblings in certain situations. They come to appreciate what a big accomplishment it is when the child with Down syndrome learns to walk, struggles to talk, or achieves a medal at a Special Olympics event. Siblings are often proud of these accomplishments. Many even volunteer to help with Special Olympics or their brother's or sister's extracurricular activities. On the other hand, they may feel jealous of the extra attention given for small successes or the way rules are changed to suit the needs of the child with Down syndrome. I have heard things like this from frustrated siblings: "She gets to eat dinner in front of the television and we can't" or "He doesn't have to make his bed and I do." They feel angry and jealous and then guilty for feeling this way about their sibling with a disability who can't help his or her limitations. What a complex mix of feelings! In more typical family settings, brothers and sisters work out some of their jealousy or frustration through aggression. They might pick a fight with their brother or sister, throw something, or hit. When the sibling has Down syndrome, some of these very natural instincts might be inhibited because it would make the child feel guilty to act out against a sibling with limitations.

Brothers and sisters of children with Down syndrome have more to worry about, too. They worry when siblings are hospitalized or need surgery. They worry about safety issues around the house. And as they get older, they worry about the child's future ability to live alone, get married, and have a happy life. Siblings are also concerned about whether the child will be teased in community settings. In the middle school years, concern about being embarrassed by a brother or sister with a disability comes into play. Children who have been the most loving and caring individuals in earlier years suddenly may not like to have their sibling hug or kiss them in front of peers or even spend as much time with him. Because "fitting in" becomes the prime motivation of the middle school years, anything or anyone who makes the student feel different can be reason enough to be embarrassed. With maturation, and sensitivity and support from parents, this difficult time can pass and comfortable relationships can be revived.

Many siblings have shared with me that having a sibling with Down syndrome has taught them many things. In general, they feel they are more sensitive and caring human beings than many of their peers at all ages. They frequently indicate that they are more responsible, patient, and tolerant of differences as well. A rather large percentage of siblings of children with Down syndrome and other disabilities find careers in the helping professions such as occupational, speech, and physical therapy, teaching, law, and medicine. One college student pointed out to me that he was pursuing a business career that had nothing to do with his brother's Down syndrome, but he was very involved with campus social service organizations. Although his career path may not have been influenced by his sibling's disability, his overall values and choice of "causes" certainly had been.

Increased empathy, patience, and sensitivity are among the gifts that growing up with a sibling with Down syndrome can provide. Dealing with all those conflicting emotions, including jealousy, embarrassment, and anger, are the challenges. What can parents do to help ensure that the gifts outweigh the challenges?

## THE ROLE OF PARENTS IN HELPING SIBLINGS GROW INTO HEALTHY ADULTS

Parents play a very important part in determining whether their other children grow up with healthy attitudes toward their sibling with Down syndrome and good feelings about their childhood. It is in the job description of the parent to attend to the emotional needs of each child in the family. This can feel like a complicated and daunting task for mothers and fathers with so many things to do in the course of life and the complication of dealing with their own emotions about their child's disability. Keeping in mind a few strategies can help parents and children live mostly happily ever after.

One of the most important things parents can do is provide their other children with information related to the disability and their sibling as often as it is necessary. Discussing the diagnosis of Down syndrome as early as possible is the first way to ensure that information is clearly conveyed. Many parents are reluctant to use the term Down syndrome early with their other children out of fear of their reaction. However, siblings seldom have any idea what the term Down syndrome actually means and have no emotional response to it. They do see parents crying and acting upset and whispering with other adults, so they are aware, without the parent saying anything, that there is something amiss. Explaining Down syndrome in simple terms to young children serves to clear up some of the mystery and the fear. Simply saying something like this is helpful: "The new baby has something called Down syndrome, which means that she will learn more slowly than other children and will need some extra help." Children's books like *We'll Paint the Octopus Red* by Stephanie Stuve-Bodeen is another way to help share the news. Children usually embrace the information matter-of-factly and without the concerns that adults exhibit. Parents can further explain that they feel sad about the news but that the family will love the baby and do everything possible to help her learn and grow.

However, the need for information about the disability continues beyond the initial facts shared after the child's birth. Sam was 10 when his sister Sara was born. In addition to having Down syndrome, she also had a serious heart problem that required surgery. His parents were aware that Sam was very worried. They arranged for him to meet the cardiologist, who explained the procedure to Sam with simple drawings. Sam then shared the information with his friends. He felt more comfortable receiving the facts first-hand from a very sensitive doctor. Sam continued to be very involved in many aspects of his sister's life. He liked to listen to what was going on with his sister and to share his point of view with his parents regarding her educational placements and recreational outlets as well. For children with disabilities aged birth to three, early intervention services are frequently provided in the home. As a result, young siblings have the opportunity right from the start to participate actively in the education of their brother or sister. One young woman, who has a sister with Down syndrome two years her junior, fondly recalls how much she enjoyed the therapists' visits to her home. Playing with all the new toys and being actively included in the sessions with her sister in a positive, helpful way lessened the potential for any sibling rivalry. With a sensitive approach, therapists and parents can help make home-based therapy an opportunity for learning and inclusion for all family members.

As children with Down syndrome reach the teen years, parents often begin to formulate a plan for their child's future. That plan might include the hope that their child could live alone in a supervised setting or in a group home. Ideas for future employment might also be part of their vision for the future. Older siblings need to know this information, too. Knowing that their parents have a plan reduces their worry and keeps the lines of communication open. Siblings can then help ensure that their parents' vision becomes a reality in the not-so-distant future.

Helping siblings express their feelings and concerns is another important way parents can help all of their children grow into healthy adults. As mentioned above, all sibling relationships include their share of negative feelings like embarrassment, anger, frustration, and occasional moments of hatred. Acknowledging that those feelings are normal and allowable is critical. If a child says he hates his sibling, parents are often quick to say something like "Of course you don't hate your sister. You love her." A child who is experiencing that extreme emotion now is forced to keep the hatred inside along with new feelings of guilt as a result of the parent's comments. If the parent instead acknowledged the intense feelings, a discussion of the troubling event might take place. A more helpful response might be to say something like this: "I hear that you are *very* angry at your brother for ruining your video game. I know you wish you could always play the game without your brother getting in the way." In this scenario, the child's feelings are respected and heard. Instead of bottling up negative feelings, they are allowed to be let out and set free. One 8-year-old boy named Jake had exactly this problem with his 5-year-old brother Jon, who has Down syndrome. Jake's mother made it a habit of acknowledging his feelings about his very important video games. Together, they developed a couple of solutions that were useful at least some of the time. They would let Jon play with a broken controller so he would think he was playing with his brother. At other times, Mom would keep Jon occupied so Jake could play video games with a friend. Although Jake still wishes he were an only child on certain days, he is very good about sharing the game with Jon on other days! Acknowledgement of extreme feelings, then, can often lead to good communication and creative solutions.

Parents should also be aware that there are certain sensitive times for siblings, particularly around events involving peers. When Lisa was in middle school, she expressed to her mother that she was uncomfortable with her sister coming into the school building to pick her up at the end of the school day. Rather than being hurt and making her daughter feel badly, this very astute mother realized that Lisa's need to fit in with her peers at that time in her life needed to be respected. She arranged to wait out in the car for Lisa instead. A few years later when the girls were in the same high school, it was no problem when the girls encountered each other in the hallway. They would even give each other a quick hug! The issues of embarrassment that were of great concern in the middle school years became less of an issue with maturity. Being able to share her needs with her mother helped Lisa cope at a very sensitive time and probably helped her to move through that stage more quickly.

Today, children with Down syndrome are often included in community activities along with their nondisabled siblings. From an early age, siblings' friends literally "grow up" with the child with Down syndrome as well. When friends are comfortable with their sibling, brothers and sisters can be more relaxed and less worried about the reactions of others. Parents can help by making their home a welcome place for friends to gather. Being that house on the block where children can feel comfortable helps both the child with Down syndrome and his or her brothers and sisters feel supported and included.

There is a great tendency for parents and other family members to highly value the accomplishments, both large and small, of the child with Down syndrome. It is critical for parents to value the things that their children without disabilities master as well. Praising each child for his or her uniqueness and abilities goes a long way toward keeping children happy. Shifting the spotlight from child to child makes everyone shine. In her book, *Special Siblings: Growing Up with Someone with a Disability,* Mary McHugh talks about growing up with a brother with mental retardation in a time when disabilities were not spoken about and children with special needs were not extensively included in the community. Mary remembers how hard she tried to please her mother when she was a child. As an accomplished writer in adulthood, she brought her published books to show her parents. They simply said, "That's nice, dear," and never read them. In contrast, her mother would speak glowingly of her brother's bowling games and other small accomplishments. Even as an adult, Mary felt extreme hurt and even anger. We all need to feel valued and loved by those who love us. Taking the time to do exactly that saves a great deal of struggle and conflict for the other children in the future.

It is important, too, for parents to expect some level of responsibility from each child in the family. Every child should be expected to do chores on the level he or she is capable of handling. All children, even children with Down syndrome, can take turns setting and clearing the table or making their beds (although not very neatly) from an early age. And although parents can expect brothers and sisters to help out with the child who has Down syndrome, expecting too much responsibility can be trying. One teen named Patricia told me that she was expected to come directly home after high school each day so she could get her younger brother Mike off the school bus and watch after him. In general she didn't mind this, but occasionally, she would have liked to stay after school for a sporting event. She wished her mother had a back-up plan in place to make this possible. Patricia also told me that she didn't mind babysitting when her parents went out on a Saturday night, but if she were missing another babysitting job as a result, she wanted to be paid her for her trouble. This was fair, Patricia felt, because everyone benefited from the situation, including Mike, who loved the extra attention from his sister.

Just as in the above example, it is often quite valuable for parents to listen to the perspective of their other children. Siblings will happily offer their ideas about age-appropriate clothing for their sibling with Down syndrome as well as ideas for after-school activities. Brothers and sisters also have a unique perspective on the behavior of their sibling. They often know, for example, when the parents are underestimating the capabilities of the child with Down syndrome. Billy, age 8, and his sister Molly, age 10, explained that their 16-year-old sister Martha with Down syndrome had a clever way of getting out of chores. On nights when it was her turn to clear the table and load the dishwasher, Martha would eat her dinner very slowly. When she was still sitting at the table, long after dinner was over, their parents would tell Molly or Billy to do Martha's job. Molly and Billy knew exactly what was going on, but their parents were clueless! How valuable it would have been for there to be a family discussion around the subject of chores.

Each child in the family needs the opportunity to do something special with one or both of their parents and no other sibling in sight. One-on-one time with one child at a time is truly priceless. It is often a time when serious discussions take place and memorable moments are created. The one-on-one opportunity doesn't need to be an elaborate full-day experience. Just driving to the store together to get milk or taking a quick walk after dinner can be a boost for any relationship at any age.

Not only do siblings need time alone with a parent, they also need time to themselves and time to be with friends without their sibling always being around. Brothers and sisters require even a small "sacred space" where they can keep things that belong just to them and that they do not have to share with anyone else. Respecting privacy and possessions is part of learning to share. In the story of Jake and the video games, Jake's mother allowed him to play video games with a friend without his brother around. This was a gift for Jake, one he'll always remember. Jake has also learned that playing video games at his friend's house works out well, too, until his friend's younger brother without Down syndrome gets in the way!

Parents who have a good understanding of Down syndrome, have a good support system for themselves, and are coping well with their child's disability tend to have children who cope effectively as well. Children mirror their parents' emotions and concerns. They know when things are not right. The greatest gift, then, that parents can give to all their children is to take care of their own emotional needs. Local support groups, one-to-one peer support, and national organizations like the National Down Syndrome Society are excellent sources. Local libraries and bookstores are filled with a growing selection of books for parents about coping with a child with special needs at all ages. Taking advantage of existing resources is an important step all parents should take.

Beyond supports for parents, there are many supports available for brothers and sisters as well. The most widely available is found in local libraries and bookstores. There are many wonderful books written specifically for children with siblings who have Down syndrome or other disabilities. These books address the full range of feelings siblings feel. Books like *We'll Paint the Octopus Red* address the worry and confusion of very young children, and stories like *My Sister Annie* by B. Dodds focus on the embarrassment and frustration siblings can feel when they are in the vulnerable middle school years. Reading about the feelings and experiences of other children goes a long way toward helping the child feel more comfortable with his or her different experience growing up with a sibling with a disability. Other books look at disabilities on a factual level, providing an understanding of chromosomes, diagnoses, Special Olympics, and group homes. They can provide valuable reference material at critical times. Many siblings eventually do science projects or term papers on the subject of a particular disability. This educates not only themselves but classmates as well.

Although not as widely available as books, sibling groups, where they exist, are a wonderful way to help brothers and sisters cope with their specialized sibling relationship. Having coordinated sibling groups for a variety of age groups over the years, I have witnessed the almost immediate benefit of such an experience time and again. When children meet other children who have a brother or sister with a disability they realize that they are not alone. Other students have the same feelings and concerns. I recently witnessed the surprise and relief 10-year-old Melissa expressed when another student shared that he pretends he's not with his sister and his mother when his sister acts up in a store. Melissa laughed and said, "You mean you do that too?" Any guilt she ever had about that behavior melted away in an instant. It was a beautiful thing to witness. Although regular access to a sibling group would be very valuable, even one session can provide a never-to-be-forgotten opportunity. In the course of sibling groups, brothers and sisters can ask questions they may not be comfortable asking their parent. One 7-year-old boy told me he worried that he might catch his sister's disability. The relief he expressed when he found out that this was not possible was visible. It served as a reinforcing lesson for every child present.

In areas where sibling groups do not exist, simply getting together as a family with another family who has a child with Down syndrome can provide a mini-sibling group experience. Meeting even one other child with a sibling with a disability can be a help. Sibling newsletters like *For Siblings Only* and *Sibling Forum* or pen pal opportunities provide another valuable option. Through these vehicles, children have the opportunity to share their thoughts and feelings with other students on paper. Reading about the real-life experiences of others and writing back to see their name and ideas in print is gratifying for children of all ages.

Although the challenges are numerous and unavoidable, the rewards are priceless. With love, support, and sensitivity to detail, parents can help ensure that their other children thrive with the added benefit of a child with

Down syndrome in their lives. Each challenge becomes an opportunity to learn and to grow. Mary, Sam, Jake, Lisa, and so many others are living proof.

## REFERENCES

### RESOURCES FOR PARENTS

Klein, S.D., and Schleifer, M.J., ed., It Isn't Fair! Siblings of Children with Disabilities, Bergin and Garvey, Westport, CT, 1993.

McHugh, M, Special Siblings: Growing Up with Someone with a Disability, Hyperion, New York, 1999.

Naseef, R.A., Special Children, Challenged Parents: The Struggles and Rewards of Raising a Child with a Disability, Carol Publishing Group, Secaucus, NJ, 1997.

Powell, T.H., and Ogle, P.A., Brothers and Sisters: A Special Part of Exceptional Families, Paul H. Brookes Publishing Co., Baltimore, 1985.

### RESOURCES FOR CHILDREN

Dodds, B., My Sister Annie, Honesdale, PA, Boyds Mills Press, 1993.

Levine, S., ed., For Siblings Only, published by Family Resource Associates, 35 Haddon Ave, Shrewsbury, NJ. A newsletter for children aged 4–10 with siblings with developmental disabilities.

Levine, S., ed., Sibling Forum, published by Family Resource Associates, 35 Haddon Ave., Shrewsbury, NJ 07702. A newsletter for children aged 10 through teens with siblings with developmental disabilities.

Meyer, D., Vadasy, P., and Fewell, R., Living with a Brother or Sister with Special Needs: A Book for Sibs, University of Washington Press, Seattle, WA, 1985.

Meyer, D., ed., Views from Our Shoes, Woodbine House, Bethesda, MD, 1997.

Rabe, B., Where's Chimpy? Albert Whitman, Morton Grove, IL, 1988.

Stuve-Bodeen, S., We'll Paint the Octopus Red, Woodbine House, Bethesda, MD, 1998.

# THE SPECIAL NEEDS PROGRAM: ESTATE PLANNING FOR FAMILIES WITH CHILDREN WITH DISABILITIES

## DAVID A. WEINGARTEN

## ESTATE PLANNING FOR FAMILIES WITH CHILDREN WITH DISABILITIES

When caring for a child with a disability, parents and family members are concerned with the child's emotional well being, financial needs, and financial security. These are not short-term issues. As persons with disabilities live longer and fuller lives, changes in family and personal circumstances are inevitable. With such changes come many questions.

- Is there a plan in place that will ensure that the child with a disability will lead a full and complete life after the death or disability of the primary caregivers?
- Who will become the primary caregiver for the child with the disability?
- Is the new primary caregiver prepared to provide the child with basic support that may run the gamut from providing living arrangements to actual physical care?

*Down Syndrome*, Edited by William I. Cohen, Lynn Nadel, and Myra E. Madnick.
ISBN 0-471-41815-3   Copyright © 2002 by Wiley-Liss, Inc.

- Is the new primary caregiver able to provide emotional support as well as any financial assistance that may be needed?
- Have government programs or charitable organizations been considered as sources of assistance?

This information is intended to be an introduction to some of the questions, issues, and possible estate planning solutions for parents with children with disabilities. The questions above are some indication of what must be considered in the planning process.

## Who Is Affected?

Although the focus of this chapter is estate planning for families with children with disabilities, physical and mental disabilities can strike at any age. The goals for families of any person disabled at any stage in life are similar in nature: to create a more certain future for the individual with a disability as well as the entire family. The specific opportunities available will vary according to the type of disability and the family's emotional and financial situation.

## Estate Planning?

Although the term "estate planning" may bring to mind families with great wealth, that is not what is meant in this context. Parents must plan their estates, regardless of size, to secure continued care and well-being of their child. Estate planning simply means organizing an estate, whatever its size, to meet the needs of the entire family as efficiently and economically as possible. Although there are many alternatives and decisions, there is no single magic formula for creating the appropriate estate plan. Every estate plan should be custom-fit to the family's circumstances.

## Identifying the Source of Assistance

### The Family

Most often, the parents of a child with a disability are his or her primary caregivers. Depending on the child's needs, the parents *directly* provide as much of the physical, emotional, and financial assistance as they are capable of giving. Other family members, particularly siblings, may also be involved in the child's care. If one or both parents die or become disabled, other family members will often assume primary care.

## THE STATE AND FEDERAL GOVERNMENTS

The government, through a variety of programs, may provide assistance to the family. The assistance may take such forms as educational programs, care institutions, medical facilities, and financial assistance. Both federal and state governments provide these programs, which are often means based.

State-based programs, even those federally underwritten but state managed, may differ significantly from one state to another. The benefits provided, the means test, and other issues will depend on state rules. Three of the most well-known government programs are:

1. *Social Security* is a benefit program provided by the federal government. The child's assets or income does not generally affect this program. Social Security will make payments directly to the child with a disability. The amount paid is based either on the parent's earnings record or on the earnings record of the child with a disability.

2. *Medicaid* is a state-run, federally underwritten program designed to pay for the medical expenses of, among others, disabled persons. This program is generally means based and designed to help those persons who need government assistance. The means test varies from state to state.

3. *Supplemental Security Income* (SSI) provides funds to those persons with disabilities who fall below a certain level of resources and income. If the child qualifies for payments, those payments may be reduced under certain situations. For example, the benefit may be reduced if funds are received by the child for his or her basic needs from other sources—it may even be reduced if the child receives free room and board.

All three of these programs may help with the care of an individual with a disability. Because the rules are complex, vary from state to state, and may change according to the whims of the state and federal government, it's important to contact the appropriate state or federal agency for up-to-date information on the programs. These are only three of the more familiar programs available; there are others, such as state programs that may provide living facilities, legal assistance, and/or special education.

## NONPROFIT ORGANIZATIONS

These organizations may also help the family. Counseling, aid, medical assistance, home care assistance, and other such services may be provided by a nonprofit organization.

The coordination of these three sources of assistance is very important. If these streams of assistance flow together in an organized fashion, the person with the disability—as well as the entire family—will be better cared for and more secure. In addition, the estate plan should focus on two further issues: 1) who should care for the child's physical and emotional needs and 2) how to ensure the financial security of the child.

## ORGANIZING THE ESTATE PLAN TO ENSURE THE CONTINUED CARE OF THE CHILD

### SELECTING A NEW PRIMARY CAREGIVER

No one is in a better position to understand the day-to-day obligations a primary caregiver faces than the parents of a child with a disability. One of the first items parents should consider is who will assume their role when they are gone. The parents must consider what their everyday role is and weigh who or what organization can fulfill the physical and emotional needs of the child.

This may be a difficult question to answer; if there are adult brothers or sisters, the parent must carefully judge whether any one or all of the siblings will be able to take charge of the day-to-day needs of the child with a disability. Although they might not attend to the daily physical requirements of the child, the remaining family will still be concerned with the emotional well-being and financial needs of the child with a disability.

An important aspect to consider is whether the care responsibilities should be made formal or informal. If the responsibility is to be formalized, guardians will have to be named. The guardian may be nominated through a will and formally appointed through a court proceeding. Keep in mind that, legally, there are separate guardians of the person and that person's property. The guardian of the person is that individual charged with the responsibility for the personal care of the child. The guardian of the property is that person charged with managing the child's finances. The same person can act as a guardian of both the person and property. If the child with the disability does not have the legal capacity to act on his or her own, then the parents should have guardians appointed.

### PLANNING FOR FINANCIAL SECURITY

A pivotal issue is ensuring that the person with the disability's financial requirements are met. When both parents are gone, the question of paying for the child's care will confront the remaining family members. The financial issues may arise as soon as the first parent dies.

The parents must decide how much, if any, direct financial support should be left to the child with the disability. In addition, there may be other family members whom the parents want to include in the estate distribution.

There are a number of estate plans that can be used; the selection will depend on many issues, including the actual financial condition of the family, the character of the disability, the level of care needed, and the reliance on government and charitable assistance. Let's review the three estate plans most often used in these situations.

ESTATE PLAN #1: LEAVE ALL THE ASSETS TO THE PERSON WITH THE DISABILITY.   The parents may leave all of their property to the child with the disability, either outright or in trust. If the funds are left outright to the child, all control over the funds falls to the child. If the funds are left in trust, the trustee will be *required* to expend the trust assets for the child's care. The trustee is not given the discretion over this matter; he or she must distribute income or principal for the child's care.

*Benefits of Estate Plan #1*
- Theoretically, depending on the size of the estate, the child may be able to lead an independent financial existence.

*Negative Aspects of Estate Plan #1*
- What is the child's legal capacity? The disability may leave the child without the capacity to manage funds or even to take legal title. Placing the funds in trust will resolve this problem. If no trust is used and the child does not have legal capacity, a guardian must be appointed.
- Providing the child with a disability with direct control of the assets could endanger his or her ability to access two of the main sources of care: government and charitable programs. Because government assistance is often means based, making the child the outright beneficiary of the estate may be unwise. In addition, placing the assets in a trust that is directed to provide ordinary care to the child will not solve this problem. The government and many charities will view the trust as an asset for the purpose of means testing.
- The assets themselves could be subject to attachment to reimburse government agencies for expenses they have incurred on the child's behalf.
- Providing all the assets to the child with a disability disinherits the other children. If the siblings are charged with the care of the child, this could lead to family discord. In addition, if the other siblings are minors, the parents must also consider their care in addition to the care of the child with the disability.
- If funds are left to a legally incompetent child, a guardian will control those funds. Guardianships are very restrictive forms of ownership,

and the guardian may be limited by state investment and distribution laws.

ESTATE PLAN #2: DISINHERIT THE CHILD WITH A DISABILITY AND RELY ON FAMILY AND GOVERNMENTAL PROGRAMS FOR ALL NEEDS. This is the complete opposite of the first plan—here, nothing is left to the child with the disability, either outright or in trust. The theory behind this plan is that the remaining family will contribute to the care of the child with the disability.

*Benefits of Estate Plan #2*

- Generally, the child should qualify for government programs, allowing the family to take advantage of resources, funds, or programs that might otherwise be lost if the child had his or her own assets. The remaining family might then supplement the child's financial needs from their own funds or from the assets received from the parents. This plan is often viewed as the only effective tool for many families. Caution must be exercised, because the government may, under some circumstances, count family gifts in means testing.

*Negative Aspects of Estate Plan #2*

- The child will depend on other family members for *all financial support* not provided by the government or charities. Given that this is an informal arrangement, there is no way to be sure that funds will be used to benefit the child with a disability. There is no way to be certain that the funds will even be there when the child with a disability needs them. Divorce, other family obligations, death, inheritance laws, bankruptcy, judgments, and other unforeseen situations can quickly deplete assets.
- If the child is left impoverished, it is more than likely that he or she will qualify for government and charitable programs. However, relying on those programs for the total financial and physical care of the child, without any backup position, is a perilous tactic to take. There's no way to be confident that government or private programs will be available to provide adequate assistance to the child.
- Will the child with the disability be able to live as the parents wish? In an era of reduced federal and state funding, what happens if the programs are eliminated or significantly reduced?

ESTATE PLAN #3: THE SPECIAL NEEDS PROGRAM.

*USING GOVERNMENT PROGRAMS AND A SPECIAL NEEDS TRUST.* Using a special needs trust in an estate plan can help accomplish a number of goals and may be the best solution to the long-term needs of the entire family.

A carefully structured trust may provide the child with the disability with security while allowing the child to qualify for government benefits. This plan provides the family with maximum flexibility, which allows the new primary caregivers to take those actions necessary for the child with a disability's social, emotional, physical, and financial needs.

*How Does This Plan Work?* Let's review the estate planner's goals: to ensure the support of the child with a disability by using governmental and charitable sources to the greatest extent possible, but also to provide a separate source of funds to assist the child when and as needed. To use governmental programs, the child with a disability must not have any significant income or resources. So, as in Estate Plan #2 above, the parents will not give the child with a disability or the child's guardian any direct control over estate assets.

The parents will generally want the child with the disability to receive a level of care that might be superior to that which can be obtained through government programs alone. In Estate Plan #2, the child must rely on other family members for such treatment. In the special needs program, a special needs trust will be created by the parents and the trustee will be instructed (via the trust instrument) to provide for the child with the disability's supplemental needs.

Remember that a trust is simply a device for holding, managing, and distributing property. It's a traditional means of managing property for beneficiaries who are unable to do so for themselves. The trust described in Estate Plan #1 above is different from the *special needs* trust. In Estate Plan #1, the trustee is to provide the child with the disability with funds for *primary care*. This type of trust is considered by government agencies to be the child's asset and could disqualify the child under a means test.

The use of special needs trust should help circumvent this problem. The special needs trust is designed to prevent inclusion of trust assets or payments from the trust in the government means test.

What is different in the special needs trust? Special needs language and discretionary distribution language is placed in the trust. The trustee is given *absolute and sole uncontestable discretion* as to whether the trust assets will be used for the care of the child with a disability and when the assets are used. The trustee is *not* required to expend any funds. The trustee is even authorized to accumulate income if distributions are not currently needed. In addition to the discretionary power, the trustee is given instructions as to which expenditures the caregivers feel are most appropriate.

It is anticipated that primary care will be provided through government and charitable programs. Therefore, the special needs trust is intended to serve as a "supplement" to public assistance. The trust is designed to ensure that the person with the disability receives those "extras," such as additional clothing, travel opportunities, and medical choices, that might not be provided through public programs. Where a government program might provide only enough funds for the child to receive one type of rehabilitative therapy, the funds in a special needs trust can be used to defray the cost of a more advanced facility. Where a government program might provide one level of medical care, the funds in a special needs trust can be used to defray the cost of more aggressive or simply different treatment. These are just two examples; the possibilities are endless.

*STATE LAW CONTROLS.* The effectiveness of a special needs trust will depend on state law. Therefore, it is vital that local counsel, experienced in this area of the law, be an integral part of this entire process. This plan is most appropriate in those states that allow these trusts protection from the claims of the federal and state governments. In many instances, asset protection and government benefits can be protected during the lifetime of the child with the disability. In some instances, however, states may require a "payback" provision in the trust. Payback language provides that the trustee "pay back" the government for benefits received before any distributions to other beneficiaries of the trust.

*FUNDING A SPECIAL NEEDS TRUST.* In designing the estate plan, keep in mind that this trust becomes the "family bank," available for the benefit of the continued care of the child with a disability. The need is triggered most often at the death of both parents—although finances can become an issue on one spouse's demise.

The issue then becomes how to ensure that there will be a reliable source of funds delivered at the death of the parents for use in the trust. The parents may also wish to provide funds for the rest of the family. Three questions become relevant to this phase of the plan:

1. How much is needed in the trust to ensure the continued financial support of the child with the disability?
2. How can these funds be made available and delivered to the trust at the death of the parents?
3. How can funds be provided to other family members?

The first issue is how much money is needed in the trust. There is no hard and fast rule here; there are, however, some ways of gauging the child's possible financial needs. First, consider that these funds must last the child's lifetime. This is, of course, totally unpredictable. However, some average life expectancy numbers should be available. Most planners take that number and add a safety factor. It's best to plan for the child to survive longer than the expected so that sufficient funds will be placed in the trust.

If you use the current cost of care in your calculation, examine whether the level of care will increase on the demise of the primary caregivers and factor in increases in the cost of living and how many years the child will survive. You should then arrive at an estimate of the size of the fund needed. This number is likely to change over the years and should be reviewed annually.

Life insurance is often used as a solution to these problems. If insurance is placed on the primary caregiver's life, the receipt of proceeds on his or her death will allow the trust to be funded at precisely the moment that the financial need arises. Life insurance also permits the creation of an estate plan that allows bequests to the family members without disabilities while guaranteeing the financial security of the disabled. In addition, the death benefits paid to the trust should be received income- and estate tax free.

Life insurance products of all kinds are available and should be tailored to the particular needs of the family. The types of policies to review include ordinary single life coverage, second-to-die protection, and even first-to-die coverage. As with the entire design of the special needs program, including your life insurance professional along with your other advisors in the process will be most advantageous.

LEGAL AND TECHNICAL ASPECTS OF THE SPECIAL NEEDS TRUST. When drafting a special needs trust, counsel should review the following technical issues:

1. *State Law Restrictions.* Do state statutes specifically exempt discretionary trusts, such as the special needs trust, from the means test to qualify for Medicaid, SSI, and other governmental programs? If there is no specific statute, have the regulatory authorities expressed an opinion?

2. *Termination of the Trust.* Consideration should be given to allowing the trustee to terminate the trust if it is challenged by a government agency or if there is a substantial change in state or federal law; an alternate beneficiary can be named to receive the trust property in the event of termination. This same alternate beneficiary is often named to receive the trust property after the death of the individual with the disability.

3. *Spendthrift Provisions.* To provide further insulation from reimbursement claims by public agencies, a special needs trust is usually designed with spendthrift language that, subject to the provisions of state law, expressly prohibits the use of the beneficiary's interest to satisfy the claims of ordinary creditors. *Some states do not recognize spendthrift clauses.* If state law is not entirely clear on the effectiveness of this language, additional instructions to the trustee setting forth the purposes of the trust and stating that its assets may not be used to provide basic (rather than supplemental) needs should be included.

On termination, amounts left in the trust may be subject to state Medic-aid reimbursement laws. Federal and state regulations are constantly chang-ing and may be interpreted differently by state courts. Some states require payback provisions in special needs. Payback language provides that bene-fits received by the person with the disability be reimbursed to the state before any distributions are made to alternate beneficiaries.

SELECTION AND RESPONSIBILITIES OF A TRUSTEE.    The selection of the appropriate trustee is vital, as he or she will make many judgments about the care of the person with the disability. The trustee will also have financial management responsibility. Sometimes more than one trustee is selected; one trustee will manage the trust assets, and the other will serve as advocate for the beneficiary.

The individual trustee, in particular, should be acquainted with the skills and needs of the beneficiary with the disability. If the person with the dis-ability is in a group home, for example, the trustee should make several visits every year to the facility to determine the appropriateness of the care being provided and any progress being made. The trust instrument itself should require the trustee to make at least an annual evaluation of the beneficiary's physical and emotional condition, educational programs, work opportuni-ties, and social needs. If the trust distribution language is drafted broadly enough, the trustee will be able to take advantage of new programs. The key to any plan is to make sure the right person is selected as trustee of your child's trust.

## SUMMARY

The estate planning process can be long and can often be heart wrenching. No matter what the family circumstances, an intelligent estate plan should provide the survivors with maximum flexibility, the appropriate level of management intervention that is necessary, and the greatest possible probate avoidance and tax advantages. In addition, the estate plan should be de-signed to ensure that the testator's wishes will be carried out to provide for his or her family's continued well-being.

Fundamentally, a program should be implemented that will provide the level of care that the child with the disability needs. As family's needs and issues change in the future, the program should be evaluated. A special needs trust may help to accomplish many of the family's financial goals. When the special needs trust is integrated into an overall plan, the parents may rest assured that all of their children will be well cared for and finan-cially secure in their future.

## NOTE

Individuals other than professional advisors should consider the material in this chapter educational in nature, not as tax or legal advice. As always, this information is designed to be of general nature. It is given with the understanding that if legal, accounting, or other professional advice is required, the service of a competent professional should be sought.

## ACKNOWLEDGMENT

The Guardian Life Insurance Company of America, New York, NY.

# HEALTH AND CLINICAL CARE

# Pediatric Health Update on Down Syndrome

## Len Leshin, M.D., FAAP

### Introduction

One of the hallmarks of Down syndrome (DS) is the variability in the way that the condition affects people with DS. With the third 21st chromosome existing in every cell, it is not surprising to find that every system in the body is affected in some way. However, not every child with DS has the same problems or associated conditions. Parents of children with DS should be aware of these possible conditions so they can be diagnosed and treated quickly and appropriately.

With all the different associated conditions and diseases seen with DS, full textbooks can be written—and have been—on this topic. The goal of this chapter is to point out the most common problems of which parents should be aware, with emphasis on newer research, in the different body systems.

### Neurology

A large effect of DS on the individual child is mental retardation, although the severity of the mental retardation varies greatly from child to child. At this time, the exact anatomic cause in the brain is still unknown, although researchers have listed such possibilities as errors during brain development

*Down Syndrome*, Edited by William I. Cohen, Lynn Nadel, and Myra E. Madnick.
ISBN 0-471-41815-3   Copyright © 2002 by Wiley-Liss, Inc.

in the fetus, atrophy of brain cells in the frontal area of the brain, and dysfunction of the individual brain cells. Recent research has focused on the *DYRK* gene, located on the 21st chromosome. This gene is very active in the fetal brain, and disruption of this gene in trisomy mice has been found to cause learning difficulties.

Hypotonia is another feature common to almost all children with DS. Hypotonia is defined as low tone of the muscle in its resting state and should not be confused with muscle strength. The low muscle tone affects all muscles, including the smooth muscle of the intestinal tract. Hypotonia may be the cause not only of delayed gross motor development (such as crawling and walking) but also constipation and gastroesophageal reflux.

Seizures occur in 5–10% of people with DS. They tend to arise most often in the first 2 years of life and then in the third decade of life. In infants with DS, the most common type of seizure seen is the infantile spasm, but other types can also occur. In adults with DS, the most common type is the tonic-clonic seizure, which causes the extremities to jerk and then stiffen up. Children with DS who develop seizures are treated with the same anticonvolsent medications as children without DS, and they usually respond better to the medications.

One feature of DS is an apparent decreased tactility. Several studies have noted a decreased tendency of children and adults with DS to react to pain, and a recently published study noted a decreased ability of adults with DS to localize painful stimulation. This does not mean they are insensitive to pain but that they express their pain differently. This decreased tactility may also have an impact on fine motor control if people with DS have less internal feedback as to objects they are holding.

Moyamoya is a condition in which one or more blockages occur in the blood vessels in the brain. Although more common in people with DS, it is still an uncommon occurrence overall. It is mostly seen in children with DS in the first decade of life and adults with DS in their 30s. The cause is unknown. Moyamoya is essentially a stroke, with the same symptoms: decreased ability to move one arm and leg on the same side of the body, decrease in or loss of speech, and sometimes loss of vision. This is diagnosed by examining the brain blood vessels by X rays with dye, called angiograms.

Although autistic-like behaviors have long been noted in some children with DS, the actual diagnosis of autism in children with DS has been overlooked until recently. It is now estimated that 7–10% of children with DS may also fit the diagnosis of one of the autism spectrum disorders. These children have more problems with speech and learning and need to be identified so as to increase their ability to succeed in school settings.

Although the main concern of this article is with pediatric care, I want to mention Alzheimer disease because it has been closely connected with DS.

It has been known for decades that almost all adults with DS have findings in the brain that are associated with Alzheimer disease. Yet only 20–25% of all adults with DS show any of the dementia or cognitive decline that is the hallmark of Alzheimer disease. The cause of the decline in these adults still is not known. Studies are currently underway on drugs that may alleviate the cognitive decline in adults with DS.

## IMMUNOLOGY

Over the years, several defects in the immune system have been found in people with DS. Decreased immunoglobulins and decreased ability of T-cells to find and kill germs have been documented. These defects are not severe enough to cause recurrent infections requiring hospitalizations, but are enough that people with DS get frequent respiratory and skin infections. A decrease in serum zinc and selenium have been theorized to be a part of this suppressed immune function, and supplementing the diet with these minerals may improve the immune system of people with DS.

Allergies to foods or environmental causes do not appear to be more common in people with DS than in the general population.

People with DS are at greater risk for a group of diseases called autoimmune disease, in which the body makes antibodies against itself. Included in this group are hypothyroidism, celiac disease, and diabetes. The reason for this increased risk is not known.

## GASTROENTEROLOGY

One aspect of DS is the increased number of birth defects involving the gastrointestinal tract. Partial or total blocks in the part of the intestine just beyond the stomach, called the duodenum, are common and require surgery. These babies have frequent vomiting that becomes more forceful over time. Another common problem is a connection between the esophagus and trachea, called a fistula. There can be several different types of these fistulas, all requiring surgery. These babies often get formula or breast milk in their lungs and are frequently coughing; in severe conditions, the esophagus does not connect to the stomach at all and surgery is required immediately.

A very common condition in infants and children with DS is gastroesophageal reflux (GER). The cause is most likely the decreased muscle tone where the esophagus meets the stomach. This decreased tone allows stomach contents to move back up the esophagus, causing indigestion and spitting up or even vomiting. Medications are often used to control the reflux until such time as the child outgrows the condition.

Another problem seen in infants at birth is constipation. This is most likely also caused by decreased muscle tone. The intestine moves stool along the gastrointestinal tract more slowly, allowing more water from the stool to be reabsorbed by the colon. This can sometimes be overcome by introducing stool softeners in the diet of infants and roughage in the diets of children.

The biggest concern in the first weeks of life in children with DS who are chronically constipated is the possible presence of the condition called Hirschsprung disease. This condition, which is more common in infants with DS than in other infants, is due to the lack of nerve cells in the part of the colon just above the rectum. This lack of nerve cells impairs the intestine's ability to move stool to the rectum and stimulate a bowel movement, causing severe constipation. If not diagnosed in a timely manner, the chronic constipation could cause the lower colon to stretch to the point that it becomes useless in moving stool at all. When suspicions arise that an infant has Hirschsprung disease, a barium enema is performed to see how well the barium moves through the lower colon. If the X ray shows any abnormalities, then a surgeon will biopsy the rectum looking for nerve cells. If there are no nerve cells, the diagnosis of Hirschsprung disease is made and the part of the colon without nerve cells is surgically removed.

One topic that has been getting much attention recently is the increased risk of children and adults with DS to develop celiac disease. Celiac disease is a disease of the small intestine in which the lining has been injured by long-term exposure to gluten, a protein found in oats, barley, rye, and wheat. The injury is caused by an inappropriate immunologic reaction in the lining of the intestine. The injured lining can no longer absorb certain nutrients, causing a number of different symptoms. The ultimate cause of celiac disease is unknown, but there appears to be a genetic predisposition to the disease. Why children with DS are more susceptible to celiac disease is not clear, but it is often assumed to be part of the overall risk to autoimmune diseases. The signs are variable, but celiac disease may cause decrease in weight gain, decrease in height, bloated stomach, chronic diarrhea, vomiting, decreased appetite, and irritability. In a small percentage of cases, there may be few symptoms. The standard way to diagnose celiac disease is to obtain a biopsy of the small bowel. However, there are ways to screen for this disease by blood tests. The most sensitive test appears to look for anti-endomysium IgA antibodies. Because of the increased risk in children with DS and the lack of obvious symptoms in some children, the DS Medical Interest Group (DSMIG) recommends that every child with DS be tested with this screen between the ages of 2 and 3 years. The need for repeated screens is still being investigated.

There is no evidence of any other diseases of malabsorption that are more common in people with DS or any decrease in the ability to digest milk over that in the general population.

## CARDIOLOGY

It has been estimated that 40–60% of all infants with DS have some type of heart defect. The most common defects are those of the septa, or walls, of the chambers of the heart. There are atrial septal defects and ventricular septal defects. The most extreme version is the atrioventricular canal. These defects can vary from severe, requiring immediate surgery, to mild, requiring no surgery at all. Although most cases of heart defects can be found on physical examination of the newborn, some newborns with serious heart defects may show no signs at all for weeks after birth. Because of this lack of signs and symptoms, it is recommended that every newborn with DS be evaluated by a cardiologist soon after birth, including an echocardiogram examination.

Another concern regards young adults with DS. There is an increased risk for disease of the heart valves in these individuals, even those who had no heart defects at birth. These conditions include mitral valve prolapse and aortic regurgitation. It is recommended that all young adults with DS be evaluated for possible valvular conditions by approximately 18 years of age.

## ORTHOPEDICS

Most of the problems encountered in this area are due to the laxity of ligaments, causing bones to move in ways that they are not supposed to move.

The best-known problem in DS is atlantoaxial instability (AAI), which is caused by excess movement between the first and second vertebrae in the neck. This is estimated to occur in about 15% of youths with DS. The presence of AAI is a concern because of a potential risk of spinal cord damage if there is impingement on the spinal cord from one of the vertebrae. Most of the time AAI impingement is without symptoms; however, impingement on the spinal cord may cause any of the following symptoms: easy fatigability, difficulties in walking, abnormal gait, neck pain, limited neck mobility, head tilt, incoordination and clumsiness, sensory deficits, spasticity, and/or hyperreflexia. Children with DS who exhibit these symptoms, whether or not they have a previous diagnosis of AAI, need immediate evaluation. The treatment for this condition is surgical fusion of the two vertebrae.

However, there is still controversy in the medical community over the likelihood of a child with nonsymptomatic AAI becoming symptomatic. Until this is known, it is still recommended that all children with DS be screened for AAI. The best way to screen presently is by lateral X rays of the neck in the normal position, flexed, and extended. The first X ray should be done at the third birthday; X rays before this point may be misleading because of the lack of enough calcification of the vertebrae to get accurate measurements. X rays should be repeated at 10–12 years of age. Any children with AAI by X ray should have an MRI of the neck to determine whether there is any injury to the spinal cord from the vertebrae and whether surgical treatment is necessary. Children with documented AAI by X ray but normal MRI scans may be managed by restrictions on activities that may cause neck strain: diving, gymnastics, and contact sports, for example.

A variant of AAI is atlantooccipital instability (AOI), which involves the first vertebra and the skull. This is not as common as AAI, and recommendations for treatment with surgical fusion are even more vague. However, AOI should be considered in children with the same symptoms as in AAI.

Another problem involving the vertebrae is scoliosis, or curvature of the spine. This is also due to lax ligaments of the spine. Scoliosis may be corrected by braces if caught early enough, but severe cases require surgical correction.

Other orthopedic problems common to children and adults with DS include instability of the hip joints, instability of the patellae (knee caps), and flat feet. There is also a slight increase of joint pain.

## OTOLARYNGOLOGY

Many of the problems faced by children with DS are due to variations in the anatomy of the upper airway. Specifically, children with DS have smaller midfacial areas, including nasal and sinus passages, which may contribute to frequent upper respiratory infections. The decreased immune response to bacteria and viruses is also a factor in the increased number of upper respiratory infections.

Another common problem is obstruction of the upper airway by large adenoids and/or tonsils. This obstruction may be constant or intermittent and may lead to mouth breathing as well as sleep apnea. Obstructive sleep apnea (OSA) is the condition in which a child's airway is so blocked that the child does not get enough oxygen during sleep. Children with OSA will often snore, and parents can sometimes notice periods in which the child appears to stop breathing for 5–10 seconds at a time. This can cause restless sleep and irritability in the mornings. This can also be dangerous because chronic decreases in oxygenation of the blood during sleep can cause high blood pressure in the lungs, called pulmonary hypertension. This hypertension is bad for the heart, causing chronic damage.

Many times OSA can be diagnosed by a careful history and examination of the child. However, in some cases where the diagnosis is not certain, it can be made by the use of polysomnography, or a "sleep study." This takes place overnight in a hospital or other monitoring center where it can be determined whether the child is actually having periods during which he or she stops breathing while sleeping.

OSA is often successfully treated by removal of the adenoids, often with the tonsils as well. Some children may require more extensive surgical procedures.

Hearing loss is more common in children with DS than in other children. This hearing loss can be from chronic fluid in the ears ("conductive"), dysfunction of the transfer of sound from the inner ear to the brain ("sensorineural"), or a mixture of both types. For this reason, hearing studies should be done on all newborns with DS and should also be done yearly on children up through 12 years of age. The newborn test should be done using a test called auditory brain stem response (ABR), which is also called the brain stem auditory evoked response (BAER). This test should continue to be used until the child is developmentally able to give adequate responses to more behavioral hearing tests. Children can be tested with pure tone audiometry tests by testing each ear separately.

Because of this increased risk of hearing loss, children with DS who have chronic or recurrent middle ear infections should be treated aggressively. Although placement of tympanostomy tubes (also called "P-E tubes") may be technically difficult because of the smaller ear canals of children with DS, the procedure is usually very successful at preserving hearing.

Another common airway problem in children with DS is recurrent croup. Croup is the term given to inflammation and swelling of the trachea and larynx, with its resultant "barking" cough. Croup can be either viral or allergic in nature. Children with DS appear to be more prone to croup because of their smaller airway, so any swelling is more likely to cause breathing problems than in other children. Croup is treated with antihistamines and humidity, and moderate to severe cases may require treatment with steroids.

## HEMATOLOGY AND ONCOLOGY

Leukemia is more common in children with DS, being seen anywhere from 10 to 30 times more often than in the general population of children. The vast majority of cases occur in the first 5 years of life. In the first 3 years of life, nonlymphoid leukemia is the most common form of leukemia in children with DS; after age 3, approximately 80% with leukemia have acute lymphocytic leukemia (AML) and 20% have nonlymphocytic leukemia (ALL). The actual treatment of leukemia is beyond the scope of this article, but it is worth noting here that children with DS who develop AML seem to respond to chemotherapy much better than do children without DS; for ALL, the response rate appears to be about the same.

Newborns with DS have an increased risk of having a condition called transient leukemia (also called transient abnormal myelopoiesis, transient blastemia, or myeloproliferative syndrome). This condition resembles leukemia but disappears on its own without treatment in just a few weeks or months. One study found that up to 10% of newborns with DS had evidence of transient leukemia on blood tests. On the blood test, the number of white blood cells is greatly above normal and immature white blood cells, or "blasts," are present. Although this condition resolves without treatment, there is an increased risk of these infants to develop leukemia later in childhood. In one study of 85 infants with transient leukemia, 30% went on to develop a type of leukemia called "nonlymphoid" (also called "myelocytic," or AML) within the next 3 years. The reason for the development of transient leukemia is not understood but is definitely linked to the extra 21st chromosome.

Another abnormal finding in newborns with DS is a low platelet count, called thrombocytopenia. The platelets are the blood cells that assist in clotting blood. Rarely, the platelet count may be so low that transfusions of platelets may be needed to prevent bleeding problems. The reason for the thrombocytopenia is unknown. Newborns with thrombocytopenia should be watched carefully for any other signs of transient leukemia.

On the other hand, some infants with DS show an increase in platelet numbers, called thrombocytosis. One research team found that 20% of all the infants they studied had thrombocytosis, but none had any complications from the condition and all had normal platelet counts 1 month later. The cause here is also unknown.

In people with DS, types of cancer other than the leukemias are rare, with the exception of testicular cancer. Men with DS have an almost 50-fold increase in cases of testicular carcinoma and should be monitored for this with regular physical exams.

## GROWTH AND ENDOCRINOLOGY

People with DS are well known to have short stature, and much research has been performed looking for the exact cause. Children with DS appear to produce less growth hormone in response to certain chemical stimuli, so some researchers believe that the stimulation of the production of growth hormone is impaired in DS. Other research indicates that there is a deficiency of insulin-like growth factors, which are the mediators between the growth hormone and the tissues of the body. With less insulin-like growth factor, the growth hormone cannot stimulate bones and other parts of the body to grow at a normal rate.

Special growth charts have been devised for children with DS. These have been reprinted in several medical journals and books and are also available on the Internet at *http://www.growthcharts.com*. These growth charts evaluate not only height and weight but also head circumference.

There has been some question as to whether human growth hormone (hGH) supplementation could be of any use in DS. Studies have shown that hGH injections can improve the height and head circumference of children with DS, but it has no effect on cognitive functioning. Although the use of hGH is definitely indicated for children with documented growth hormone deficiencies, its use in other children, even with short stature, is still controversial in the medical community. The administration of hGH is through repeated injections, and there are still concerns over possible long-term side effects including the induction of leukemia.

Thyroid disorders are common in people with DS. Hypothyroidism, or low thyroid levels, is the most common and can be found at any age. In infants and newborns with hypothyroidism, the most common cause is failure of the thyroid gland to develop correctly. In older children and adults, the most common cause is an autoimmune reaction, in which the body makes antibodies against thyroid tissue. The symptoms of hypothyroidism can be subtle, especially in people with DS: decreased growth rate, weight gain, constipation, lethargy, decreased muscle tone, and dry skin. Because it is easy to miss these symptoms, it is recommended that infants with DS be tested for hypothyroidism by blood tests at 6 months and 1 year of age and once a year thereafter for life. Hypothyroidism is treated by administration of thyroid hormone replacement orally.

A common condition found in screening children with DS for hypothyroidism is normal thyroid hormone blood levels along with abnormally elevated thyroid-stimulating hormone levels. This state may represent either a temporary condition or the first step of hypothyroidism. Often, the finding of anti-thyroid antibodies in the blood can help diagnose early hypothyroidism. However, the treatment of this situation has not been established; some doctors may choose to treat with just enough thyroid hormone to bring the levels of thyroid-stimulating hormone to normal, and other doctors choose to wait and retest 3–6 months later.

Recent research indicates that zinc may be a necessary component of thyroid function. Children with elevated thyroid-stimulating hormone levels, normal thyroid levels, and low blood zinc levels may benefit from a trial of oral zinc supplementation.

Hyperthyroidism, or high thyroid hormone levels in the blood, is also more common in people with DS, although not as common as hypothyroidism. The cause is, again, autoimmune disease, referred to as Graves disease. The symptoms include rapid heart rate, nervousness, sweating, decreased attention span, flushed skin, always feeling hot, and loss of hair. The diagnosis is made through blood tests and thyroid imaging studies.

There are three possible treatments of hyperthyroidism. One treatment is aimed at blocking the action of the thyroid hormone on body tissues, which involves the use of antithyroid drugs. This is often the first treatment used; however, almost all of these drugs can cause significant side effects. A second treatment is surgery to remove part or all of the thyroid;

the child or adult is then started on thyroid replacement, if needed. The third treatment is the use of radioactive iodide, which destroys the thyroid's ability to produce thyroid hormone. The patient then takes replacement thyroid hormone. There is some concern over the use of radioactive iodide in people with DS because of the increased risk of leukemia, but no cases of leukemia traceable to this treatment have been published to date. At the present time, there is no clear consensus on the best way to treat hyperthyroidism in children with DS.

Diabetes mellitus is another common finding in children and adults with DS. Diabetes is another autoimmune disease, causing the body to stop making insulin and resulting high blood sugars. Initial signs of diabetes are increased urination followed by increased thirst, along with increased hunger and decreased energy levels. After a few weeks, if untreated, the child may suffer weight loss and vomiting. Diabetes is diagnosed through urine and blood tests and is treated by regular insulin injections.

## OPHTHALMOLOGY

The earliest eye abnormality seen in DS is the presence of dense congenital cataracts, which are opacifications of the lens of the eye and may be present at birth. All newborns should be examined carefully for cataracts, which must be surgically removed immediately to preserve eyesight.

A common finding in infants with DS is dacryostenois or blocked tear duct. The infant will present with one or both eyes tending to tear up frequently and frequent eye infections. Blocked tear ducts are managed initially by tear duct massage and antibiotic eye drops, but if they do not clear up by 9–12 months of age, the ducts may need to be opened by an ophthalmologist.

Strabismus, or the lack of alignment of the eyes, is frequent in infants with DS. When this occurs, young children will see double images. They can suppress the image from the deviating eye, but that may cause a loss of vision in the suppressed eye, called amblyopia. Early treatment involves patching the stronger eye and sometimes glasses. Surgery is needed for large deviations. However, the broad nasal bridge in infants with DS will often cause a child to appear as though one or both eyes are turning inward toward the nose when in fact the eyes are normal. An ophthalmologist will be able to determine whether strabismus truly exists.

Errors in visual acuity, such as nearsightedness (myopia), farsightedness (hyperopia), and astigmatism are highly common in children with DS. For this reason, it is recommended that children with DS be evaluated for their vision between 6 and 9 months of age and once a year after that for life.

Blepharitis is a chronic infection of the edge of the eyelid and occurs frequently in children and adults with DS. Treatment requires antibiotic ointments to be applied to the lids along with lid scrubs and, occasionally, steroid drops.

## Traditional Therapies

Besides medical therapies aimed at any of the conditions or diseases that may arise in people with DS, there are other therapies of which parents should be aware. Speech, occupational, and physical therapies are all important parts of treating the child with DS, although emphasis may vary at different times of his or her life. Nutritional guidelines may be required to help an infant with feeding problems or, later, to prevent obesity.

## Alternative Therapies

Over the decades, many different therapies have been advocated for alleviating certain aspects of the condition. These include cell therapy, DMSO, and nootropics ("smart drugs"). To date, none of these has been found to be useful in any rigorous scientific testing in children with DS.

Nutritional supplements have also been championed in various forms since the 1950s. Repeated studies have shown that there are no nutritional deficiencies common to all children with DS, and no study has ever documented the need for any of these supplements, with the possible exception of the minerals zinc and selenium mentioned above.

Plastic surgery has been popular in certain areas such as Europe and Israel. One type of plastic surgery is strictly cosmetic and is aimed at "correcting" such features as epicanthal folds and the flattened nasal bridge. Another type of surgery is designed to decrease the size of the tongue, in an effort to improve speech. However, studies have shown that reduction of tongue size has little to no effect on the speech of children with DS.

## Health Supervision for Children with Down Syndrome

The DSMIG, a group of physicians and other health care professionals with a personal interest in this topic, has produced guidelines for physicians caring for people with DS. The 1999 version was printed in the Down Syndrome Quarterly (Sept. 1999 issue) and is reprinted elsewhere in this book. This is a useful item for parents as well, to ensure that the medical needs of their children continue to be met. (See Chapter 17, Healthcare Guidelines for Individuals with Down Syndrome—1999 Revision.)

## REFERENCES

### A. NEUROLOGY

Burt DB et al. (1998): Dementia in adults with Down syndrome: diagnostic challenges. Am J Ment Retard 103(2):130–145.

Brandt BR, Rosen I (1995): Impaired peripheral somatosensory function in children with Down syndrome. Neuropediatrics 26:310–312.

Cramer SC et al. (1996): Moyamoya and Down syndrome: clinical and radiological features. Stroke 27:2131–2135.

Howlin P et al. (1995): The recognition of autism in children with Down syndrome—implications for intervention. Dev Med Child Neuro 37:398–414.

Kishnani PS et al. (1999): Cholinergic therapy for Down's syndrome. Lancet 353: 1064.

Pueschel SM et al. (1991): Seizure disorders in Down syndrome. Arch Neurol 48:318–320.

Smith DJ et al. (1997): Functional screening of 2 Mb of human chromosome 21q22.2 in transgenic mice implicates *minibrain* in learning defects associated with Down syndrome. Nat Genet 16:28–36.

Stafstrom CE et al. (1991): Seizures in children with Down syndrome: etiology, characteristics and outcome. Dev Med Child Neuro 33:191–200.

Stafstrom CE, Konkol RJ (1994): Infantile spasms in children with Down syndrome. Dev Med Child Neuro 36:576–585.

### B. IMMUNOLOGY

Magnusson CG et al. (1997): Differential effect of selenium supplementation on immunoglobulin levels in Down's syndrome. Acta Paediatr 86(12):1385–1386.

Nespoli L et al. (1993): Immunological features of Down's syndrome. J Intellect Disabil Res 37:543–551.

### C. GASTROENTEROLOGY

Gale L et al. (1997): Down's syndrome is strongly associated with celiac disease. Gut 40:492–496.

Levy J (1992): Gastrointestinal concerns. In: Pueschel SM and Pueschel JK (eds.), Biomedical Concerns in Persons with Down Syndrome, Baltimore: Paul H. Brookes, pp 119–125.

Quinn FMJ et al. (1994): The influence of trisomy 21 on outcome in children with Hirschsprung's disease. J Pediatr Surg 29(6):781–783.

Zachor DA et al. (2000): Prevalence of celiac disease in Down syndrome in the United States. J. Pediatr Gastroenterol Nutr 31:275–279.

## D. Cardiology

Marino B (1992): Cardiac aspects. In Pueschel SM and Pueschel JK (eds.), Biomedical Concerns in Persons with Down Syndrome, Baltimore: Paul H. Brookes, pp 91–103.

## E. Orthopedics

American Academy of Pediatrics Committee on Sports Medicine (1984): Atlantoaxial instability in Down syndrome. Pediatrics 74(1):152–154.

American Academy of Pediatrics Committee on Sports Medicine (1995): Atlantoaxial instability in Down syndrome: subject review. Pediatrics 96:151–154.

Brockmeyer D (1999): Down syndrome and craniovertebral instability. Pediatr Neurosurg 31(2):71–77.

Cohen WI (1998): Atlantoaxial instability. What's next? Arch Pediatr Adolesc Med 152(2):119–122.

Mendez AA et al. (1988): Treatment of patellofemoral instability in Down's syndrome. Clin Orthop 234:148–158.

Pueschel SM (1998): Should children with Down syndrome be screened for atlantoaxial instability? Arch Pediatr Adolesc Med 152(2):123–125.

Shaw ED, Beals RK (1989): The hip joint in Down's syndrome: a study of its structure and associated disease. Clin Orthop Relat Res 278:101–107.

Uno K et al. (1996): Occipitoatlantal and occipitoaxial hypermobility in Down syndrome. Spine 21(12):1430–1434.

## F. Otolaryngology

Carroll JL, Loughlin GM (1995): Obstructive sleep apnea in infants and children: clinical features and pathophysiology. In: Ferber R and Kryger M (eds.) Principles and Practice of Sleep Medicine in the Child, Philadelphia: WB Saunders, pp 163–191.

Marcus CL et al. (1991): Obstructive sleep apnea in children with Down syndrome. Pediatrics 88(1):132–139.

Shott SR (2000): Down syndrome: common pediatric ear, nose and throat problems. Down Syndrome Q 5(2):1–6.

## G. Hematology and Oncology

Homans A et al. (1993): Transient abnormal myelopoiesis of infancy associated with trisomy 21. Am J Pediatr Hematol Oncol 15(4):392–399.

Hord JD et al. (1995): Thrombocytopenia in neonates with trisomy 21. Arch Pediatr Adolesc Med 149:824–825.

Kivivuori SM et al. (1996): Peripheral blood cell counts in infants with Down's syndrome. Clin Genet 49:15–19.

Ragab AH et al. (1991): Clinical characteristics and treatment outcome of children with acute lymphocytic leukemia and Down's syndrome. Cancer 67:1057–1063.

Satge D et al. (1997): An excess of testicular germ cell tumors in Down's syndrome. Cancer 80:929–935.

Zipursky A et al. (1997): Leukemia and/or myeloproliferative syndrome in neonates with Down syndrome. Semin Perinatal 21(1):97–101.

## H. GROWTH AND ENDOCRINOLOGY

Ali FE et al. (1999): Treatment of hyperthryoidism in Down syndrome: case report and review of the literature. Res Dev Disabil 20(4):297–303.

Anneren G et al. (1999): Growth hormone treatment in young children with Down's syndrome: effects on growth and psychomotor development. Arch Dis Child 80:334–338.

Anwar AJ et al. (1998): Type 1 diabetes mellitus and Down's syndrome: prevalence, management and diabetic complications. Diabet Med 15(2):160–163.

Christina GS et al. (1992): Head circumference of children with Down syndrome. Am J Med Genet 42:61–67.

Cronk CE (1988): Growth charts for children with Down syndrome. Pediatrics 81(1):102–110.

Cronk CE, Anneren G (1992): Growth. In: Pueschel SM and Pueschel JK (eds.), Biomedical Concerns in Persons with Down Syndrome, Baltimore: Paul H. Brookes, pp 19–37.

Ivarsson S-A et al. (1997): The impact of thyroid autoimmunity in children and adolescents with Down syndrome. Acta Paediatr 86:1065–1067.

Pueschel SM, Bier JB (1992): Endocrinologic aspects. In: Pueschel SM and Pueschel JK (eds.), Biomedical Concerns in Persons with Down Syndrome, Baltimore: Paul H. Brookes, pp 259–272.

Sustrova M, Strbak V (1994): Thyroid function and plasma immunoglobulins in subjects with Down's syndrome during ontogenesis and zinc therapy. J Endocrinol Invest 17: 385–390.

## I. OPHTHALMOLOGY

Courage ML et al. (1994): Visual acuity in infants and children with Down syndrome. Dev Med Child Neurol 36(7):586–93.

Da Cunha RP, Moreira JB (1996): Ocular findings in Down's syndrome. Am J Ophthalmol 122(2):236–244.

Rozien NJ et al. (1994): Ophthalmic disorders in children with Down syndrome. Dev Med Child Neuro 36:594–600.

Woodhouse JM et al. (1996): Visual acuity and accommodation in infants and young children with Down's syndrome. J Intellect Disabil Res 40(1):49–55.

## J. TRADITIONAL THERAPIES

Bruni M (1998): Fine Motor Skills in Children with Down Syndrome: A Guide for Parents and Teachers. Bethesda, MD: Woodbine House.

Kumin L. (1994). Communication Skills for Children with Down Syndrome: A Guide for Parents. Bethesda, MD: Woodbine House.

Winders PC (1997): Gross Motor Skills in Children with Down Syndrome: A Guide for Parents and Professionals. Bethesda, MD: Woodbine House.

## K. ALTERNATIVE THERAPIES

Ani C et al. (2000): Nutritional supplementation in Down syndrome: theoretical considerations and current status. Dev Med Child Neuro 42:207–213.

Heggarty HJ et al. (1996): Amino acid profile in Down's syndrome. Arch Dis Child 74(4):347–349.

Lobaugh NJ et al. (2001). Piracetam does not enhance cognitive functioning in children with Down syndrome. Arch Ped Adol Med 155(4):442–448.

Margar-Bacal F et al. (1987): Speech intelligibility after partial glossectomy in children with Down's syndrome. Plastic Reconstr Surg 79:44–47.

Parsons CL et al. (1987):. Effect of tongue reduction on articulation in children with Down syndrome. Am J Ment Defic 91:328–332.

Pruess JB et al. (1989): Vitamin therapy and children with Down syndrome: a review of research. Except Child 55(4): 336–341.

Van Dyke DC et al. (1990): Cell therapy in children with Down syndrome. Pediatrics 85: 79–84.

## L. HEALTH SUPERVISION

American Academy of Pediatrics Committee on Genetics (2001): Health supervision for children with Down syndrome. Pediatrics 107(2):442–449.

Cohen, WI (1999): Health care guidelines for individuals with Down syndrome. Down Syndrome Q 4(3):1–15.

# THE GOAL AND OPPORTUNITY OF PHYSICAL THERAPY FOR CHILDREN WITH DOWN SYNDROME[1]

## PATRICIA C. WINDERS, PT

*The appropriate goal of physical therapy for children with Down syndrome is not to accelerate their rate of gross motor development as is commonly assumed. The goal is to minimize the development of abnormal compensatory movement patterns that children with Down syndrome are prone to develop. Early physical therapy makes a decisive difference in the long-term functional outcome of the child with Down syndrome. Beyond this goal, there is an additional opportunity that physical therapy makes available to parents. Because gross motor development is the first learning task that the child with Down syndrome encounters, it provides parents with the first opportunity to explore how their child learns. There is increasing evidence that children with Down syndrome have a unique learning style. Understanding how children with Down syndrome learn is crucial for parents who wish to facilitate the development of gross motor skills as well as facilitating success in other areas of life including language, education and the development of social skills.*

The mother of an infant with Down syndrome recently asked about beginning physical therapy for her child. She began the meeting by asking: "If we start physical therapy now, what difference will it make when my child is

[1]Reprinted with permission from *Down Syndrome Quarterly*, Volume 6, Number 2, June 2001, pg. 1–5.

9 or 10 years old?" **What a great question!** It is exactly how she should be thinking about physical therapy, and, in fact, it is exactly how she should be thinking about all the services for her child. She has focused on **the long-term functional outcome** for her child. That question and that focus have guided my work for many years. This paper will answer her question. What difference, indeed, will it make years from now, when a child is an adolescent or an adult, whether or not he or she had physical therapy as a child? This article will address the goal of physical therapy for children with Down syndrome, and then looking beyond that goal, will discuss an additional opportunity that is available to parents while their child is receiving physical therapy.

## THE GOAL OF PHYSICAL THERAPY

Before discussing what the goal of physical therapy for children with Down syndrome **is**, it is necessary first to understand what the goal **is not**. The goal of physical therapy **is not** to accelerate the rate of gross motor development. This statement is more controversial than it may initially seem to be. Many parents, many physical therapists and many insurance companies assume that the value of physical therapy can be measured by whether or not a child is achieving motor skills more quickly. Some therapeutic techniques promote themselves by saying that children who are treated with that technique develop motor skills earlier. If, however, one begins with the premise that the goal of physical therapy is to accelerate the rate of gross motor development, then one needs to answer the question posed by that mother. What difference will it make in 9 or 10 years that a child with Down syndrome walked at 21 rather than 24 months of age? How will that three-month difference affect a child's long-term functional outcome? I do not believe that it will make any difference whatsoever, and, therefore, I do not believe that it is the appropriate goal for physical therapy for children with Down syndrome. The rate of gross motor development in children with Down syndrome is influenced by a number of factors, including:

- hypotonia
- ligamentous laxity
- decreased strength
- short arms and legs.

These factors are determined by genetics, and although some may be influenced by physical therapy, they cannot be fundamentally altered.

So then, what is the goal of physical therapy for children with Down syndrome? Children with Down syndrome attempt to compensate for their hypotonia, ligamentous laxity, decreased strength and short arms and legs by developing compensatory movement patterns, which, if allowed to persist, often develop into orthopedic and functional problems. **The goal of physical therapy is to minimize the development of the compensatory movement patterns that children with Down syndrome are prone to develop.**

Gait is a primary example. Ligamentous laxity, hypotonia and weakness in the legs lead to lower extremity posturing with hip abduction and external rotation, hyperextension of the knees, and pronation and eversion of the feet. (See Figure 14.1.) Children with Down syndrome typically learn to walk with their feet wide apart, their knees stiff, and their feet turned out. They do so because hypotonia, ligamentous laxity and weakness make their legs less stable. Locking their knees, widening their base, and rotating their feet outward are all strategies designed to increase stability. The problem is, however, that this is an inefficient gait pattern for walking. The weight is being borne on the medial (inside) borders of the feet, and the feet are designed to have the weight borne on the outside borders. If this pattern is

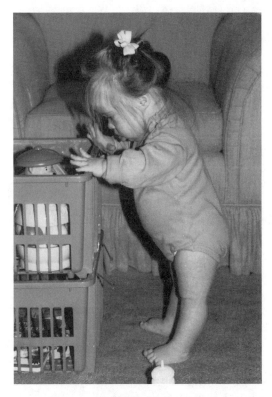

FIGURE 14.1.

allowed to persist, problems will develop with both the knees and the feet. Walking will become painful, and endurance will be decreased. Physical therapy should begin teaching the child with Down syndrome the proper standing posture (i.e., feet positioned under the hips and pointing straight ahead with a slight bend in the knees) when he is still very young. (See Figure 14.2.) With appropriate physical therapy gait problems can be minimized or avoided. (See Figure 14.3.)

Trunk posture is another example. Ligamentous laxity, hypotonia, and decreased strength in the trunk encourage the development of kyphosis, which is often first seen when the child is learning to sit. Children with Down syndrome typically learn to sit with a posterior pelvic tilt, trunk rounded and the head resting back on the shoulders. (See Figure 14.4.) They never learn to actively move their pelvis into a vertical (upright) position, and therefore, cannot hold their head and trunk erect over it. If this posture is allowed to persist, it will ultimately result in impaired breathing and a decreased ability to rotate the trunk. Physical therapy must teach the child the proper sitting posture by providing support at the proper level even

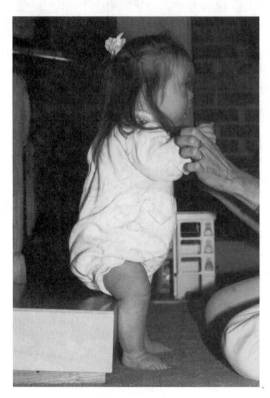

FIGURE 14.2.

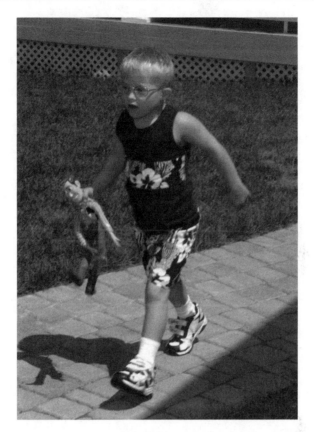

FIGURE 14.3.

before the child is able to sit independently. (See Figure 14.5.) First, the therapist provides upper trunk support, then middle trunk support, then support between the scapula and the waist, then support at the waist and finally pelvic support. The support provided at each level keeps the spine and pelvis in proper alignment until the child develops the strength to hold that segment in alignment himself. Appropriate physical therapy can minimize problems with trunk posture. (See Figure 14.6.)

PHYSICAL THERAPY SERVICES:

- should be concerned with the child's long-term functional outcome;

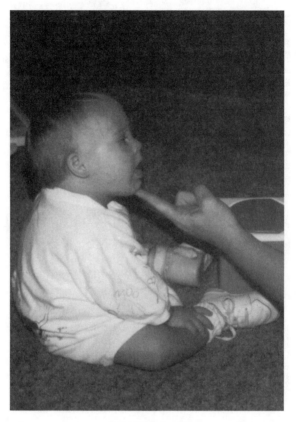

FIGURE 14.4.

- should seek to minimize the development of compensatory movement patterns;
- should be based on a thorough understanding of the compensatory
  movement patterns that children with Down syndrome are prone to
  develop;
- should be strategically designed to proactively build strength in the
  appropriate muscle groups so that the child with Down syndrome
  develops optimal movement patterns;
- should focus on gait, posture and exercise.

So the answer to that mother's question is that physical therapy for the
young child with Down syndrome will make an enormous difference not
only when the child is 9 or 10 years of age, but also when he or she is an
adolescent and an adult. It can and should result in adults who are healthier and more functional.

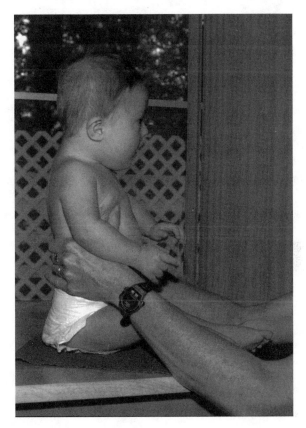

FIGURE 14.5.

## THE OPPORTUNITY OF PHYSICAL THERAPY

If physical therapy has achieved the goal of minimizing the development of abnormal movement patterns, it will have influenced the health of the child with Down syndrome throughout the course of his or her life. But there is actually an opportunity beyond the development of motor skills of which parents may wish to take advantage while their child is receiving physical therapy.

There is mounting evidence that children with Down syndrome do not learn in the same manner that typical children do. They have a different style of assimilating information, and, therefore, the usual methods of instruction are less effective. The development of gross motor skills is the first learning task that the child with Down syndrome and his parents will face together. There are many other challenges to come including language, education, and the development of social skills, but learning gross motor skills is the first

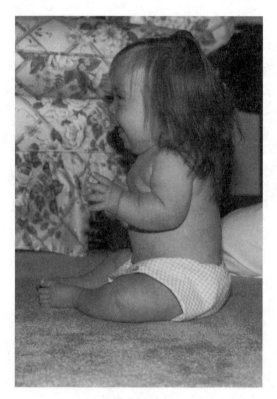

FIGURE 14.6.

developmental challenge. **The opportunity is for parents to use the arena of gross motor development to begin to understand how their child learns.** Knowing how to facilitate their child's learning will be critical to their success in collaborating will their child throughout his or her lifetime.

Wishart (1991), a psychologist at the University of Edinburgh in Scotland, has done leading edge work in studying how children with Down syndrome learn. She writes:

> Despite the absence of an adequate developmental database, theory and practice in this area have nonetheless continued to assume that the process of learning in children with DS is essentially a slowed-down version of normal cognitive development. An increasing number of recent studies are suggesting that this 'slow development' approach may be ill founded and that learning may differ significantly in structure and organization from that found in ordinary children . . . (pp. 28–29).
>
> Infants with DS consistently showed evidence of underperforming, with avoidance routines being produced on many of the tasks presented, regardless of whether these were above or below the infant's current developmental level.

New skills, even once mastered, proved to be inadequately consolidated, often disappearing from the infant's repertoire in subsequent months. Follow-up studies using a wider range of tasks provided additional evidence of this tendency to 'switch out' of cognitive tasks, with many children failing on items which should have been well within their capabilities and which had been passed in earlier sessions . . . (p. 29).

Regardless of whether these irregular performance profiles reflect genuine developmental instability or are the result of fluctuating motivation in assessment-type situations, it remains that if test behaviour is typical of behaviour in other, everyday situations, development itself must be compromised. (p. 29).

Investigation into the learning style of children with Down syndrome is in its early stages. Kumin (2001) and Oelwein (1995) also have made important contributions in this area. In her book, *Classroom Language Skills for Children with Down Syndrome: A Guide for Parents and Teachers*, Kumin discusses how the insights of Howard Gardner can be applied to children with Down syndrome. Gardner's book, *Frames of Mind* 1983, presents the theory of multiple intelligences, which postulates that intelligence is multi-faceted. The theory holds that besides linguistic and mathematical intelligences, there are also spatial, interpersonal and musical intelligences, to mention only a few. Kumin notes that it has been her experience that many children with Down syndrome learn well using music. She has also written about the unique learning style of children with Down syndrome, and how it pertains to learning speech and language in her book, *Communication Skills in Children with Down Syndrome: A Guide for Parents* (Kumin, 1994).

Oelwein (1995) also has written about the learning style of children with Down syndrome and how it impacts education. She has highlighted the need to consciously assist children with Down syndrome with how information can be effectively filed, stored and retrieved. Her book, *Teaching Reading to Children with Down Syndrome: A Guide for Parents and Teachers*, provides a comprehensive, step-by-step guide to teaching reading to children with Down syndrome. All of this work points to how important it is for parents to have an understanding of how their child assimilates information so that they can be successful partners in their child's learning.

It has been my experience in 21 years of providing physical therapy to children with Down syndrome that they do indeed learn differently and that it is necessary to modify my approach if I wish to obtain the best result. I consider it an important opportunity of my work to help parents begin to understand how their child learns. The following "tips" were derived from many years of working with children with Down syndrome. They are offered to provide a starting point for both parents and therapists to begin to explore the unique learning style of the child with Down syndrome.

1. Children with Down syndrome have a decreased ability to generalize. This means that a skill learned in one setting does not

necessarily transfer to another setting. For instance, a child may be quite competent climbing the stairs at home, but when confronted with stairs at the clinic, he or she may regress to a much more primitive stair-climbing strategy until he or she has relearned the skill in the new setting.

2. Children with Down syndrome need information to be delivered in small bite-sized pieces. It has been my experience that if a child appears to have plateaued, the problem is most likely to be that the next piece of information is too large and needs to be further broken down.

3. The setup is crucial and needs to be as close to perfect as possible. Children with Down syndrome need structure, consistency and a familiar environment if you hope to get their best performance. Do not try something new or challenging when the child is tired, hungry or not at his best for some reason. The quality of the work you do together is more important than the quantity. Minimize distractions in the environment.

4. Follow the child's lead. The child must be motivated to perform a particular skill. Trying to impose your will on a child with Down syndrome is a losing game. I often try to model my style of interaction after the parent's. It is familiar to the child and most likely to be successful.

5. Be attentive to how the child reacts when learning new gross motor skills. Some children are cautious, and others are risky. A cautious child prefers to stay in one position, while the risky child prefers to be in motion. For example, when learning to walk, the cautious child will want lots of support and will be upset if he or she falls. The risky child will like walking because it involves movement and will not be concerned about support or care how many times he or she falls.

6. Know when to quit. Some children will only give you two repetitions at a particular skill and then insist on moving on. Other children will gladly give you a dozen repetitions. Set up the game so that the child is successful and avoid frustration.

7. Be strategic in planning your session. Practice what the child is ready to learn. Tackle the most difficult skills first before the child becomes tired. Alternate difficult skills with easier ones to give the child time to recover his strength.

8. Be strategic in providing support. Children with Down syndrome tend to become quickly dependent on support. Provide as little support as possible while still allowing the child to succeed and remove the support as soon as possible.

9. Skills will be learned grossly at first and then refined. For instance, children will initially learn to walk with a wide base and their feet externally rotated. This is not the optimal gait pattern, but it needs to be allowed initially and then refined through the post-walking skills.

10. Do not interfere with an established skill in which the child has achieved independence. You will not be successful in introducing change and the child will only experience you as nagging. Changes will need to be made at the next level of motor development. For instance, some children, instead of learning to creep on both knees, learn to creep on one knee and one foot. Once this pattern has been established and the child is proficient in its use, you will not be successful in altering it and will succeed only in angering the child. Teach the child to use both knees in climbing up stairs rather than interfering with this established pattern.

11. Children with Down syndrome learn best through a gradual process.
    a. Introduction of the new skill is the first step. The new skill needs to be introduced slowly and carefully with the goal being simply to have the child tolerate the movement.
    b. Familiarity is the second step. In this step the child becomes accustomed to the skill and how it feels physically. This is the "I get it" phase in which the child understands the game and what is being asked of him or her.
    c. Collaboration is the third step. The child increases his collaboration and cooperation, and at the same time support is decreased.
    d. Independence is the final step where the child has mastered the skill and can perform it independently without support.

These tips are offered tentatively, knowing that they are far from definitive answers. Much more research is needed to begin truly to understand the learning style of children with Down syndrome. It is crucial, however, that parents gain skill in facilitating the learning of their child. Otherwise, as Wishart (1995) says, we "could run the risk of changing slow but willing learners into reluctant, avoidant learners." (p. 62).

Parents who are newly assuming the responsibility of caring for a child with Down syndrome are confronted with a confusing array of treatment options and opportunities. It can be difficult to know where to focus limited time and resources. It is hoped this article will provide parents and caregivers with a starting point and a framework for making decisions about what is important. They should think about proposed therapies just like the mother described in the first paragraph, from the perspective of the child's long-term functional outcome. Physical therapy is a crucial service, not because it will accelerate a child's rate of development, but because it will improve a child's long-term functional outcome by preventing the development of abnormal movement patterns that are likely to become even more serious problems in adolescence and adulthood. Secondly, because gross motor development is the first learning task a child faces, it provides parents and other caregivers with the opportunity to learn how a given child learns. Let the long-term functional outcome guide decisions about *what* to work on, and let understanding of the child's learning style guide decisions about *how* to work on them.

## REFERENCES

Gardner, H. (1983). *Frames of Mind: the theory of multiple intelligences.* New York: Basic. Books.

Kumin, L. (2001). *Classroom Language Skills for Children with Down Syndrome: A Guide for Parents and Teachers.* Bethesda, MD: Woodbine House.

Kumin, L. (1994). *Communication Skills in Children with Down Syndrome: A Guide for Parents.* Rockville, MD: Woodbine House.

Oelwein, P. (1995). *Teaching Reading to Children with Down Syndrome: A Guide for Parents and Teachers.* Bethesda, MD: Woodbine House.

Winders, P. (1997). *Gross Motor Skills in Children with Down Syndrome: A Guide for Parents and Professionals.* Bethesda, MD: Woodbine House.

Wishart, J. G. (1995). Cognitive Abilities in Children with Down Syndrome: Developmental Instability and Motivational Deficits. In: C. J. Epstein, T. Hassold, I. T. Lott, L. Nadel, & D. Patterson (Eds.), *Etiology and Pathogenesis of Down Syndrome.* New York: Wiley-Liss, Inc.

Wishart, J. G. (1991). Taking the initiative in learning: a developmental investigation of infants with Down syndrome. *International Journal of Disability, Development, and Education, 38,* 27–44.

# BEHAVIORAL CONCERNS IN PERSONS WITH DOWN SYNDROME

## BONNIE PATTERSON, M.D.

Behavioral studies from the 1960s, '70s, and '80s variously described children with Down syndrome as good tempered, affectionate, placid, cheerful, stubborn, sullen, withdrawn, and defiant (Pueschel et al., 1991). In 1972, Barron published a study looking at the temperament of individuals with Down syndrome and concluded that behavior in his study group was similar to the general population if mental age was taken into account (Pueschel et al., 1991). In recent years, it has become evident that the old stereotypes are incorrect and that children and adults with Down syndrome have the same range of temperament and behavior as the general population.

Physicians and other professionals involved in the care of people with Down syndrome are often asked by parents and teachers for help in understanding the behavior difficulties that impact on the social and educational development of their children and can be disruptive in the home and the classroom. The definition of what a behavior problem is varies from person to person, but certain guidelines can be helpful in determining when a simple "problem" becomes a "behavior problem." These would include behaviors that interfere with development/learning; that are disruptive to the family/school; that are harmful to the child or others; and that are discrepant from what might be typically displayed by someone of comparable development.

*Down Syndrome*, Edited by William I. Cohen, Lynn Nadel, and Myra E. Madnick.
ISBN 0-471-41815-3   Copyright © 2002 by Wiley-Liss, Inc.

When evaluating children and adults with Down syndrome for behavioral concerns, it is important to determine whether there are acute or chronic health problems impacting on development and/or behavior. Vision and hearing problems can have a significant effect on a person's ability to function both at home and in the school/workplace setting and should be monitored closely as recommended in the *Healthcare Guidelines for Persons with Down Syndrome* (Cohen, 1999). Other medical problems that can be associated with behavioral changes include: hypo- and hyperthyroidism, celiac disease (sensitivity to oats, wheat, barley, and rye), sleep apnea, anemia, gastroesophageal reflux, and constipation. Evaluation by the primary care physician to assess for medical/neurological problems is an important component of the workup for behavioral concerns in persons with Down syndrome of any age.

Parents, teachers, and therapists frequently report compliance issues or oppositional behaviors in children and adults with Down syndrome. When evaluating these behaviors, it is important to clarify the frequency, duration, and intensity. Descriptions of the child's behavior during a typical day both at home and at school can help determine the antecedent event that may have precipitated the oppositional or noncompliant behavior. Some people with Down syndrome who are described as oppositional, stubborn, or aggressive are in actuality using behavior as a means to communicate secondary to their significantly impaired verbal expression. It is important when evaluating a person for behavioral problems to have a clear understanding of their language and cognitive development. Because people with Down syndrome often have strong social adaptive skills, it is sometimes mistakenly assumed that receptive and expressive language skills are at that same level of functioning. This misperception can lead to difficulties in the classroom or workplace, particularly if the person is not provided with support services to help develop socially appropriate nonverbal responses. Children with Down syndrome are very adept at distracting parents and teachers when they are challenged with a difficult task. This is done to remove themselves from a frustrating situation and may be interpreted as oppositional or stubborn. When evaluating a child or adult with Down syndrome for compliance issues, it is important to assess speech-language abilities, hearing status, and general cognitive development. Understanding how their developmental strengths and weaknesses are related to the perceived difficult behavior will help in development of an intervention plan for home, school, or workplace.

The definition of attention deficit hyperactivity disorder (ADHD) includes attention problems being present for at least 1 year occurring in more than one setting and behavior characterized by inattention, distractibility, overactivity, and impulsivity. Attention problems are often reported in children with Down syndrome by parents or teachers but should be evaluated with the child's developmental age in mind rather than chronological age. The use of parent and teacher rating scales, such as the Conner's Rating Scale or the Achenbach Child Behavior Checklist, can aid in making the diagnosis. (The scales used must be appropriate for the child's developmental level.) If children with Down syndrome are diagnosed with ADHD, the interventions are the same as those for children of a similar developmental age without Down syndrome. Behavioral strategies will need to be instituted both at home and at school, and if a psychostimulant medication, such as Ritalin or Adderall, is prescribed it is important to remember that children with Down syndrome may be more sensitive and require a lower dose. Children with language processing problems are sometimes misdiagnosed with ADHD because of their difficulty in processing verbal information, which can manifest itself as inattention and distractibility. Anxiety disorders can also present as problems with attention and impulsivity. A multifactored evaluation including observation in the classroom or home setting is helpful in the assessment of children with suspected ADHD.

Parents of adolescents and young adults with Down syndrome sometimes report regression of self-care skills, reduced motivation or energy, social withdrawal, and functional decline. Many parents and professionals fear that these changes in behavior may be early signs of Alzheimer disease; however, in most situations that is not the case. These changes can be signs of depression and/or anxiety. Transitions at home and at school, such as siblings leaving for college or marriage, changes in parent's health status, and graduation from high school, can often be related to the onset of feelings of anxiety and sadness. The evaluation of behavior changes should include a thorough medical examination to rule out chronic or acute health problems that could be impacting on day-to-day function at home and in the workplace. If depression and/or anxiety is diagnosed, medical management is often successful in treating the symptoms. Behavioral counseling by an experienced professional can be beneficial for both the adult with Down syndrome and the family. Self-talk is common in adolescents and young adults with Down syndrome and is not an indication of serious psychiatric illness. Young adults with Down syndrome may also continue to have imaginary friends.

Obsessive-compulsive behaviors are often reported in children and adults with Down syndrome. A study by Evans and Gray published in April 2000 reported that children with Down syndrome had similar mental age-related changes and compulsive-like behaviors compared with mental age-matched controls. Younger children (both typical and those with Down syndrome) exhibited significantly more compulsive behaviors than older children. Children with and without Down syndrome did not differ from each other in the number of compulsive behaviors they engaged in, although children with Down syndrome engaged in these behaviors more frequently and more intensely.

Intervention strategies for treatment of behavioral problems are quite variable and dependent on the child's age, the severity of the problem, and the setting in which the problem is most commonly seen. Local parent support groups can often help by providing suggestions, support, and referral to community treatment programs. Psychosocial services in the primary care physician's office can be used for consultative care regarding behavior and developmental issues. As noted above, when evaluating behavior problems it is important to have a clear understanding of the person's developmental and language skills, particularly when noncompliant behaviors are reported. Medical assessments should include vision and hearing screens and thyroid tests if they have not been done within the past year. Chronic behavioral problems often warrant referral to a behavioral specialist experienced in working with children and adults with special needs. The use of medication for help in behavior management must be discussed with the primary care physician and specialists involved in the child's care. Children with Down syndrome may be more sensitive to certain medications. In older adults who present with new-onset behavioral changes, assessment for Alzheimer disease should be part of the medical work-up. Reports of loss of memory for activities of daily living skills, familiar routines or places, and people may also be helpful in the diagnostic process. In the older adult it is important to provide support and education for the person's caregivers whether they be family members or the staff of a nursing home.

Guidelines for development of a behavioral support plan include the following:

- What function does the behavior serve for the person?
- What behavior could meet that need in an acceptable way?
- What are the antecedents of the behavior?
- What are the consequences of the behavior?
- What are the frequency and duration of the target behaviors?
- What are the reinforcers for the individual?
- Have all medical factors been investigated? (Disability Solutions, 1999)

If at all possible, family members and caregivers should try to reduce stress when dealing with a child or adult with significant behavioral problems. Suggestions include increasing the number of people in the person's life who provide direct care, giving the caregiver permission to be angry/sad/upset, etc., and anticipating situations that result in behavioral outbursts and trying to prevent them before the behavior occurs.

## References

Cohen W.I., Healthcare Guidelines for Individuals with Down Syndrome: 1999 Revision (Down Syndrome Preventive Medical Check List) is published in Down Syndrome Quarterly (Volume 4, Number 3, September, 1999, pp. 1–16), and these excerpts are reprinted with permission of the Editor. Information concerning publication policy or subscriptions may be obtained by contacting Dr. Samuel J. Thios, Editor, Denison University, Granville, OH 43023.

Disability Solutions (1999): Practical approaches to behaviors that drive you crazy. 4:1–14.

Evans DW, Gray FL (2000): Compulsive-like behavior in individuals with Down syndrome: Its relation to mental age level, adaptive and maladaptive behavior. Child Dev 71:288–300.

Pueschel SM, Bernier JC, Pezzullo JC (1991): Behavioural observations in children with Down's syndrome. J Ment Def Res 35:502–511.

# LIFE ISSUES OF ADOLESCENTS AND ADULTS WITH DOWN SYNDROME

## DENNIS E. MCGUIRE, PH.D., AND BRIAN A. CHICOINE, M.D.

At the turn of the twentieth century, a person with Down syndrome (DS) was expected to live only about 9 years. Today, life expectancy is about 56 years—more than a sixfold increase (Eyman et al., 1991). As professionals and caregivers working with people with DS, we must do our best to ensure that this longer life is also a full and healthy one, both in terms of general health as well as emotional wellness and social functioning.

In this chapter, we will share with you what we have learned from our endeavors in a multidisciplinary center serving more than 1200 adolescents and adults with DS. (See Chicoine et al., 1995, for details on this center.) We will focus on the medical and psychosocial aspects of our work (Chicoine and McGuire, 1996), with the hope that our findings will help caregivers and other professionals as they strive to better serve the needs of people with DS.

## PSYCHOSOCIAL ISSUES: ADAPTIVE LIVING SKILLS

If adults with (DS) are to achieve a measure of independence and proficiency in their daily lives, helping them develop adaptive skills is essential. However, we believe that in addition to mastering these activities of daily

*Down Syndrome*, Edited by William I. Cohen, Lynn Nadel, and Myra E. Madnick. ISBN 0-471-41815-3   Copyright © 2002 by Wiley-Liss, Inc.

living (ADLs), other abilities also play a critical role in successful adaptation for people with DS. These include learning expressive language, sustaining positive personal beliefs and attitudes, understanding social and interpersonal issues, and developing creative and flexible approaches to dealing with changes in their lives.

## ACTIVITIES OF DAILY LIVING (ADLs)

To assess a person's daily-living skills, we use the Developmental Disability Profile. This is a quick and reliable measure (Brown et al., 1986) of a person's basic abilities and degree of independence. It also helps us determine whether a loss or change of function can be attributed to normal aging or whether its cause is a physical or mental health condition.

## ASSESSING BASIC SKILLS

We have found that most people with DS can carry out routine grooming and personal hygiene activities, housekeeping chores, and food preparation. Many can also use a stove or microwave, do laundry, and choose appropriate clothes with guidance. Among the skills that require more hands-on help are using public transportation, planning meals and going grocery shopping, getting around in the community, and managing money.

## ASSESSING INDEPENDENCE

Through our work with people with DS, we have learned what they should be able to do on their own. If a person who is capable of certain tasks is not doing them, it may be because he or she is not challenged. It also may be the result of being overprotected by caregivers. Deliberate overprotection may stifle a person's natural drive toward independence and could cause behavioral problems or depression.

We often see unintentional overprotection—cases in which caregivers do things that the person with DS could do, but less quickly and efficiently. It's important to find a balance between the needs of the household and the needs of the person with DS. For example, in families where both parents work, there often is not time for the person with DS to do tasks at his or her own speed, such as helping to get dinner on the table or doing laundry. So whenever possible, people with DS should be allowed to manage their own daily living tasks, particularly when these tasks help them develop new skills or use a trial-and-error approach. Successfully completing new tasks will build their experience and increase their confidence when dealing with new and challenging situations, such as the difficult transition from school to work.

On the other hand, sometimes the problem is too much independence, and a person's health, safety, and self-esteem are at risk. We know of one example in which an older woman in an agency-run apartment was unable to manage on her own. Her home and her life were in shambles. Besides allowing her apartment to become littered with spoiled food, unpaid bills, and dirty laundry, she was frequenting a local tavern, which created an alcohol addiction and an extreme safety risk. She was pleased to be moved into a small, supervised group home because it allowed her to regain her feelings of competence and self-esteem.

Appropriate levels of supervision are helpful in resolving problems with independent living. People with DS should be allowed challenge and independence, but never at the risk of their health and safety.

## Assessing Skill Loss

When people with DS have difficulty expressing themselves, a loss of daily living skills can be a very telling indicator of problems, concerns, or life issues. Normal aging, mental health conditions, sensory difficulties, or medical conditions may cause skill loss. It is important that caregivers consider underlying causes and, when indicated, seek assistance in making the correct assessment.

The normal aging process is accelerated in adults with DS, who age some 10–20 years earlier than the general population. Caregivers often perceive this premature aging as a shortened middle age or a rapid onset of aging; accordingly, a 40- or 50-year-old person may be more like someone who is 60 or 70. Skill loss at what would be considered an early age can actually be the result of the normal aging process associated with DS.

We tell caregivers that, like retirees in the general population, adults with DS who remain active are more likely to live longer and healthier lives. Those in a community setting can maintain their skills and even slow the aging process. Even when they lose interest in formal work pursuits or retire from them, aging adults with DS should still be involved in many social and recreational activities.

Some care providers may not understand how a person with DS ages and may misinterpret a slowdown in work or other activities as a symptom of Alzheimer disease or a behavior problem. This may lead to a consideration of discharging the person with DS from his work setting or transferring him to a different living setting. An improved knowledge of the aging process should help families and care providers and encourage them to develop new programs and services to meet the needs of the aging person with DS.

Other conditions may cause a significant loss in daily living skills. Vision or hearing loss, which occurs more frequently than in the general population, could be at the root of the problem. Depression or other mental health disorders could be a factor, as well as medical conditions such as hypothyroidism. Treatment for these conditions is readily available and could help forestall loss of skills.

Alzheimer disease is often blamed as the cause of skill loss in older people with DS. On the basis of the findings of studies (Dalton and Crapper-McLachlan, 1984; Lai and Williams, 1989; Oliver and Holland, 1986), a decline in a person with DS was commonly believed to always be secondary to Alzheimer disease, a progressive and irreversible condition. Recent research has found that when Alzheimer disease develops in a person with DS, it often occurs at a younger age, possibly because of premature aging, (Devenny et al., 1996; Wisniewski and Rabe, 1986). However, when a person with DS declines, with a thorough evaluation, the diagnosis is often found to be something else that is potentially reversible (Chicoine et al., 1999). Misdiagnosis and consequent ineffective treatment are often the result of an assumption that a decline in function in a person with DS is Alzheimer disease.

The thorough evaluation of a person whose skills are declining is critical. In our own clinical sample of 443 people, 148 (33%) showed loss of skills. Of those 148, only 11 people—just 7%—were diagnosed with Alzheimer disease. For those over 40—the age group most at risk for Alzheimer's—11 of 53 people with skill loss were diagnosed with the disease. The remaining 42 people responded positively to medical or mental health treatments or to remedial treatment for sensory impairment.

The message for caregivers is obvious: Insist on a comprehensive evaluation before accepting a diagnosis of Alzheimer disease.

## EXPRESSIVE LANGUAGE

People with DS often find it difficult to speak clearly and to express their thoughts and feelings effectively. Many engage in self-talk, which is described as a conversation with oneself that is spoken out loud.

Intelligibility is the degree to which others understand spoken language. Most adults with DS experience some degree of difficulty being understood by anyone other than their caregivers. This situation can lead to dependence on the people who best understand what is being said, and problems can arise when those "interpreters" are unavailable. A person who loses an understanding listener can feel lost and disoriented, which in turn may lead to adjustment problems and depression. We have found that people with a wide circle of family and friends have fewer difficulties adjusting to the loss of one such person. Learning sign language or an alternative way to communicate can also help to prevent dependence on just a few people.

Even if they can speak intelligibly, it is our experience that many adults with DS have a difficult time telling others about their personal thoughts and feelings. Even when they can convey strong emotions through facial expressions and body language, often their caregivers cannot understand and respond to what is being communicated. This is particularly true on the job and in other outside settings with people who are less familiar with the person with DS.

To remedy this, family or caregivers can teach staff at work and in residential settings how to better interpret the nonverbal expressions of the person with DS. This will help the person feel more confident and competent. And the more people there are who understand him or her, the less likely the person with DS is to suffer when one of them moves out of his or her life.

Families tell us they often hear their relative with DS talking out loud about the events of the day, much as we would review our day in our minds (McGuire et al., 1997). One parent responded to his son's particularly loud self-talk by knocking on his bedroom door and asking, "WHO are you talking to in there?" This answer was fired back: "MYSELF! Who do you think?"

Given the cognitive level of most adults with DS, we believe that self-talk is not inappropriate. In the general population, self-talk is usually internalized between the ages of 5 and 7, but self-talk in adults with DS continues to serve as an adaptive mechanism. It helps them to plan action and practice alternatives, review daily occurrences, entertain themselves when they are alone, and vent feelings they cannot readily express to others.

It's important to know that when self-talk changes dramatically in tone and incidence, it may signal a psychological problem such as depression, anxiety, physical pain, or illness. Conversations may become angry and animated. Other indications are hallucinatory-like conversations with imagined others, self-absorption, and increased self-talk in public. Fortunately, antidepressants are very effective in treating this and other symptoms of depression or anxiety. It has been noted that because this behavior may be misdiagnosed as a psychosis (McGuire and Chicoine, 1996; Sovner, 1986), it may be treated with antipsychotic medications. These carry a greater risk of side effects than antidepressants (Sovner and DesNoyers, 1993). If a person with DS requires treatment, caregivers and practitioners should be aware of this issue to ensure that appropriate medications are prescribed.

## BELIEFS

How people with DS view themselves and how confident they are in dealing with the world are fundamental to successful adaptiveness (Bandura 1971; Beck, 1976). However, it is difficult for adults with DS to generate positive feelings about themselves. Within the two key areas of self-esteem and competence, we have identified three beliefs that affect adults with DS— stigmatization, accepting disability, and demoralization.

## STIGMATIZATION

People with DS are minority members of society, and because they are easily identified, they are often defined and treated as different. This stigma that society attaches to DS may profoundly influence the self-esteem of people with DS (Gibbons, 1985; Reiss et al., 1982). Stigmatization may not be obvious in young children, but when they reach adolescence, people with DS often become aware of the realities of their lives, particularly when they compare themselves to siblings who go to college, move out on their own, or get married. For example, for a long time after her younger sister's wedding, one young woman with DS was cross, moody, and withdrawn. In time, she was able to explain that she was upset because she would probably never marry, live independently, or have an "important job" like her sister.

Some people with DS are not able to verbalize these feelings and become frustrated and demoralized. They may withdraw into anger or depression. It is our experience that although some reaction to these stigmatizing realities is inevitable, people who have more choices and opportunities in their work, social, and recreational spheres are less likely to be seriously affected by limitations and stigma in their lives.

## ACCEPTING DISABILITY

At some point in their adult lives, most people with DS deal with the usual identity issues of who they are. However, we have found that many people have not been given an opportunity to discuss the most basic issue of their identity—the fact that they have DS. Encouraging dialogue at the appropriate time can help people with DS better understand and accept their condition. Bolstered by self-acceptance, they are often happier. Additionally, they are more likely to make the best use of their resources and abilities and to advocate more effectively for their rights and needs.

A second issue in the arena of acceptance is the attitude of a person with DS toward others with disabilities. Some feel an aversion to associating with people with disabilities. This can be problematic, as it severely limits their opportunities to make friends. Because everyone tends to associate with others at the same cognitive level, people with DS who refuse to have anything to do with those who are disabled can find themselves in a "social no-man's land": Some in the general population do not accept them, and they deliberately disengage from peers with disabilities.

This attitude can be relatively short lived, but we have found it to be more lasting in "higher-functioning" individuals, who may be more sensitive to the stigmatizing realities of life with DS. Assuming this aversion is driven by a negative self-image, we have learned that giving these people opportunities to become peer leaders or assistants often leads to their feeling better about themselves and others.

## Demoralization in the Workplace

Studies have shown that many people with disabilities are deeply frustrated and demoralized in the workplace (Zetlin and Turner, 1985; Weyman et al., 1988). Moreover, their sense of competence can be adversely affected by the limited number of jobs available to them and by the lack of independence and control they have over their own lives (Weyman et al., 1988). These studies also indicate that many people fall far short of meeting their life goals. Our own clinical sample has shown some evidence of demoralization, which we have found to be a contributing factor to a diagnosis of depression.

Studies suggest ways to decrease demoralization in the workplace (Weyman et al, 1988). Research shows that people who are most likely to get and keep a community job after graduating from school are those who had previous work experience in the community (Hasazi et al., 1985). It is important to note, however, that job success does not necessarily depend on getting a paycheck. Volunteer work can bring meaning and purpose to many people's lives.

Most people are demoralized when they have had no say in where they work. Meeting family expectations is not nearly as important as meeting the needs and wants of the person with DS. For example, the family may suggest a community job, but the person with DS would be happier working with his friends in a more sheltered work setting. Conversely, a family preference for the relative safety of the workshop setting may feel stifling to a person with DS who wants to work in the community. As we know, it often is not easy for a person with DS to express thoughts and feelings, so discontent may be communicated inappropriately. One young man working in a grocery store tossed carts into the road; another simply sat down on the job. Caregivers, although well meaning, should avoid imposing their wishes or need on people with DS. An ideal approach would be to offer a choice of work situations, even if among only a few options.

## Social and Interpersonal Skills

There is a great deal of research on the importance of social and interpersonal skills for adaptation and well-being (Greenspan and Grandfield, 1992). A lack of these skills is associated with adjustment difficulties and mental health problems, and a strong association has been demonstrated between poor social skills and depression (Reiss and Benson, 1985).

Poor social skills also play a role in job failure (Greenspan and Shoultz, 1981; Martin et al, 1986). Unfortunately, most job coaches do not teach the skills that help people keep their jobs. Workers with DS should be taught how to restrict self-talk on the job, how to get ready and dress appropriately for work, and how and when to address their fellow employees as well as their supervisor.

In our clinical group, we have experienced relatively few instances of rude or offensive behavior. More often, inappropriate displays of affection—primarily hugging—have been the issue. For most people, this conduct is easily corrected with training and social experience.

Social interaction presents a much larger problem for people with DS. It is often difficult for them to start and participate in a conversation, to show interest in another person, or to take another person's perspective in a social setting (Greenspan and Grandfield, 1992). These limitations have given rise to some questions on the quality of friendships among people with disabilities (Clegg and Standen, 1991). However, caregivers report that for the most part, peer relationships are strong, long-lived, and critically important. They say these friendships develop over a period of time and familiarity, such as when people share a job site or school program for many years. The value of time and familiarity has been demonstrated even for people with severe cognitive disabilities, who may have been considered to have few or no relationships.

Consequently, life changes that separate friends can be devastating. A person with DS may become overwhelmed when faced with starting over with unfamiliar people. This can hinder his or her adjustment and can lead to depression. It is possible, however, to minimize personal losses by ensuring that people have other sources of friends besides work or school. Ideally, these should be ongoing social and recreational programs that foster relationships over time with a consistent group of people.

## MENTAL AND BEHAVIORAL FLEXIBILITY

The reason that many adults with DS find life changes difficult is that they need consistency, repetition, and order in their lives. We call this tendency "the groove" (McGuire, 1999). In the general population this tendency may be considered an obsessive-compulsive behavior, but for people with DS grooves can help them manage and cope with the stress and strain of daily life.

When tasks are clearly laid out and schedules are routine, most people with DS do very well. Their grooves provide them with a sense of order and structure. Grooves also help people who process things slowly in a fast-moving world have more control over their lives. In addition, because they help people organize and manage daily tasks, grooves actually promote independence.

Although many adults with DS will adapt to major changes when given adequate time and preparation, those who do not can develop an obsessive-compulsive disorder (Vitello et al, 1989). Among the signs of this disorder are extremely repetitious activities, a slowdown in behavior, and an over-reliance on a precise way of doing things (McGuire and Chicoine, 1995).

To prevent a groove from becoming a disorder, it is important that people with DS be encouraged to deal with and surmount day-to-day challenges. This will better equip them to handle significant changes they will inevitably face.

## Promoting Health

Being healthy means much more than not being sick. Health is a state of physical and mental well-being that can only be achieved when we make intelligent and informed choices about how we care for ourselves. This is as true for people with DS as it is for the general population.

### Nutrition

Although people with DS are less likely to develop heart disease and high blood pressure (Brattstrom et al., 1987), nutritional recommendations for them are much the same as for the general population. In a nutshell, this means following a diet that is high in complex carbohydrates and low in fat (the familiar food pyramid model).

Obesity is common in people with DS, and recent research (Rubin et al., 1998) suggests that it be considered a major public health concern that warrants continuing research. Other studies indicate that children with DS have a slower metabolism (Luke et al., 1994) than the general population. On average, people with DS burn 200–300 fewer calories per day while at rest. In addition, trying to correct for the slower metabolism by only reducing calories can lead to nutritional deficiencies, and, therefore, adults with DS need to increase their physical activity to keep from gaining weight.

In our clinical sample, restricting deserts and snacks is not as successful as offering healthy, low-fat alternatives such as fruit, vegetables, popcorn, and pretzels. The traditional medical advice still holds true today—in the long run, the best health results are achieved not by dieting, but by eating sensible, nutritious meals and getting regular exercise.

### Exercise

What do we mean by regular exercise? Generally, this consists of 20–30 minutes of aerobic exercise at least 3 days a week. Aerobic exercises include brisk walking, jogging, swimming, bicycling, and cross-country skiing. However, we have found that access to social activities, not necessarily exercise, helps people with DS stay closer to their ideal body weight (Fujura et al., 1997). Drama groups, gardening, trips to museums and other activities are all beneficial.

Doctors often suggest that anyone contemplating an exercise program get a physical exam first. This is particularly important for people with DS, who may have certain physical conditions that can be affected by exertion.

Some 40–50% of babies born with DS have congenital heart disease (Greenwood and Nadas, 1976). This may be corrected before adulthood, but not all people with DS have undergone this surgery. Furthermore, a few studies show that in later life adults with DS may develop valvular heart disease. Obviously, it is important that a doctor evaluate the person's condition before he or she begins an exercise regime. It may be necessary to restrict the length or intensity of exercise.

Exercise restrictions may also be necessary if a person has atlantoaxial instability, a condition in which the first vertebra in the neck slips onto the second. It is more common in people with DS (Pueschel and Scola, 1987), and contact sports and activities that might jar the neck could be dangerous. That's why Special Olympics requires that children with DS undergo a diagnostic lateral neck X ray before they participate in their program.

Researchers have not delved very far into the subject of exercise and people with DS. It is well known that in the general population exercise helps to improve people's fitness, self-esteem, and overall sense of well-being (Simon, 1985). Moreover, it is an excellent mechanism to help people deal with stress and minimize its effects.

## SLEEP

Getting enough sleep is critical to good health. How much is enough varies from person to person, but after a good night's sleep people should feel energetic all day long.

Many families have commented on the sleeping position of their son or daughter with DS—bent at the waist, with the head resting on the legs. In itself, this does not appear to be a significant problem. However, an unusual sleeping position could be a sign of sleep apnea. People with DS have a higher incidence of sleep apnea, which is characterized by restless sleeping, irregular breathing, snoring or snorting, and daytime sleepiness. It is most often caused by an obstruction in the airway and may cause heart disease and other health problems. An evaluation through a comprehensive sleep study has proven helpful with many individuals with DS.

## SOCIAL OPPORTUNITIES

We have already demonstrated that adults with DS tend to be healthier when they are active socially—with friends, family, and co-workers. By taking advantage of social opportunities, they bolster their sense of self-esteem, well-being, and happiness. Studies in the general population, as well as our study of persons with DS, support the notion that these feelings contribute to general good health. In the general population, studies link depression and stress to decreased immunity and increased illness.

## PREVENTIVE MEASURES

### IMMUNIZATIONS

We recommend that all adults with DS receive appropriate immunizations. A diphtheria-tetanus booster every 10 years is advised. People over 65 and those with certain chronic illnesses should get a flu shot each year, as well as a one-time pneumonia vaccine. Some researchers suggest that adults with DS be given flu and pneumonia vaccines in their fifties because of their relatively weaker immune systems. Additionally, all people living in residential facilities and those with a high potential of exposure to influenza should get an annual flu shot. Other children and young adults with DS do not necessarily need to receive these immunizations unless they have congenital heart problems or recurrent pneumonia.

The hepatitis B immunization, a three-shot series, is recommended for people living in residential facilities. Some studies have found adults with DS to be at greater risk of contracting hepatitis B, possibly in workshops and other group settings. Although the risk of transmission of hepatitis B virus is greater in people who share needles and have multiple sexual partners, the virus can be shed in all body secretions. This means that people can get hepatitis B in settings where hygiene practices are not up to par or where they might come in contact with the secretions of an infected person.

Varicella (chicken pox) vaccine is recommended for those who have not previously had chicken pox. We recommend checking a blood test to see whether the person is already immune to chicken pox. Apparently many people who do not recall having chicken pox have had an unrecognized mild case. If the blood test demonstrates immunity, the vaccine is not needed.

### ANTIBIOTIC PROPHYLAXIS

Antibiotic prophylaxis simply means taking an antibiotic before certain medical procedures to prevent infection. Some people with congenital heart disease need to take antibiotics before going to the dentist, even for a routine cleaning. This will avert an infection in the heart. They also will take medication when undergoing gastrointestinal or urinary tract procedures.

### SEX EDUCATION

Adults with DS often lack information about sexuality and reproduction. Men with DS are usually sterile, although there is one reported case of a man with DS fathering a child. Women with DS have a slightly reduced fertility rate, but they can conceive and bear children. Roughly half of the children born to women with DS will also have the condition.

In terms of birth control, oral contraceptives, Depo-Provera, and Norplant have fewer medical complications than tubal ligation. Barrier methods—condoms and diaphragms—are often ineffective because of the limitations of the person to use them correctly each time.

Sexual abuse is a serious concern and should be addressed even if a person is using birth control or has been sterilized.

## HEALTH SCREENING AND TREATING MEDICAL PROBLEMS

The same routine health screening recommended for the general population is advised for adults with DS as well. Currently, this includes mammograms, Pap smears, testing for colorectal cancer, and cholesterol screening. Further study of the frequency of these diseases in people with DS could alter these recommendations.

During the medical history and physical exam, the doctor should pay special attention to conditions more common in adults with DS. The Down Syndrome Medical Checklist (Cohen, 1999) suggests an annual physical, including a thyroid screening for both hypothyroidism and hyperthyroidism (underactive or overactive thyroid gland). We also recommend neck X rays to screen for atlantoaxial instability if not previously done. Hearing and vision tests are recommended every year or two.

### EYESIGHT

Poor eyesight is as common among people with DS as it is in the general population. However, it may be difficult for a person with DS to perceive the problem or communicate it to someone who can help. If work or daily skills deteriorate, the fix could be as simple as a pair of glasses.

### HEARING

Hearing loss is more common in adults with DS (Evenhuis et al., 1992). This can be the result of fluid behind the eardrum or a buildup of wax in the ear canal, both of which are relatively easily corrected. More serious problems would be an inner ear condition common to people with DS that affects their ability to hear high-pitched sounds, including many speech consonants. If hearing loss is suspected, an evaluation by an audiologist is recommended.

### TEETH AND GUMS

Cavities are less common in people with DS, but there is a tendency toward periodontal (gum) disease. Gum disease can lead to tooth loss. Good oral hygiene and regular dental visits can keep gum disease under control.

## GYNECOLOGIC HEALTH

General gynecologic care includes daily care and hygiene as well as routine medical care. It is important that a woman with DS learn proper self-care and that she be well prepared for her gynecologic examination. Sometimes a pelvic ultrasound can yield information if an exam is not possible.

Like the general population, women with DS can experience painful menstrual periods as well as premenstrual syndrome (PMS). Because she might not be able to communicate her pain, a change in behavior at the time of her period might be the only sign her caregivers will perceive. Caregivers also should be alert to behavior changes that occur cyclically, which could signal PMS.

## ORTHOPEDIC ISSUES

We have discussed atlantoaxial instability as an issue in exercise. It also must be considered in a presurgical examination. People with this condition can receive a severe neck injury when their neck is extended to insert the endo-tracheal (breathing) tube. It is critical for the anesthesiologist to make adjustments to prevent injury to the patient. Even if the surgical patient with DS has not been shown to have atlantoaxial instability, special care should be given to his neck during anesthesia. In addition, as joints age and degenerate, even in a person who did not previously have atlantoaxial instability, increased mobility may occur. This can lead to spinal cord compression. Symptoms of weakness of the arms and/or legs, onset of incontinence of urine or stool, unsteady gait, pain in the neck, and tilting of the head can be symptoms of instability of the cervical spine and should be evaluated with neck X rays and possibly computed tomography (CT) and/or magnetic resonance imaging (MRI) scans.

## MENTAL HEALTH

Several critical aspects of a healthy life foster good mental health in both people with DS and in the general population.

Being able to communicate with others significantly impacts one's mental health. Besides speech therapy, tools such as communication boards and sign language can augment weak communications skills. However, we have noted that people with DS can find it difficult to convey their emotions adequately even when verbal skills are good. Sometimes it is helpful for people with DS to gather with other adults with developmental disabilities to share their experiences.

Living in a place that is comfortable and safe and having a job that is interesting and stimulating bolster self-esteem and feelings of accomplishment. Opportunities for recreation and relationships with family and friends promote both physical and mental health.

It is important to assess a person's mental health within the framework of his or her life and skills. Then, if evaluation reveals mental illness, it may be easier to isolate the problem and develop a treatment plan.

## Depression

Depression, which occurs slightly more often than in the general population, can be difficult to identify in people with DS. Lack of verbal skills, as in other situations, contributes to the difficulty in diagnosing and treating depression. Untreated, depression can last for years. Fortunately, treatment can bring about remarkable improvement in daily living skills, motivation, and interaction with others.

Antidepressants, group or individual therapy, and taking part in daily activities—particularly exercise—are all beneficial in lifting a patient out of depression. Occasionally, the patient will need additional help from occupational therapists, respite workers, and others to recover fully.

## Obsessive-Compulsive Disorder

Obsessive-compulsive disorder (OCD) can occur with depression or on its own and is probably more common in people with DS. In addition to medication, a person with OCD will often respond to a restructured environment that reduces the frustration of the compulsion.

## Other Mental Health Disorders

Although people with DS can develop psychological problems such as attention-deficit hyperactivity disorder (ADHD) and bipolar disorder (manic-depression), there is no evidence that these occur with any more frequency than in the general population. As a matter of fact, schizophrenia is thought to be uncommon in people with DS.

## Conclusion

Most adults with DS can live healthy lives. Caregivers and the professionals who work with them can help people with DS follow the multifaceted approach to good health recommended in this article. That approach includes having a healthy lifestyle, following certain preventive measures, participating in appropriate health screening, and treating health problems early in their course. We know that some disorders occur more frequently in people with DS, but some occur less frequently, too. Being aware of the health and psychosocial issues unique to people with DS is the first step toward helping them live a full and happy life.

## Acknowledgments

Work for this chapter was partially funded by the Research and Training Center on Aging with Mental Retardation, Institute on Disability and Human Development, the University of Illinois at Chicago, funded by the U.S. Department of Education National Institute on Disability and Rehabilitation Research, Grant No. H133b30069.

## References

Bandura A (1971): "Social Learning Theory." New York: General Learning Press.

Beck AT (1976): "Cognitive Therapy and Emotional Disorders." New York: International Universities Press.

Brattstrom L, England E, Bun A (1987): Does Down syndrome support homocysteine theory of arthersosclerosis? Lancet I:391–397.

Brown MC, Hanley, AT, Nemeth C, Epple W, Bird D, Bontempo T (1986): The developmental disability profile. New York State Office of Mental Retardation and Developmental Disabilities.

Chicoine B, McGuire D (1996): Promoting health in adults with Down syndrome. Document available through the Clearinghouse on Aging and Developmental Disabilities of the RTC on Aging in Persons with Mental Retardation, The Institute on Disability and Human Development, the University of Illinois at Chicago.

Chicoine B, McGuire D, Hebein S, Gilly, D (1995): The development of a clinic for adults with Down syndrome. Ment Retard 32:100–106.

Chicoine B, McGuire D, Rubin, S (1999): Specialty Clinic Perspectives. In Janicki, M. and Dalton, A. (eds.), Dementia, Aging, and Intellectual Disabilities: A Handbook. (pp 278–293). Philadelphia: Taylor and Francis.

Clegg JA, Standen PJ (1991): Friendships among adults who have developmental disabilities. Am J Ment Retard 95:663–672.

Cohen WI (ed.) (1999): Health Care Guidelines for Individuals with Down Syndrome—1999 Revision. Down Syndrome Q 4(3):1–16.

www.denison.edu/dsq/health99.htm

Dalton, AJ, Crapper-McLachlan DR (1984): Clinical expression of Alzheimer's disease in Down's syndrome. Psychol Clin North Am 9:659–670.

Devenny DA, Silverman WP, Hill AL, Jenkins E, Sersen EA, Wisnewshi KE (1996): Normal aging in adults with Down's syndrome: a longitudinal study. J Intellect Dis Res 40:208–221.

Evenhuis HM, Van Zanten GA, Brocaar MP, Roerdinkholder WHM (1992): Hearing loss in middle-age persons with Down syndrome. Am J Ment Retard 97:47–56.

Eyman R, Call T, White J (1991): Life expectancy of persons with Down syndrome. Am J Ment Retard 95:603–612.

Fujura GT, Fitzsimons N, Marks B, Chicoine B. (1997): Predictors of BMI among adults with Down syndrome: The social context of health promotion:. Res Dev Disabil 18(4): 261–274.

Gibbons FX (1985): Stigma perception: social comparisons among mentally retarded persons. Am J Ment Defic 90:98–106.

Greenspan S, Grandfield JM (1992): Reconsidering the construct of mental retardation: implications of a model of social competence. Am J Ment Retard 96:442–453.

Greenspan S, Shoultz J (1981): Why mentally retarded adults lose their jobs. Social competence as a factor in work adjustment. Appl Res Ment Retard 2:23–38.

Greeswood RD, Nadas AD (1976): The clinical cause of cardiac disease in Down's syndrome. Pediatrics 58:278–281.

Hasazi SB, Gordon LR, Roe CA, Finck K, Hull M, Salembier G (1985): A statewide follow-up on post high school employment and residential status of students labesed "mentally retarded." Educ Training Ment Restard 14:222–234.

Lai F, Williams RS (1989): A prospective study of Alzheimer disease in Down sundrome individuals. Arch Neurol 46:377–385.

Luke A, Rozien NJ, Sutton M, Schoeller DA (1994): Energy expenditure in children with Down syndrome: correcting metabolic rate for movement. J Pediatr 125:829–838.

Martin JE, Rusch FR, Lagomarcino T, Chadsey-Rusch JR (1986): Comparisions between workers who are nonhandicapped and mentally retarded: why they lose their jobs. Appl Res Ment Retard 7:476–474.

McGuire D. (1999): The Groove. NADS Newsletter, 6–7.

McGuire D, Chicoine, B (1996): Depressive disorders in adults with Down Syndrome. Hab Ment Healthcare Newsl 1:1–7.

McGuire D, Chicoine B, Greenbaum E. (1997): "Self-talk" in adults with Down syndrome. Disability Solutions 2(1): 1–4.

Oliver C, Holland AJ (1986): Down sydrome and Alzheimer's disease: a review. Psychol Med 16:307–322.

Pueschel SM, Pezzullo JC (1985): Thyroid dysfunction in Down syndrome. Am J Disease Child 139:636–639.

Pueschel SM, Scola FH (1987): Atlantoaxial instability in individuals with Down syndrome: epidemiologic, radiographic, and clinical studies. Pediatrics 80:555–560.

Rubin SS, Rimmer JH, Chicoine B, Braddock D, McGuire DE (1998): Overweight prevalence in persons with Down syndrome. Ment Retard 36(3): 175–181.

# HEALTH CARE GUIDELINES FOR INDIVIDUALS WITH DOWN SYNDROME—1999 REVISION[1]

## WILLIAM I. COHEN, M.D.

[Author's Note: The vagaries of book publishing are such that this chapter, which consists of the 1999 Revision of the "Health Care Guidelines [HCG] for Individuals with Down Syndrome" will be published close in time to the expected publication of the next revision of the HCG due in 2002. The Down Syndrome Medical Interest Group (DSMIG), which is responsible for the guidelines, anticipates only minor revisions of the guidelines. DSMIG is currently developing parallel guidelines for motor development, speech and language development, education, and behavior. Like the HCG themselves, they will be published in *Down Syndrome Quarterly* and likewise, they will be available on the World Wide Web at *www.denison.edu/dsq/*.

This version of the Guidelines is significant because it coordinates closely with "Health Supervision for Children with Down Syndrome" published by the Committee on Genetics of the American Academy of Pediatrics

[1] Health Care Guidelines for Individuals with Down Syndrome: 1999 Revision (Down Syndrome Preventive Medical Check List) is published in *Down Syndrome Quarterly* (Volume 4, Number 3, September, 1999, pp. 1-16), and these excerpts are reprinted with permission of the Editor. Information concerning publication policy or subscriptions may be obtained by contacting Dr. Samuel J. Thios, Editor, Denison University, Granville, OH 43023 (E-mail: thios@denison.edu).

*Down Syndrome,* Edited by William I. Cohen, Lynn Nadel, and Myra E. Madnick.
ISBN 0-471-41815-3   Copyright © 2002 by Wiley-Liss, Inc.

(AAP) in 2001. The only substantial difference is the fact that the AAP does not currently recommend screening for celiac disease.

What follows is a summary of the key points of the Health Care Guidelines, grouped by age.]

## NEONATAL (BIRTH TO 1 MONTH)

### HISTORY

Review parental concerns. Was there a prenatal diagnosis of Down syndrome (DS)? With vomiting or absence of stools, check for gastrointestinal tract blockage (duodenal web or atresia, or Hirschsprung disease); review feeding history to ensure adequate caloric intake. Any concerns about hearing or vision? Inquire about family support.

### EXAM

Pay special attention to cardiac examination, cataracts (refer immediately to an ophthalmologist if the red reflex is not seen), otitis media, subjective assessment of hearing, and fontanelles (widely open posterior fontanelle may signify hypothyroidism). Exam for plethora, thrombocytopenia.

### LAB AND CONSULTS

Chromosomal karyotype; genetic counseling; hematocrit or complete blood count to investigate plethora (polycythemia) or thrombocytopenia (possible myeloproliferative disorders); thyroid function test: check on results of state-mandated screening; evaluation by a pediatric cardiologist including echocardiogram (even in the absence of a murmur); reinforce the need for subacute bacterial endocarditis (SBE) prophylaxis in susceptible children with cardiac disease; refer for auditory brain stem response (ABR) or otoacoustic emission (OAE) test to assess congenital sensorineural hearing loss at birth or by 3 months of age. Refer for a pediatric ophthalmological evaluation by 6 months of age for screening purposes. Refer immediately if there are any indications of nystagmus, strabismus, or poor vision. If feeding difficulties are noted, consultation with a feeding specialist (occupational therapist or lactation nurse) is advised.

### DEVELOPMENTAL

Discuss value of early intervention (infant stimulation) and refer for enrollment in local program. Parents at this stage often ask for predictions of their child's abilities: "Can you tell how severe it is?" This is an opportunity to discuss the unfolding nature of their child's development, the importance of developmental programming, and our expectation of being able to answer that question closer to 2 years of age.

## RECOMMENDATIONS

Referral to local DS parent group for family support, as indicated.

## INFANCY (1–12 MONTHS)

### HISTORY

Review parental concerns. Question about respiratory infections (especially otitis media); for constipation, use aggressive dietary management and consider Hirschsprung disease if resistant to dietary changes and stool softeners. Solicit parental concerns regarding vision and hearing.

### EXAM

General neurological, neuromotor, and musculoskeletal examination; must visualize tympanic membranes or refer to ear, nose, and throat (ENT) specialist, especially if suspicious of otitis media.

### LAB AND CONSULTS

Evaluation by a pediatric cardiologist including echocardiogram (if not done in newborn period): remember to consider progressive pulmonary hypertension in DS patients with a ventricular septal defect or atrioventricular septal defect who are having few or no symptoms of heart failure in this age group. ABR by 3 months of age if not performed previously or if previous results are suspicious. Pediatric ophthalmology evaluation by 6 months of age (earlier if nystagmus, strabismus, or indications of poor vision are present). Thyroid function test (TSH and $T_4$), at 6 and 12 months of age. Evaluation by ENT specialist for recurrent otitis media as needed.

### DEVELOPMENTAL

Discuss early intervention and refer for enrollment in local program (if not done during the neonatal period). This usually includes physical and occupational therapy evaluations and a developmental assessment.

## Recommendations

Application for Supplemental Security Income (SSI) (depending on family income); consider estate planning and custody arrangements; continue family support; continue SBE prophylaxis for children with cardiac defects.

## Childhood (1 Year to 12 Years)

### History

Review parental concerns; current level of functioning; review current programming (early intervention, preschool, school); ear problems; sleep problems (snoring or restless sleep might indicate obstructive sleep apnea); constipation; review audiologic and thyroid function tests; review ophthalmologic and dental care. Monitor for behavior problems.

### Exam

General pediatric and neurological exam including evaluation for signs of spinal cord compression: deep tendon reflexes, gait, Babinski sign. Include a brief vulvar exam for girls. Use DS growth charts as well as growth charts for typically developing children. Be sure to plot height for weight on the latter chart.

### Lab and Consults

Echocardiogram by a pediatric cardiologist if not done previously; Thyroid function test (TSH and $T_4$) yearly; behavioral auditory testing every 6 months until 3 years of age, then yearly. Continue regular eye exams every year if normal, or more frequently as indicated. Between 3 years and 5 years of age, lateral cervical spine X rays (neutral view, flexion and extension) to rule out atlantoaxial instability: have the radiologist measure the atlanto-dens distance and the neural canal width. X rays should be performed at an institution accustomed to taking and reading these X rays. Initial dental evaluation at 2 years of age with follow-ups every 6 months. At 2–3 years of age, screen for celiac disease with IgA anti-endomysium antibodies as well as total IgA.

### Developmental

Enrollment in appropriate developmental or educational program; complete educational assessment yearly, as part of individualized family service plan (IFSP) for children from birth to 3 years of age, or individualized educational plan (IEP) from age 4 until the end of formal schooling. Evaluation by a speech and language pathologist is strongly recommended to maximize language development and verbal communication. An individual with significant communication deficits may be a candidate for an augmentative communication device.

## Recommendations

Twice-daily teeth brushing. Total caloric intake should be below recommended daily allowance (RDA) for children of similar height and age. Monitor for well-balanced, high-fiber diet. Regular exercise and recreational programs should be established early. Continue speech therapy and physical therapy as needed. Continue SBE prophylaxis for children with cardiac defects. Monitor the family's need for respite care, supportive counseling and behavior management techniques. Reinforce the importance of good self-care skills (grooming, dressing, and money handling skills).

## Adolescence (12 Years to 18 Years)

### History

Review interval medical history, questioning specifically about the possibility of obstructive airway disease and sleep apnea; check sensory functioning (vision and hearing); assess for behavioral problems; address sexuality issues.

### Exam

General physical and neurological examination (with reference to atlantoaxial dislocation). Monitor for obesity by plotting height for weight on the growth charts for typical children. Pelvic exam if sexually active only. (See Consults, below.) Perform a careful cardiac exam in adolescents, looking for evidence of valvular disease.

### Lab and Consults

Thyroid function testing (TSH) yearly. Hearing and vision evaluations every year. Repeat screening cervical spine X rays as needed for Special Olympic participation. Echocardiogram if evidence of valvular disease on clinical exam. Consult with adolescent medicine practitioner or a gynecologist experienced in working with individuals with developmental disabilities to address issues of sexuality and/or for pelvic examination for sexually active teenager. Continue twice-yearly dental exams.

## Developmental

Repeat psychoeducational evaluations every 2 years as part of IEP. Monitor independent functioning. Continue speech/language therapy as needed. Health and sex education, including counseling regarding abuse prevention. Smoking, drug, and alcohol education.

## Recommendations

Begin functional transition planning (age 16). Consider enrollment for SSI depending on family income. SBE prophylaxis needed for individuals with cardiac disease. Continue dietary and exercise recommendations (see Childhood, above). Update estate planning and custody arrangements. Encourage social and recreational programs with friends. Register for voting and Selective Service at age 18. Discuss plans for alternative long-term living arrangements such as community living arrangements (CLA). Reinforce the importance of good self-care skills (grooming, dressing, and money handling skills).

## Adults (Over 18 Years)

### History

Interval medical history. Ask about sleep apnea symptoms. Monitor for loss of independence in living skills, behavioral changes, and/or mental health problems. Symptoms of dementia (decline in function, memory loss, ataxia, seizures, and incontinence of urine and/or stool); this may also represent spinal cord compression from atlantoaxial subluxation.

### Exam

General physical and neurological examination (with reference to atlantoaxial dislocation). Monitor for obesity by plotting height for weight. Cardiac exam: listen for evidence of mitral valve prolapse and aortic regurgitation; confirm suspicions with echocardiogram. Sexually active women will need Pap smears every 1–3 years after the age of first intercourse. For women who are not sexually active, single-finger bimanual examination with finger-directed cytology exam. Screening pelvic ultrasound every 2–3 years for women who refuse or have inadequate follow-up bimanual examinations. This may require referral to an adolescent medicine practitioner or a gynecologist with experience with individuals with special needs. Otherwise, pelvic ultrasound may be considered in place of pelvic examinations. Breast exam yearly by physician.

## LAB AND CONSULTS

Annual thyroid screening (TSH and $T_4$). Ophthalmologic evaluation every 2 years (looking especially for keratoconus and cataracts). Repeat cervical spine X rays as needed for Special Olympic participation. Continue auditory testing every 2 years. There are two different suggestions for mammography: Dr. Heaton recommends yearly study after age 50 or beginning at age 40 for women with a first-degree relative with breast cancer. Dr. Chicoine suggests a mammogram every other year beginning at 40 and yearly beginning at 50. Continue twice-yearly dental visits. Mental health referral for individuals with emotional and behavioral changes.

## DEVELOPMENTAL

Continue speech and language therapy, as indicated. For individuals with poor expressive language skills, consider referral for augmentative communication device. Discuss plans for further programming/vocational opportunities at age 21 or when formal schooling ends. Be aware that accelerated aging may affect functional abilities of adults with DS, more so than Alzheimer disease.

## RECOMMENDATIONS

Discuss plans for alternative long-term living arrangements such as CLA. SBE prophylaxis needed for individuals with cardiac disease. Continue dietary and exercise recommendations (see Childhood, above). Update estate planning and custody arrangements. Encourage social and recreational programs with friends. Register for voting and Selective Service at age 18. Reinforce the importance of good self-care skills (grooming, dressing, and money handling skills). Bereavement counseling for individuals who have experienced the loss of an important person in their life, either via death or by other circumstances, for example, sibling moves away after marriage or goes off to college.

[A discussion of each of the above recommendations is included in the full guidelines, which is available on the World Wide Web at www.denison.edu/dsq/health99.htm.]

## ANTICIPATED CHANGES AND CLARIFICATIONS

### FORMAT

In response to requests from parents and professionals, we will simplify the format, to make it easier to follow.

## CELIAC DISEASE

The recommended test for screening for celiac disease will be tissue transglutaminase antibody along with total IgA level. Tissue transglutaminase will detect 95–100% of cases of celiac disease, and this replaces the IgA anti-endomysial antibody.

The next revision will clarify the frequency of retesting individuals who are negative at the time of the first screen.

Note that the diagnosis of celiac disease is made only on the basis of an intestinal biopsy. Dietary changes should not be made until the intestinal biopsy is obtained.

## EAR, NOSE, AND THROAT AND AUDIOLOGY

The only way to be certain that a child has adequate hearing is to obtain a pure tone audiogram using headphones, to test each ear individually. (Sound field audiometry tests both ears at the same time.) Periodic hearing tests should be performed until the child is developmentally able to cooperate with this procedure.

We are becoming increasingly aware of how common sleep abnormalities are in children with Down syndrome. These abnormalities appear to occur even in those individuals without evidence of obstruction and/or sleep apnea (snoring, cessation of breathing.)

## ATLANTOAXIAL INSTABILITY

A recent study highlighted the value of including the neural canal width in decision making during screening for atlantoaxial instability (Brockmeyer, 1999). In addition, our colleagues who care for adults with DS report that cervical spine abnormalities appear to occur commonly perhaps related to arthritic changes that occur in this group of individuals.

## PNEUMOCOCCAL VACCINE

The seven-valent conjugated pneumococcal vaccine (Prevnar) was licensed in January 2000 and became incorporated in the standard recommendations for immunizations for infants in the United States. There is a dosage schedule for administration of this vaccine to children older than 24 months and younger than 5 years. Twenty-three-valent pneumococcal vaccine (Pneumovax) should be considered for individuals older than 5 years. These vaccines prevent serious bacterial infections that can affect the ears, nose, and throat as well as causing pneumonia.

## Cognitive Enhancements

Recent studies have looked at the use of anticholinesterase inhibitors to improve cognitive function in adults with DS.

## References

Brockmeyer D (1999): Down syndrome and craniovertebral instability: Topic review and treatment recommendations. Pediatr Neurosurg 31(2):71–77

Committee on Genetics, AAP (2001): Health supervision for children with Down syndrome. Pediatrics 107(2):442–449.

Cohen WI (ed.) (1999): Health Care Guidelines for Individuals with Down Syndrome—1999 Revision. Down Syndrome Q 4(3):1–16.

Available on the Internet at: www.denison.edu/dsq/health99.htm

DS Growth Charts: www.growthcharts.com

# RESEARCH

# Sequencing of Chromosome 21/The Human Genome Project

## David Patterson, Ph.D.

## A Brief Description of the DNA Sequence Data

In May of 2000, the DNA sequence of the long arm of chromosome 21 and a catalog of the genes on the chromosome was published (Hattori et al., 2000). The length of this chromosome arm is 33,546,361 base pairs (bp) of DNA. Only about 100,000 base pairs, distributed in three small gaps, remained unsequenced. In addition, 281,116 bp of the short arm was sequenced. This was a seminal event in research about Down syndrome, because, for the first time, we had a reasonably complete list of all the genes on the chromosome. The number of known genes and gene predictions was 225. Of these 225 genes, 127 correspond to known genes and 98 represent novel genes. Since the publication of the sequence, analysis of its content continues, and the precise number of genes is changing as is the categorization of genes as more experimentation is carried out. One good source of information on the current status of the annotation of chromosome 21 is the Eleanor Roosevelt Institute Chromosome 21 website (*http://eri.uchsc.edu/chromosome21/index.html*).

The number of genes found was considerably lower than the number previously thought to be on chromosome 21 on the basis that this chromosome (technically, the long arm of the chromosome) comprised 1% of

*Down Syndrome,* Edited by William I. Cohen, Lynn Nadel, and Myra E. Madnick.
ISBN 0-471-41815-3   Copyright © 2002 by Wiley-Liss, Inc.

the total human genome. This had led to predictions that 500–1000 genes would be found on chromosome 21. In addition, chromosome 22, which was roughly the same size as chromosome 21, had been found to have 545 genes (Dunham et al., 1999). This finding was consistent with hypotheses that chromosome 21 might be relatively gene poor. However, now that the entire human genome sequence has been determined and analyzed, we see that the estimate for the total number of human genes is about 27,000 (Venter et al., 2001; International Human Genome Sequencing Consortium, 2001). Therefore, the number of genes on human chromosome 21 may be closer to the average gene density than was previously thought.

In addition to the gene catalog, the chromosome 21 DNA sequence has been analyzed and compared with other human genome regions, with some intriguing results. For example, a number of clusters of related genes have been found on the chromosome, suggesting tandem duplication events early in evolution. In addition, regions of chromosome 21 have been duplicated both within the chromosome and on other chromosomes. These duplicated regions may be associated with various forms of chromosome abnormality.

A notable feature of the chromosome is the asymmetric distribution of genes. Thus roughly 10 million base pairs (mbp) of the chromosome, one region of 7 mbp and three regions of 1 mbp each, contain only one gene. It is not yet clear why these gene-poor regions exist.

At the time of publication, three small gaps remained in the DNA sequence of the long arm of chromosome 21, and less than 300,000 bp of the short arm had been sequenced. It is anticipated that these gaps will be closed rather quickly by individual research groups interested in these particular regions of the chromosome. The short arm of chromosome 21 poses difficult challenges for DNA sequencing. It is highly repetitive and is very similar to the short arms of chromosomes 13, 14, 15, and 22. Nevertheless, a high-resolution physical map of this chromosome arm has been published (Wang et al., 1999). This should prove useful for structural and functional studies of this region of the chromosome and perhaps eventually for sequencing of this difficult region. Fortunately, this region is likely to have little relevance for Down syndrome or for other human health problems, because individuals with either too many or too few short arms appear to be indistinguishable from people with the typical number. So far, only one gene encoding a protein, *TPTE*, has been located on the short arm of chromosome 21 and the functionality of this gene remains to be determined (Guipponi et al., 2000).

Thus the remaining tasks with regard to completion of the DNA sequence are to close the remaining gaps in the sequence of the long arm and to complete the sequence of the short arm of the chromosome.

## Assessment of the Gene Content of Chromosome 21

It must be noted that there is a great deal of work to do before we truly understand the gene content of chromosome 21. Thus, at the time of the initial publication, 98 genes or predicted genes were only computer predictions. Of these, only 13 had similarity to known proteins. Even for the known genes, their pattern of expression in the body or during development remains largely unknown. Until there is experimental verification that any particular gene prediction is actually expressed in the body, no firm conclusions can be drawn about whether the prediction is actually a true gene. In addition, considerably more computer-assisted analysis of the sequence remains to be done.

## New Research Opportunities Offered by the DNA Sequence

Having the DNA sequence of human chromosome 21 promises to revolutionize research about Down syndrome. For example, in the past, many investigators had chosen particular genes on chromosome 21 for study because rational hypotheses could be made linking them potentially to one or more of the phenotypes seen in individuals with Down syndrome. This has been a fruitful line of research, and knowing all of the genes may enhance this effort, because there are now more genes to choose from (Chrast et al., 2000a; Smith et al., 1997).

However, for the first time, the DNA sequence of chromosome 21, as well as the complete human genome sequence, allows a more direct and comprehensive approach to understanding Down syndrome. It is now well within our experimental capability to assess directly where in the body and when during development every gene or presumed gene on chromosome 21 is active. This is most easily done in the mouse, considering that it is difficult or impossible to obtain the necessary human tissue samples. Fortunately, the mouse genome will be completely sequenced very shortly, and already many research groups are comparing the mouse and human DNA sequences.

Thus one could undertake the following empirical approach to deciding which genes are most likely to be important for Down syndrome. First, one isolates the cognate mouse gene. Then one determines where during embryonic development and during aging of the animal this gene is actually active. If the gene is active during the life of the animal in a tissue thought to be important for the phenotype of Down syndrome, then this gene becomes a more attractive candidate for study. For example, a gene expressed in the mouse in brain regions known to be anatomically different in persons with Down syndrome would be a high priority for study. This information can be obtained using well-known and robust experimental procedures such as tissue in situ hybridization (TISH) to assess expression patterns in time and place in mice (Neidhardt et al., 2000). Another approach, which is being taken by several research groups, is to use one of the new genomics-based approaches to assess levels of gene expression, for example, DNA microarrays (DNA "chips") or serial analysis of gene expression (SAGE) to assess alterations in levels of gene expression (Le Naour et al., 2001; Chrast et al., 2000b). In this case, one can compare samples from individuals with and without Down syndrome or one can examine one or more of the various mouse models of Down syndrome. Also, one can study just genes on chromosome 21 (or the equivalent mouse chromosomes, 16, 17, and 10), or one can examine expression of genes on all chromosomes. The latter is important because it is almost certainly true that the presence of three copies of chromosome 21 influences the expression of genes on other chromosomes.

Given that there are about 225 genes on chromosome 21, all of these experiments are feasible. In this way, we can generate lists of chromosome 21 genes whose expression is indeed altered in Down syndrome and whose expression is altered in, for example, brain regions affected morphologically or by other criteria in Down syndrome.

These techniques measure the transcription of genes, that is, they measure the presence and/or levels of mRNA. They do not measure protein levels, and for most genes it is their encoded proteins that actually perform relevant biological functions, for example, as enzymes or as structural molecules or molecules important for controlling cellular metabolism and, indeed, the activities of other genes. Fortunately, it is becoming possible to analyze the proteins themselves on a global scale (Lopez, 2000). This is the new field of proteomics, which is highly complementary to genomics and functional genomics (Ideker et al., 2001). The current standard approach to global analysis of protein expression combines the ability of gel electrophoresis to separate proteins with the ability of advanced mass spectrometry techniques to identify the separated proteins. In a single experiment, it is in principle possible to identify over 1000 proteins, although in practice this has not yet been achieved. Nonetheless, the technology exists. Again, in principle, it should be possible, in less than 100 experiments, to gain some understanding of the actual protein levels and locations in body tissues of proteins corresponding to the genes on chromosome 21.

This approach becomes all the more necessary because of the emerging realization that each gene can encode the production of more than one form of any particular protein. In fact, some estimates indicate that on average there may be two forms of protein produced by each gene, vastly increasing the ability of a genome with 27,000 genes to generate additional complexity in the organism (Corthals et al., 2000). These different forms of protein are difficult to detect by DNA array technology, TISH, or even standard mRNA quantitation experiments. Analysis of the proteins themselves offers a direct answer to these questions of complexity.

## New Opportunities for Understanding Down Syndrome

The DNA sequence of chromosome 21 by itself reveals new complexities that must be dealt with when studying Down syndrome. Thus the presence of several related genes very close to each other raises some interesting questions. Even more perplexing is the finding that in many cases closely related genes exist on other chromosomes in addition to chromosome 21. If this is so, how are we to interpret increased expression by gene dosage, that is, to 150% of what one sees in a person with two chromosome 21s, in a person with Down syndrome? If the gene in question is unique in function, then we can truly expect that 150% of that gene's product may have significance. However, what if there are genes with similar or identical function on, for example, three other chromosomes? Then, in typical people, there will be eight total copies of these genes, whereas a person with Down syndrome will have nine copies, and the difference in functional expression will be much less than 50%. Solving this problem will require much more sophisticated understanding of the function of closely related genes.

As mentioned above, this problem is even further complicated because many genes encode for different forms of the same protein that may have quite different functions. Comparison of the genomic sequence containing the gene with the sequence of various forms of mRNA produced by the gene and with the various forms of protein produced by the mRNA will allow understanding of these complexities.

## Mouse Models and the DNA Sequence

One of the most notable new advances in research about Down syndrome is the recent production and characterization of mouse models trisomic for significant regions of mouse chromosomes that are homologous to human chromosome 21 (Davisson and Costa, 1999). The genes on human chromosome 21 are found on three mouse chromosomes, 16, 17, and 10. So far, the order of genes in the mouse is the same as the order in the human. This conservation of chromosomal regions has led to attempts to produce mice trisomic for the parts of mouse chromosomes 16, 17, and 10 that are homologous to human chromosome 21. The first of these, trisomy 16 (Ts16) in the mouse, leads to lethality during embryogenesis or shortly after birth. Even so, during embryonic development, these mice show anatomic features that are reminiscent of what one observes in persons with Down syndrome (Lacey-Casem and Oster-Granite, 1994).

To overcome the problem of early lethality, investigators have produced mice that are trisomic for part of mouse chromosome 16 (Davisson et al., 1990; Sago et al., 2000). The most widely used of these is the Ts65Dn mouse, which contains an extra copy of a large fraction of mouse chromosome 16 that appears to contain many of the genes found on human chromosome 21 and no mouse genes whose human homologs are not located on chromosome 21 (Davisson and Costa, 1999). This mouse has behavioral and developmental features reminiscent of certain features seen in persons with Down syndrome (Hyde et al., 2001). However, the boundaries of the homologous region of chromosome 16 trisomic in this mouse line to human chromosome 21 are not yet precisely known. Given the sequence of human chromosome 21, this situation is likely to change rapidly as the DNA sequence of the mouse is completed. This will have direct relevance for understanding which genes found on chromosome 21 in humans actually are trisomic in this mouse model and therefore may play a role in the altered phenotype of this mouse.

In addition, questions bearing on the evolution of mammalian chromosomes can be addressed when the mouse chromosome 16 sequence becomes available. For example, are duplications like those seen on human chromosome 21 also seen in the mouse? Are there large regions of mouse chromosome 16 that are devoid of genes? Is there conservation of regions of mouse chromosome 16 and human chromosome 21 sequence that do not encode genes? If so, what is the nature of these conserved regions? Are the genes in the mouse homologous region in the same precise order and orientation as on human chromosome 21?

This information will have important implications for the creation of additional mouse partial trisomies for the study of Down syndrome. For example, this knowledge should greatly ease the production of mice with Cre recombinase-based technology (Zheng et al., 2000). This promising approach requires integration of two loxP DNA sequences at precise positions in the mouse genome. Recombination can then occur between the two loxP sites, resulting in either deletion or duplication of the regions between the loxP sites. In this way partial, or segmental, trisomies can be made for any desired region of the mouse genome. However, the loxP DNA sequences must be integrated in the same orientation for this experiment to work. Knowledge of the human and mouse DNA sequences will aid this experiment in two ways. First, it will allow precise positioning of the loxP sites so that researchers will know exactly what is present in an extra copy. Second, by knowing the sequence, researchers will be able to control the orientation of the integrated loxP sites, allowing a very significant savings in time and resources.

A second approach to production of mouse models is the introduction of individual genes or defined gene regions into the mouse genome by DNA injection, resulting in transgenic mice containing extra copies of one or a few genes (Hogan et al., 1994). In this way, the effects of small numbers of genes or even individual genes can be studied in mouse models. To carry this approach out, researchers need to isolate the particular human DNA region containing the gene or genes of interest. If the goal is to study the effect of a single gene, then one must be sure that the entire gene and its regulatory regions are contained in the isolated DNA region. In addition, one needs to know whether other genes are present in the DNA clone isolated. Now that the DNA sequence of chromosome 21 is known, this information can be obtained rapidly and precisely simply by determining the DNA sequence of the ends of each cloned region. This will result in a huge savings of time and effort, because production of mice with incomplete genes or unwanted genes can be avoided.

## CLINICAL IMPLICATIONS OF THE DNA SEQUENCE OF CHROMOSOME 21

The knowledge of the DNA sequence of chromosome 21 by itself will not have immediate clinical implications for people with Down syndrome. Its major effect is likely to be a marked enhancement of the rate of progress in understanding how the presence of an extra chromosome 21 leads to Down syndrome. The ability to screen all the genes on the chromosome for altered expression in Down syndrome and/or in mouse models of Down syndrome will focus efforts on the genes most likely to be involved, namely, those with altered expression in affected tissues and cell types. Knowledge of the DNA sequence of all of the genes should allow much more rapid determination of what the functions of the proteins encoded by each gene are. Knowledge of the DNA sequence of chromosome 21 will greatly enhance our ability to produce important mouse models expressing genes most likely to lead to the phenotype of Down syndrome. The production of these models not only promises to help us understand the basic mechanisms by which extra copies of genes lead to Down syndrome, but they provide an ideal system in which to test interventions with medicines before use of these therapies in people.

Each gene on chromosome 21 that shows altered expression in Down syndrome represents a possible therapeutic target. The more we know about these genes and how they act, the more quickly and rationally we can devise ways to counteract the effects of the extra copy of any particular gene.

We need also to keep in mind that it is virtually certain that genes on chromosome 21 do not work alone to cause the features we recognize as Down syndrome. They must work in concert with genes on other chromosomes. This is likely to be one of the reasons for the wide diversity seen in persons with Down syndrome. That is, this diversity is likely to simply reflect the diversity of humanity as a whole. Although this would seem to further complicate the situation because it means that more genes are involved in the production of the phenotype of Down syndrome, one can turn this argument around. With the use of global functional genomics and proteomics approaches, it will be possible to identify genes on other chromosomes whose expression or function is altered by the presence of three copies of chromosome 21. These genes represent additional therapeutic targets.

Because we now have the sequence of essentially all of the human genome as well as the sequence of chromosome 21, it may be possible to use this information to help answer questions about how the nondisjunction of chromosomes occurs in the first place. If this can be done, it may be possible to minimize the occurrence of nondisjunction, most of which occurs before conception. This information would be a profound contribution to our understanding of human genetics.

Thus the sequencing of human chromosome 21, and indeed the sequencing of the entire human genome, must be seen as a beginning rather than an ending. It will profoundly change how human medical genetics research is carried out. The pace of research findings has already been markedly accelerated and indeed was accelerated as the sequence information was acquired even before the task was completed. It is now up to us to use this information as wisely and efficiently as possible for the benefit of persons with Down syndrome and indeed of all humanity.

## Acknowledgments

This is contribution #1798 of the Thomas G. and Mary W. Vessels Laboratory for Molecular Biology and the John C. Mitchell Laboratory for the Study of Genetic Diseases and Human Development of the Eleanor Roosevelt Institute. This work was supported by NIH grant HD-17449.

## References

Chrast R, Scott HS , Madani R, Huber L, Wolfer DP, Prinz M, Aguzzi A, Lipp HP, Antonarakis SE (2000a): Mice trisomic for a bacterial artificial chromosome with the single-minded 2 gene (Sim2) show phenotypes similar to some of those present in the partial trisomy 16 mouse models of Down syndrome. Hum Mol Genet 9:1853–1864.

Chrast R, Scott HS, Papasavvas MP, Rossier C, Antonarakis ES, Barras C, Davisson MT, Schmidt C, Estivill X, Dierssen M, Pritchard M, Antonarakis SE (2000b): The mouse brain transcriptome by SAGE: Differences in gene expression between P30 brains of the partial trisomy 16 mouse model of Down syndrome (Ts65Dn) and normals. Genome Res 10:2006–2021.

Corthals GL, Wasinger VC, Hochstrasser DF, Sanchez J-C (2000): The dynamic range of protein expression: A challenge for proteomic research. Electrophoresis 21:1104–1115.

Davisson MT, Costa A (1999): Mouse models of Down syndrome. In: Popko B (ed.), Advances in Neurochemistry: New York, Kluwer Academic/Plenum Publishers, pp 297–327.

Davisson MT, Schmidt, Akeson EC (1990): Segmental trisomy of murine chromosome 16: A new model system for studying Down syndrome. Prog Clin Biol Res 360:263–280.

Dunham I, Shimizu N, Roe BA, Chissoe S, Hunt AR, Collins JE, Bruskiewich R, Beare DM, Clamp M, Smink LK, Ainscough R, Almeida JP, Babbage A, Bagguley C, Bailey J, Barlow K, Bates KN, Beasley O, Bird CP, Blakey S, Bridgeman AM, Buck D, Burgess J, Burrill WD, O'Brien KP, et al. (1999): The DNA sequence of human chromosome 22. Nature 402:489–495.

Guipponi M, Yaspo ML, Riesselman L, Chen H, De Sario A, Roizes G, Antonarakis SE (2000): Genomic structure of a copy of the human TPTE gene which encompasses 87 kb on the short arm of chromosome 21. Hum Genet 107:127–131.

Hattori M, Fujiyama A, Taylor TD, Watanabe H, Yada T, Park HS, Toyoda A, Ishii K, Totoki Y, Choi DK, Soeda E, Ohki M, Takagi T, Sakaki Y, Taudien S, Blechschmidt K, Polley A, Menzel U, Delabar J, Kumpf K, Lehmann R, Patterson D, Reichwald K, Rump A, Schillhabel M, Schudy A (2000): The DNA sequence of human chromosome 21. The chromosome 21 mapping and sequencing consortium. Nature 405:283–284.

Hogan BL, Beddington R, Costantini F, Lacy E (eds.) (1994): Manipulating the mouse embryo. Plainview, NY: Cold Spring Harbor Press.

Hyde LA, Frisone DF, Crnic LS (2001): Ts65Dn Mice, a model for Down syndrome, have deficits in context discrimination learning suggesting impaired hippocampal function. Behav Brain Res 118:53–60.

Ideker T, Thorsson V, Ranish JA, Christmas R, Buhler J, Eng JK, Bumgarner R, Goodlett DR, Aebersold R, Hood L (2001): Integrated genomic and proteomic analyses of a systematically perturbed metabolic network. Science 292:929–934.

International Human Genome Sequencing Consortium (2001): Initial sequencing and analysis of the human genome. Nature 409:860–921.

Lacey-Casem ML, Oster-Granite ML (1994): The neuropathology of the trisomy 16 mouse. Crit Rev Neurobiol 8:293–322.

Le Naour, Hohenkirk L, Grolleau A, Misek DE, Lescure P, Geiger JD, Hanash S, Beretta L (2001): Profiling changes in gene expression during differentiation and maturation of monocyte derived dendritic cells using both oligonucleotide microarrays and proteomics. J Biol Chem 276:17920–17931.

Lopez MF (2000): Better approaches to finding the needle in a haystack: Optimizing proteome analysis through automation. Electrophoresis 21:1082–1093.

Neidhardt L, Gasca S, Wertz K, Obermayr F, Worpenberg S, Lehrach H, Herrmann BG (2000): Large-scale screen for genes controlling mammalian embryogenesis, using high-throughput gene expression analysis in mouse embryos. Mech Dev 98:77–93.

Sago H, Carlson EJ, Smith DJ, Rubin EM, Crnic LS, Huang TT, Epstein CJ (2000): Genetic dissection of region associated with behavioral abnormalities in mouse models for Down syndrome. Pediatr Res 48:606–613.

Smith DJ, Stevens ME, Sudanagunta SP, Bronson RT, Makhinson M, Watabe AM, O'Dell TJ, Fung J Weier HU, Cheng JF, Rubin EM (1997): Functional screening of 2 Mb of human chromosome 21q22.2 in transgenic mice implicates minibrain in learning defects associated with Down syndrome. Nat Genet 16:28–36.

Venter JC, Adams MD, Myers EW, Li PW, Mural RJ, Sutton GG et al. (2001): The sequence of the human genome. Science 291:1304–1351.

Wang SY, Cruts M, Del-Favero J, Zhang Y, Tissir F, Potier MC, Patterson D, Nizetic D, Bosch A, Chen H, Bennett L, Estivill X, Kessling A, Antonarakis SE, van Broeckhoven C (1999): A high-resolution physical map of human chromosome 21p using yeast artificial chromosomes. Genome Res 9:1059–1073.

Zheng B, Sage M, Sheppeard EA, Jurecic V, Bradley A (2000): Engineering mouse chromosomes with cre-loxP: Range, efficiency, and somatic applications. Mol Cell Biol 648–655.

# Nonconventional Therapies for Down Syndrome: A Review and Framework for Decision making

## W. Carl Cooley, M.D.

Horatio:

    O day and night, but this is wondrous strange!

Hamlet:

    And therefore, as a stranger give it welcome.
    There are more things in heaven and earth, Horatio,
    Than are dreamt of in your philosophy.

                        Hamlet Act I; Scene V

## INTRODUCTION

In an era of evidence-based medicine and a demand for measures of educational excellence, it is possible to forget that most decisions about health remain determined as much by psychological and cultural factors as by scientific data. A growing number of Americans choose to supplement their diets and complement their doctors' advice from an enormous inventory of vitamins, minerals, herbs, and alternative health services. Approximately 11% of parents in the United States choose alternative and complementary

*Down Syndrome,* Edited by William I. Cohen, Lynn Nadel, and Myra E. Madnick.
ISBN 0-471-41815-3   Copyright © 2002 by Wiley-Liss, Inc.

therapies for their children, and over 50% of parents of children with autism use some form of unconventional therapy for their child (Spigelblatt et al. 1994; Nickel, 1996). Although catalyzed by advertising claims, the sales of these products and services continue to grow even in the face of absent or fragmentary evidence of real benefits. Most U.S. medical schools now offer alternative medicine courses, and the U.S. government has established the National Center for Complementary and Alternative Medicine within the National Institutes of Health. Recently, the American Academy of Pediatrics published a policy statement to guide pediatricians who work with families considering nonconventional therapies for a child with special health care needs (American Academy of Pediatrics, Committee on Children with Disabilities, 2001).

It should be no surprise that parents of children with Down syndrome are interested in a wider spectrum of therapeutic choices than those offered by mainstream medical and educational professionals. Doctors, therapists, and educators imply that parents should accept an inevitable baseline of challenges to health, learning, and accomplishment for their child. They offer life-saving treatments for heart defects, bowel disease, and leukemia; potent preventive health measures to avert secondary disabilities like hearing impairment; and increasingly integrative and asset-driven approaches to education. But the same professionals explain that, although the genetic mysteries of Down syndrome are gradually being solved, there remains a limited understanding of the biological basis for specific health and developmental challenges. Fueled by a mixture of hope, parental responsibility, and the fear of narrow windows of opportunity, parental interest in complementary therapies is understandable.

The dissemination among parents of theories and practices outside the mainstream has been advanced by an uncritical, sometimes sensationalizing media and the explosion of information available through electronic technology. Like an enormous library after an earthquake, the Internet provides wide access to an unannotated mixture of the knowledge, experience, wishful thinking, and promotional efforts of academic researchers, profit-oriented businesses, well-meaning theorists, and individual parents.

Names not only carry definitional value, but may also convey judgment and categorical assignment. How we name the therapies discussed in this chapter carries meaning about our understanding of or our assumptions about the truth of each therapy's claims and its place in the continuum of acceptance of interventions for a person with Down syndrome. Terms like unproven or unconventional therapy usually imply the absence of scientific evidence for or widespread belief in the therapy's benefit. Often, anecdotal or parental experience is not regarded as proof, and professionals, not families, make the determination of the conventional. Complementary therapies are nonmainstream interventions that supplement or complement conventional approaches, and alternative therapies carry the implication of interventions used in place of the conventional approach. Finally, integrative treatments, at least in the medical world, are based on thoughtful efforts to blend conventional Western medicine with nonconventional remedies and treatments. For the purposes of this discussion, the term unconventional therapy will be used to include therapies that are not widely accepted as part of the medical or educational mainstream, but without meaning to prejudge the potential of some to join that mainstream in the future.

Science has become the arbiter of truth in the training and practice of Western medical professionals, and evidence-based approaches are influencing the evaluation of developmental and educational interventions as well. Although families are generally interested in what has proven to work safely and effectively, they are in search of solutions to the challenges that confront their children. In addition to the proven and safe, families may gravitate toward what makes sense, what might work, and what other families say has worked. They are likely to reach their own conclusions about the balance between risk and benefit. They are justified in doing so.

## WHAT MAKES INTERVENTIONS "CONVENTIONAL"?

Conventional therapies, treatments, and interventions have survived a complex interplay of professional evaluation and cultural acceptance against a background of political and economic factors. The strongest scientific evidence may be insufficient to overcome strongly held cultural beliefs or powerful economic factors.

Professional evaluation generally begins with anecdotal experience or empirical assumptions. In fact, the anecdotal experience of individuals, for example, parents of children with Down syndrome, may ignite the empirical impressions of professionals attempting to serve their needs. Such impressions become the ingredients of hypothetical statements. Hypotheses in turn define the experimental design that would lead to scientific evidence for the generalizability of individual experiences. More recently, qualitative and participatory research designs have allowed a stronger connection between the experience of the beneficiaries of research and the hypothetical assumptions and parameters of the research itself.

Even when research finds evidence to support a particular therapy or intervention, widespread conventional use will not occur without cultural acceptance. Therapies must be compatible with societal or cultural values and must have achieved some credibility in the eyes of consumers. For example, there is strong scientific evidence that the distribution of sterile needles to intravenous drug users will reduce the incidence of HIV infection in this population. However, in many areas such a public health intervention is incompatible with public values about the use of illegal drugs. Mounting scientific evidence for the health risks of smoking did not become widely credible to the American public until the Surgeon General of the United States endorsed the data and declared smoking cessation a national health priority.

Recently, the influence of the media and marketing on cultural acceptance has made advertising a powerful tool both for matters of public health policy and for improved profitability of some prescription drugs. Public health officials are making increasingly sophisticated use of the media to wage wars on smoking, drug use, and head injury. Similarly, drug companies interested in the rapid transition of new drugs into the realm of conventional therapies have shown the dramatic results of direct marketing of prescription drugs to consumers. Similarly, through the use of the Internet, direct mail, and the underwriting of workshops and conferences, some marketers of unconventional therapies for Down syndrome are plying this path toward wider acceptance.

Finally, for some therapies to gain conventional status and mainstream use, there may be political and economic factors that influence the process. Available resources may affect the budget and priorities of national public and private research-funding agencies. Many therapies, particularly drugs and medical procedures, may need to negotiate a regulatory process within government entities such as the Food and Drug Administration. Payors for health and health-related products and services (public and private insurance) may not approve payment for therapies for which evidence of beneficial outcomes is not yet established. Finally, family and consumer advocacy organizations can influence the progress of a therapy toward conventional acceptance through their endorsement or their lobbying for research support.

## EVALUATING NEW THERAPIES IN A FAMILY CONTEXT

Parents or guardians generally make therapeutic choices for children with Down syndrome. Mainstream or conventional therapeutic decisions usually involve consultation with a child's primary or specialist physicians or with therapists and educational professionals. Ideally, in the context of family-centered care, these decisions result from an exchange of information and a collaborative process between parents and professionals.

When parents are considering an unconventional therapy for their child, the information-gathering process may be more challenging. Naturally, parents will have obtained information from advocates of the therapy including that obtained from direct consultation, conferences or workshops, or the Internet. Before making a decision about proceeding with a new therapy, consultation with trusted professionals or experts about Down syndrome should be sought regarding what is known about the therapy's risks and benefits. In addition, the opinions of other parents may be useful, including parents who use the therapy, parents who have used the therapy but decided to stop, and parents who made a decision not to use the therapy.

There are other considerations that parents and the professionals that advise them might take into consideration. A family or parent's personal style or values should be considered. Are parents inclined toward an active interventionist style or are they more likely to take a "leave well enough alone" position? Are they comfortable with intuitive feelings about the right path or do they prefer a more rational, scientific approach? Do they tend to approach decisions with caution or to adopt a more experimental approach?

A family's resources may also be an important consideration. Most non-conventional therapies are not covered by public or private insurance plans, so any financial burdens will most likely be the family's responsibility. There may be additional nonmonetary costs of time or absence from work. Some therapies may carry emotional costs because of the expectations or hopes placed on the therapy's outcomes or because of disagreement within the family or between the family and professionals about the advisability of using the intervention. Finally, some therapies may require such a commitment of time and effort that considerable disruption of normal family life and routines will result. The impact of these changes on all family members must be weighed against the anticipated benefits of the therapy.

In many respects, choosing any therapy or intervention can be seen as a consumer decision in which there is a product to be evaluated, advocates who are "selling" the products, data to be reviewed regarding efficacy and safety, alternatives to consider, and costs to be weighed. Parents need to know who is advocating the therapy, what claims are being made, and what rationale is proposed for the therapy's mechanism of action and effects. It is important to consider whether the rationale makes sense, whether the therapy's claims are plausible and specific for Down syndrome, and whether there are any independent scientific data to support claims of the therapy's benefits. In this regard, parents should understand that the most objective and reliable scientific information would have been published in "peer reviewed" professional journals. Research data appearing in such journals have been subjected to critical review by multiple experts who examine the research for any flaws that would make the "new" data suspect or unreliable.

## SPECIFIC NONCONVENTIONAL THERAPIES

An exhaustive review of nonconventional therapies for Down syndrome is beyond the scope of this chapter. Therapies of current interest and a few of historical interest are included. To provide a consistent approach to each therapy, the discussions are structured identically with five sections: historical background, procedures used to implement the therapy, proposed rationale for the therapy, possible risks of the therapy, and a short review of any scientific evidence related to the therapy. The review that follows will also be limited to medical interventions. A more exhaustive discussion of non-conventional therapies might include neurodevelopmental strategies such as patterning, sensory integration therapy, auditory retraining, facilitated communication, and craniosacral therapy. The reference section includes several references providing reviews of these nonmedical therapies (Pueschel and Pueschel, 1992; Nickel, 1996).

## PLASTIC SURGERY

HISTORY.    In 1977 plastic surgeons in Germany began reporting their experience with surgical procedures intended to "normalize" the facial features of Down syndrome (Lemperle and Radu, 1980). Surgeons in Israel and Australia also described similar approaches. More limited interventions have been the subject of study in Canada.

PROCEDURE.    Multiple procedures have been described including augmentation of chin and cheeks with Teflon implants, correction of epicanthal folds and upward obliquity of the eyes, tongue reduction, remodeling of ears, and removal of excess neck skin. In most instances the procedures are performed in infancy or toddlerhood, either in a single operation or in several stages.

RATIONALE.    The dual aims of plastic surgery in children with Down syndrome are to improve function and to improve appearance and acceptance. Improved speech intelligibility, swallowing, and possibly respiratory function have been suggested as consequences of tongue reduction (Parsons et al., 1987). The set of multiple procedures advocated in Germany and Israel are intended to "normalize" facial appearance, thereby reducing stigmatization and enhancing social acceptance. On the premise that the features of the Down syndrome phenotype diminish the expectations of families, friends, and teachers, plastic surgery would promote higher achievement and more natural integration of people with Down syndrome.

RISKS.    All surgical procedures involve risks including infection, poor healing, bleeding, and the complications of general anesthesia. Problems have been reported with the Teflon implants, and because they are implanted in infancy or toddlerhood, they may be outgrown and require replacement. Postoperative airway problems, usually temporary, have also occurred. A nonmedical risk has been exaggerated expectations by parents of a child transformed physically and functionally by surgery.

EVIDENCE.    The surgeons performing the operations carried out most initial studies of the effectiveness of plastic surgery in Down syndrome. In these studies 75% of the parents and nearly all of the surgeons were very satisfied with the results (Lemperle and Radu, 1980; Olbrisch, 1982). However, later studies began to include peers and teachers(Arndt 1986). Subjects were shown a mixed series of photographs of children with Down syndrome. The photographs were in random order and included children both before and after plastic surgery. Subjects were asked to judge the appearance of the children in the photographs with respect to characteristics of Down syndrome, whether the subject would choose the person as a friend, and other subjective impressions. The subjects of these studies displayed no preference for the photographs of children who had had plastic surgery, in fact, the postsurgery photographs were found to be less attractive. In addition, there has been no evidence that children who have undergone plastic surgery have achieved greater skills, integration, or happiness than those without surgery.

## SICCA CELL THERAPY

HISTORY.    Sicca cell therapy was in use in Europe for cancer and for a variety of psychiatric disorders. In Germany in the 1970s, the use of sicca cell therapy was popularized for people with Down syndrome. The application continued into the early 1980s, when the national health insurance program in Germany discontinued coverage of sicca cell therapy because of concerns about its safety and effectiveness. Subsequently, a similar therapy using human fetal tissue was offered in Russia. The therapy has never been sanctioned in the United States, but American parents have taken children with Down syndrome to Germany and Russia to obtain sicca cell treatment.

PROCEDURE.    Sicca cell treatments involve the injection of freeze-dried brain tissue from the fetuses of sheep, goats, or rabbits into young children with Down syndrome. The treatments generally start before age 3 and are repeated every 5 months.

RATIONALE.    Sicca cell advocates hypothesized that primordial tissue of fetal origin had the potential to replace, repair, or stimulate growth in the developing brain tissue of children with Down syndrome. This would result in increased brain growth and complexity, which would in turn allow for greater developmental accomplishment.

RISKS.    The injection of foreign protein into any human carries the potential for allergic and toxic reactions. In addition, animal brain tissue may harbor slow virus infections similar to the type causing "mad cow disease," resulting in a progressive, ultimately fatal infection in the recipient of the treatment. There is a theoretical risk of potentiation of seizure activity.

EVIDENCE.   In 1978, Schmid reported the results of his use of sicca cell therapy in Down syndrome (Schmid, 1978). His report describes developmental benefits but is entirely subjective and anecdotal with no controls and no citation of specific data. Subsequent double-blind studies in Germany, Canada, and the United States showed no beneficial effects for sicca cell therapy. In 1990, Van Dyke reviewed the experience of 21 Americans treated with sicca cell injection and found no evidence of benefit (VanDyke et al., 1990).

## NEUROTRANSMITTER PRECURSORS

HISTORY.   In the 1960s studies of neurochemistry in people with Down syndrome revealed diminished levels of the neurotransmitter serotonin. This prompted Bazelon to examine whether increased serotonin levels were associated with improved muscle tone (Bazelon et al., 1967). Bazelon's results prompted a series of carefully designed studies to determine whether the administration of metabolic precursors of serotonin would have any benefit.

PROCEDURE.   Supplements of 5-hydroxytryptophan were administered orally. In some instances, an additional cofactor such as vitamin $B_6$ was provided.

RATIONALE.   As a serotonin precursor, 5-hydroxytryptophan was predicted to increase the levels of serotonin in the brain. Increased serotonin, it was hypothesized, would increase muscle tone and improve muscle function. This improvement in muscle function would in turn enhance the progress of motor development and, indirectly, overall development.

RISKS.   No specific risks or adverse effects were found to occur with 5-hydroxytryptophan administration. Tryptophan is a nutritional supplement and is not subject to the same quality controls in production as pharmaceutical products. Therefore, there is the potential for contamination and imperfections in commercially obtained tryptophan.

EVIDENCE.   After Bazelon's initial promising findings, Coleman, Partington, Weise, and Pueschel conducted a number of well-designed studies during the 1970s and 1980s. None of these studies showed any developmental differences in subjects using 5-hydroxytryptophan compared with control subjects taking a placebo (Partington et al., 1971; Coleman, 1973; Weise et al., 1974; Pueschel et al., 1980).

## FREE RADICAL INHIBITORS/ANTIOXIDANTS

HISTORY.    Beginning in the 1970s, theories that oxygen free radicals might be implicated as a cause for central nervous system injury in Down syndrome began to emerge in the context of similar beliefs about the cause of a number of degenerative diseases (de Haan, 1997). Further in vitro (test tube) laboratory studies of the neuronal tissue of Down syndrome fetuses raised additional concerns about possible free radical effects (Busciglio and Yankner, 1995).

PROCEDURE.    Treatments involve the oral administration of supplementary or excess doses of antioxidant vitamins and other substances believed to have antioxidant effects. The oral administration of cofactors for the action of antioxidants such as the minerals zinc and selenium is frequently included. Antioxidants and their cofactors have been included in nutritional supplements advocated for people with Down syndrome such as Nutravene-D.

RATIONALE.    Oxidative processes in living cells produce oxygen free radicals, which in turn result in the production of hydrogen peroxide. Hydrogen peroxide is toxic and has the potential for causing increased cell death in its vicinity. A gene controlling the production of an enzyme called superoxide dismutase (SOD) has been mapped to the 21st chromosome and is located in the region of the chromosome felt to be associated with the Down syndrome phenotype. People with Down syndrome produce an excess of some gene products of the 21st chromosome including SOD. Excess SOD is hypothesized to result in an excess of oxygen free radicals and, in consequence, an excess of hydrogen peroxide. Antioxidants are believed to block or reduce this effect.

RISKS.    The risks of side effects or complications of this therapy are few. However, some vitamins, minerals, and other antioxidants can be given in quantities associated with overdose effects. As with other nutritional supplements, there is little regulation or quality control over the manufacture and marketing of products.

EVIDENCE.    Because of the interest generated in the possible benefits of supplementary doses of vitamins, minerals, and other substances during the 1960s and 1970s, a number of well-designed publicly and privately funded research studies were conducted during the 1980s (Nickel, 1996). None of these studies showed any evidence of improved developmental outcomes for individuals with Down syndrome. However, most of these studies focused more strongly on developmental rather than possible health benefits. Some laboratory-based in vitro studies have suggested that zinc and/or selenium supplementation might improve immune function in individuals with Down syndrome, but no in vivo studies have substantiated this possibility.

## COGNITION-ENHANCING DRUGS (NOOTROPICS)

HISTORY.   In 1966, a new drug called piracetam was developed for the treatment of motion sickness. By 1968, piracetam was noted to produce some enhancements of memory and further animal studies seemed to confirm the presence of these effects. This led to a series of clinical trials of piracetam for its potential therapeutic role in the treatment of traumatic brain injury, dyslexia, Parkinson disease, and in the emerging race by drug companies for effective treatments for Alzheimer-type dementia. The association between Down syndrome and Alzheimer-type dementia led to speculation that piracetam or related drugs might benefit people with Down syndrome. A number of drugs in the same class have subsequently been developed including oxiracetam, etiracetam, and aniracetam.

PROCEDURE.   The medication (piracetam or similar drug) is administered in a daily oral dose.

RATIONALE.   Through their presumed enhancement of neuronal transmission, the nootropic medications are said to augment specific cognitive functions such as memory and, thereby, to improve overall cognitive functioning. One rationale would involve the continuous use of piracetam to improve functioning ("raise the bar") on a daily basis. Another rationale would propose the administration of a drug like piracetam during the period of rapid brain growth and differentiation in early childhood. Theoretically, the enhancement of cognitive functioning during this critical period would result in permanent changes in the brain and would not necessitate a lifetime of daily use of the medication.

RISKS.   Clinical studies of a variety of potential uses for piracetam have demonstrated only sporadic possible side effects all of which were mild and disappeared when the drug was discontinued or the dosage reduced. However, there have been few well-controlled studies of use in people with Down syndrome, and no information is available about the risks of long-term use (Holmes, 1999).

EVIDENCE.   In most instances, including Alzheimer-type dementia, piracetam was found to have no observable benefits, but some studies of dyslexia seemed to show increases in reading speed but no appreciable effect on comprehension (Dilanni et al., 1985). There have been no large studies of nootropics in people with Down syndrome. A very small study of teenage boys revealed no apparent improvement in skills with piracetam use (Fialho, 1977). Preliminary data from a well-designed pilot study involving preschool-aged children with Down syndrome also failed to demonstrate a beneficial effect, but its purpose was to develop the parameters (appropriate dose protocols, duration of treatment, selection of subjects) for further studies. A recent study of 25 children (aged 6.5–13 years) concluded that piracetam therapy did not enhance cognition or behavior but was associated with adverse effects (Lobaugh et al., 2001).

## VITAMINS AND NUTRITIONAL SUPPLEMENTS

HISTORY.   Beginning in the 1940s, Henry Turkel, a Michigan physician, developed a theory based on the belief that individuals with Down syndrome experienced deficiencies of a variety of essential metabolic elements (Turkel and Nusbaum, 1985). Dr. Turkel proposed supplementing or countering these deficiencies with partially individualized formulations of vitamins, minerals, and medications. Called the "U-Series," this formulation became the basis for many subsequent variations and the subject of a number of studies of its effects from 1950 through 1980. Schmid's concept of the genetotrophic basis for the challenges resulting from genetic conditions and the orthomolecular theory of Linus Pauling provided additional theoretical frameworks for nutritional supplementation in Down syndrome (Schmid, 1978). In 1981, a study of institutionalized adults with mental retardation by Ruth Harrell reported significant improvements in cognitive abilities after the administration of a U-series-like supplement (Harrell et al., 1981). When subsequent studies failed to corroborate these claims, interest in nutritional supplements subsided until 1995. In that year, a popular network prime-time news program televised a story of a mother of a child with Down syndrome who used the Internet to gather information. She found the theories about the benefits of nutritional supplements compelling and developed her own formulation for her daughter. She also found information about the nootropic drugs like piracetam, obtained the drug outside the United States, and included it in her child's regimen. The television program portrayed the effects of these interventions as miraculous, although the accomplishments of the child were similar to those of many children with Down syndrome in the 1990s. This publicity and the energy of a number of parents launched a movement of renewed enthusiasm for nutritional supplements, on which a number of companies manufacturing supplemental formulae have capitalized.

PROCEDURE.   Vitamin and nutritional supplementation involves the oral administration of individual or blended formulae on a daily basis. Formulations include vitamins, minerals, amino acids, and other chemicals. The

U-series contained 48 different substances and included bronchodilators like theophylline and thyroid hormone stimulators. Some companies supply a standardized formula to all, whereas others require the performance of metabolic blood tests to customize or "target" the formula to each individual ("targeted nutritional intervention" or "TNI").

RATIONALE. Based on beliefs, claims, and spotty scientific evidence, supplementation is aimed at correcting presumed deficiencies of individual substances, providing an excess of some substances based on assumptions of enhanced daily requirements for people with Down syndrome and correcting specific metabolic disorders due to presumptions of specific altered enzyme actions. Once these deficiencies are corrected, it is claimed that secondary benefits to health and development will ensue.

RISKS. For most nutritional supplements, there are few risks because what is not needed is excreted or metabolized. However, a number of vitamins and minerals carry significant risks of overdosage with well-described overdose syndromes. The fat-soluble vitamins (A, D, E, and K) tend to be stored in the body and can accumulate when administered in excessive doses. One of the B vitamins can induce a peripheral neuropathy in some individuals. Because nutritional supplements are treated like food products rather than like drugs from a regulatory standpoint, there are no quality control standards to assure consumers about the quantities and quality of a formula's constituents. There is no information or data about the safety of various combinations of supplements, about their interactions with other medications, about their effects on the developing nervous system of infants and toddlers, or about their long-term effects. Some formulae are expensive, costing up to $100/month, an expense that is not covered by insurance plans.

EVIDENCE. Most current support for vitamin and nutritional supplementation has come from the testimonial stories of parents and from the manufacturers of nutritional supplement products or laboratories engaged in performing metabolic test panels. A well-designed study in 1964 by Bumbalo et al. demonstrated no beneficial effects for Dr. Turkel's U-series in comparison to a placebo. However, Ruth Harrell's 1981 study suggesting improved cognition with a nutritional supplement led to a number of well-funded and well-controlled studies during the 1980s. None of these studies demonstrated any effects of the nutritional supplements compared with controls (Smith et al., 1984; Bennett et al., 1983; Coburn et al., 1983; Golden, 1984; Coleman, 1997). In retrospect, there were serious design flaws in Dr. Harrell's study, including the repeated, frequent administration of the same intelligence test, which might have accounted for some of her results.

## FUTURE OF NEW THERAPIES

The current array of conventional and unconventional, mainstream and alternative therapies for children with Down syndrome will no doubt change and evolve as new information and knowledge is revealed. Some unconventional therapies may become mainstream while others become historical footnotes. Some new approaches may become integrated with other approaches while others remain on the fringe of standard interventions. Meanwhile, considerable research activity is targeted directly or indirectly at a better understanding of the challenges facing people with Down syndrome. The recent completion of the map of the human genome means that the 21st chromosome has been mapped. Some new therapies are likely to result from this amazing accomplishment. Simply stated, individuals with Down syndrome experience the results of an excess of 21st chromosome material. Their bodies produce and respond to the effects of an "overdose" of the proteins that are manufactured according to the genetic blueprints contained in chromosome 21. It seems likely that therapies that block or otherwise offset some of these "overdose" effects will be a possibility for persons with Down syndrome. Drug companies are devoting enormous research and development efforts to treatments for Alzheimer-type dementia. Because individuals with Down syndrome have an increased risk for this condition, they will most certainly benefit from any successful products of this research. New tools for evaluating the outcomes of therapies are also likely to appear. Much of the existing research is based on relatively crude and unreliable measures of intelligence and adaptive behavior. Methods of measuring more subtle effects on specific areas of cognitive and language processing will be developed. Newer brain imaging technologies will allow real time assessments of neuropsychological functioning as well as providing new indicators for neuropathological change such as oxidative cell injury or immunological changes. Specific elements of some unconventional therapies, for example, zinc and selenium supplements, may prove to have specific value or benefit such as improved immunological functioning (Anneren et al., 1989; Lockitch et al., 1989) The certainty of an expanded array of new, effective therapeutic resources for people with Down syndrome will no doubt be balanced by the certainty of the continued emergence of new and reconsideration of older unconventional and alternative interventions.

## REFERENCES

American Academy of Pediatrics, Committee on Children with Disabilities (2001): Counseling families who choose complementary and alternative medicine for their child with chronic illness or disability. Pediatrics 107(3): 598–601.

Anneren G., Gebre-Medhin M. et al. (1989): Increased plasma and erythrocyte selenium concentrations but decreased erythrocyte glutathione peroxidase activity after selenium supplementation in children with Down syndrome. Acta Paediat Scand 78: 879–884.

Arndt E. (1986): Fact and fantasy: Psychological consequences of facial surgery in 24 Down syndrome children. Br J Plast Surg 39: 498–504.

Bazelon M., Paine R. et al. (1967): Reversal of hypotonia infants with Down syndrome by administration of 5-hydroxytryptophan. Lancet i: 1130–1132.

Bennett F. et al. (1983): Vitamin and mineral supplementation in Down syndrome. Pediatrics 72: 707–713.

Busciglio J. and Yankner B. (1995): Apoptosis and increased generation of reactive oxygen species in Down's syndrome neurons in vitro. Nature 378: 776–779.

Coburn S., Schaltenbrand W. et al. (1983): Effect of megavitamin treatment on mental performance and plasma vitamin B6 concentrations in mentally retarded young adults. Am J Nutr 38: 352–355.

Coleman M. (1973): Serotonin in Down Syndrome. New York: Elsevier/North-Holland.

Coleman M. (1997): Vitamins and Down syndrome. Down Syndrome Q 2(2): 11–13.

De Haan J. (1997): Reactive oxygen species and their contribution to pathology in Down syndrome. Adv Pharmacol 38: 379–402.

Dilanni M., Wilsher C. et al. (1985): The effects of piracetam in children with dyslexia. J Clin Psychopharmacol 5: 272–278.

Fialho J. (1977): Dromia and piracetam: a useful association in the treatment of Down's syndrome. Tempo Medico 30: 944.

Golden G. (1984): Controversies in therapy for children with Down syndrome. Pediatr Rev 6: 116–120.

Harrell R., Capp R. et al. (1981): Can nutritional supplements help mentally retarded children—an exploratory study. Proc Natl Acad Sci USA 78(1): 574–578.

Holmes L. (1999): Concern about piracetam treatment for children with Down syndrome. Pediatrics 103: 1078–1079.

Lemperle G., Radu D. (1980): Facial plastic surgery in children with Down's syndrome. Plast Reconstruct Surg 66: 337–342.

Lobaugh N., Karaskov V. et al. (2001): Piracetam therapy does not enhance cognitive functioning in children with Down syndrome. Arch Pediatr Adolesc Med P55: 442–448.

Lockitch G. et al. (1989): Infection and immunity in Down syndrome: A trial of long-term low oral doses of zinc. J Pediatr 114: 781–787.

Nickel R. (1996): Controversial therapies for young children with developmental disabilities. Infants Young Child 8(4): 29–40.

Olbrisch R. (1982): Plastic surgical management of children with Down's syndrome: Indications and results. Br J Plast Surg 35: 195–200.

Parsons C., Iacono T. et al. (1987): Effect of tongue reduction on articulation in children with Down syndrome. Am J Ment Retard 91: 328–332.

Partington, M., MacDonald M. et al. (1971): 5-Hydroxytryptophan (5-HTP) in Down's syndrome. Dev Med Child Neurol 13: 362–372.

Pueschel S., Reed R. et al. (1980): 5-Hydroxytryptophan and pyridoxine. Am J Dis Child 134: 834–844.

Pueschel S. M., Pueschel J. K. (eds.) (1992): Biomedical Concerns in Persons with Down Syndrome. Baltimore, Paul H. Brookes.

Schmid F. (1978): Down syndrome: Treatment and management. Cytobiologische Revue 1: 25–32.

Smith G., Spiker D. et al. (1984): Use of megadoses of vitamins with minerals in Down syndrome. J Pediatr 105: 228–234.

Spigelblatt L., Laîné-Ammara G. et al. (1994): The use of alternative medicine by children. Pediatrics 94(6): 811–814.

Turkel H., Nusbaum I. (1985): Medical Treatment of Down Syndrome and Genetic Disease. Southfield, MI: Ubiotica.

VanDyke D., Lang D. et al. (1990): Cell therapy in children with Down syndrome: A retrospective study. Pediatrics 85(1): 79–84.

Weise P., Koch R. et al. (1974): The use of 5-HTP in the treatment of Down's syndrome. Pediatrics 54: 165–168.

# THE GENETIC ORIGINS OF COGNITION AND HEART DISEASE IN DOWN SYNDROME

JULIE R. KORENBERG , PH.D., M.D., GILLIAN BARLOW, PH.D., LORA S. SALANDANAN, B.S., PRANAY BHATTACHARYYA, B.S., XIAO-NING CHEN, M.D., AND GARY E. LYONS, PH.D.

## INTRODUCTION

Down syndrome (DS) is the most common cause of genetic mental retardation (Epstein, 1986) and affects the welfare of over 350,000 individuals and their families in the U.S. alone. DS is also associated with a wide variety of other clinical features, including congenital heart and intestinal disease, eye problems, deficits of the immune and endocrine systems, and increased risks for leukemia and Alzheimer disease, as well as characteristic facial and physical features.

Researchers first began to tease out the genetic basis of these cognitive and physical features in 1959 with the discovery that DS was caused by the presence of three copies of chromosome 21 (Jacobs et al., 1959; Lejeune et al., 1959). This extra *normal* genetic material resulted in the overexpression of specific genes that then subtly disturbed the biological pathways underly-

*Down Syndrome*, Edited by William I. Cohen, Lynn Nadel, and Myra E. Madnick.
ISBN 0-471-41815-3   Copyright © 2002 by Wiley-Liss, Inc.

ing the various features or "phenotypes" of DS. And by 1992, we knew that smaller slices of chromosome 21 were associated with subsets of features including congenital heart and intestinal disease, cognitive deficits, and facial features (McCormick et al., 1989; Rahmani et al., 1990, Korenberg et al., 1990, 1992). However, by 1994 (Korenberg et al., 1994) it became clear that we needed to know more about the problems of individuals with DS and more about the genes on chromosome 21. Today, with the completion of the entire DNA sequence of chromosome 21 (Hattori et al., 2000) and most of the sequence of the remainder of the human genome (Cheung et al., 2001), we can begin to relate the chromosomal aberrations observed in subjects with DS to the information in genome databases. By doing this, we can obtain clues to understanding how the imbalance of specific genes on chromosome 21 lead to the clinical features of DS.

The challenge now facing DS researchers is to understand both the genes and developmental pathways that link these genes to features of DS. Although there are many important questions, it is important to begin with problems whose solution will improve the life experience of persons with DS. Therefore, we have investigated the origins of congenital heart disease (CHD) and mental retardation (MR) in rare persons with DS and partial trisomy for 21 and have related their features to the molecular structure and genes located on their chromosomes 21. This essential step will provide a firm basis for designing and applying new therapies to improve cognition and behavior, to ameliorate CHD, to treat endocrine and immune deficits, and to decrease the risk of cancer, both in DS and in the normal population.

In this chapter, we will describe progress in relating genes to features of DS beginning with tools such as the *partial trisomy panel*. We will show how these individuals can provide insight into the relationship of specific genes to clinical aspects of DS. We will then use MR and CHD to illustrate models for understanding development.

## TOOLS FOR RELATING GENES TO FEATURES: INDIVIDUALS WITH PARTIAL TRISOMY 21

Our work began by identifying individuals with partial trisomies for chromosome 21, meaning individuals with only *distinct* triplicated regions. This is in contrast to full trisomy, commonly associated with DS, in which the *entire* chromosome is present as a third copy, instead of two copies. As a consequence of the distinct parts of chromosome 21 present in three copies, individuals with partial trisomy have sets of features different from those with full trisomy (Epstein, 1986). These rare individuals provide the opportunity to correlate clinical and molecular levels of DS, by relating specific features, such as CHD and mental retardation, to explicit subsets of chromosome 21 genes.

On the molecular level, a number of methods were used to define the regions duplicated in patients with partial aneuploidy of chromosome 21. These are quantitative Southern blot dosage analysis and fluorescence in situ hybridization (FISH), as described by Korenberg et al. (1994). Each utilizes a series of previously mapped chromosome 21 DNA markers to define the copy number and/or structural rearrangement of the aneuploid chromosome, where the approximate map positions and order for each of these loci was first indicated by physical mapping studies (Cox and Shimizu, 1991; Gardiner et al., 1990; Korenberg et al., 1989; Owen et al., 1990) and now by reference to the DNA sequence of chromosome 21 as described elsewhere in this volume. Combining the results from all methods produced information both on copy number and on structural orientation of regions on chromosome 21 duplicated and/or deleted in each of the individuals with partial trisomy 21. A summary of the molecular studies on many individuals is shown in Figure 20.1.

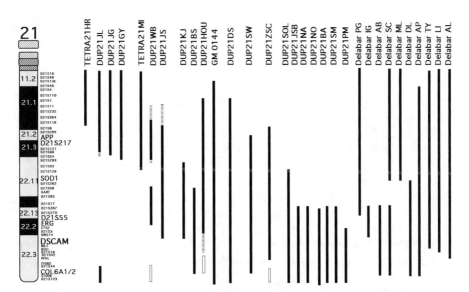

FIGURE 20.1. Panel of individuals with partial trisomy for chromosome 21. These individuals have extra copies of different regions of chromosome 21 (represented by the black lines) and have different subsets of the features of Down syndrome (DS). The open boxes represent single-copy regions. All of the DS individuals represented are described in Barlow et al. (2001a) and Korenberg et al. (1994), with the exception of TETRA21HR (Slavotinek et al., 2000). The cases on the right were described by the group of Jean Delabar.

## CHROMOSOME 21 SEQUENCE LEADS TO
## INFORMATION ON GENES

Chromosome 21, the smallest of human chromosomes, was one of the first to be sequenced in its entirety (Hattori et al., 2000). The molecular data described above were further refined by relating regions of triplications with DNA sequence to identify genes located within, a rigorous approach employing current databases [Genome Database (http://www.gdb.org), NCBI (http://www.ncbi.nlm.nih.gov), and the Wellcome Trust Sanger Institute (http://www.sanger.ac.uk)] and other available programs [Vector NTI (http://www.informaxinc.com), Emboss (http://www.hgmp.mrc.ac.uk), and Sim 4 (Florea et al., 1998)], making it possible to determine chromosome 21 rearrangements as well as duplications and deletions of specific regions and genes.

## PHENOTYPIC MAPS OF DS

### WHICH OF THE MANY GENES ON CHROMOSOME 21 ARE RESPONSIBLE FOR DS?

The summary of molecular studies seen in the partial trisomy panel (Fig. 20.1) along with clinical data collected (Korenberg et al., 1994) provide the basis for a DS phenotypic map. By "phenotype" we mean any feature or measurable parameter, including neurocognitive, neuroanatomic, clinical, physical, cellular, and physiological features. The purpose of constructing a "phenotypic map" is to define molecularly the chromosomal regions and ultimately the genes, which are responsible for the variation in particular features. Although there are approximately 250 genes (see Chapter 18 by Patterson) known on this chromosome, overexpression of only a portion of them mapping to D21S267 at band 21q22.1 through the telomere can produce many of the characteristic features seen in persons with DS (Rahmani et al., 1989; McCormick et al., 1989; Korenberg et al., 1990; Korenberg et al., 1992). Nonetheless, it is known that the overexpression of genes on chromosome 21 outside this region is also associated with many cognitive and physical features (Korenberg et al., 1994). The features (phenotypes) seen in individuals with DS may result from the interactions of a small or large number of genes, both on chromosome 21 and elsewhere in the genome. Some or one of the genes on chromosome 21 may be responsible for an overwhelming share of the variation seen in uncommon, more specific traits such as atrioventricular septal defects or duodenal stenosis (Korenberg et al., 1992; Barlow et al., 2001a). In contrast, for common, nonspecific phenotypes such as short stature, mental retardation, and upslanting palpebral fissures, many genes likely contribute (Korenberg et al., 1994). To begin to sort out which chromosome 21 genes or combinations are responsible for the phenotypes of DS, we keep these caveats in mind and use the information from the individuals with partial trisomy 21 to examine which questions can be answered now.

## Is There a Single Gene or Gene Cluster Responsible for the Features of DS?

One significant conclusion is there is *no* single gene or gene cluster whose duplication is responsible for *all* DS features, because duplication of regions *distinct from* distal 21q22 is sufficient to produce many of what have been called "typical DS features." This is illustrated in Figure 20.2 by three children with duplications for different regions of chromosome 21 all of whom, however, have developmental delay and hypotonia. We note that individual in the top panel in Figure 20.2 also has some of the facial features of persons with DS and has four copies of genes in the region indicated, which is entirely different and does not include any genes from the region that has been suggested as the "Down syndrome critical region" (Delabar et al., 1993). These additional regions expand the knowledge of the molecular-genetic basis of DS features and emphasize the necessity for the construction of detailed phenotypic maps and the need for further definition of measurable "phenotypes," particularly for the neurocognitive features.

## Could One or a Few Known Genes Be Responsible for Much or Most of the Cognitive Features of DS?

Although the overexpression of each of a small number of genes could, by itself, be responsible for aspects of the cognitive deficits, many genes must contribute. For example, we can see from the individual in the middle panel of Figure 20.2 that the region including the minibrain gene (*DYRK1A*) in the absence of other regions is not invariably associated with the facial features or with severe MR. Similarly, the gene for superoxide dismutase (*SOD1*) is not duplicated in many individuals with partial duplications, almost all of whom have moderate cognitive deficits (Korenberg et al., 1994). Nonetheless, like others with similar duplications, these individuals will provide unique opportunities to determine which aspects of cognitive function *are* associated with these genes.

## Are There Any Features That Have Been Linked to Smaller Numbers of Genes?

The increased risk of Alzheimer disease (AD) seen in persons with DS has important implications for the quality of later life, and mutations in the

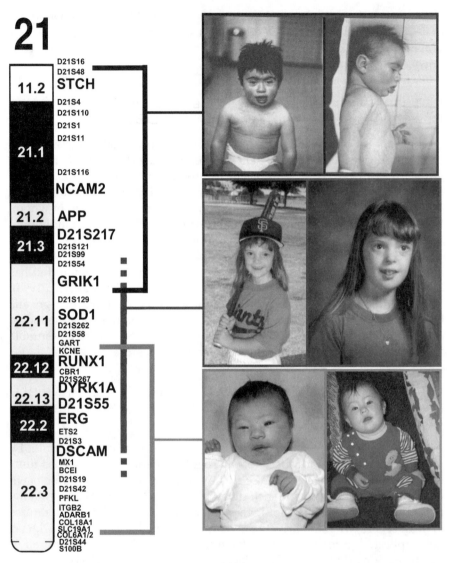

FIGURE 20.2. Three individuals with different chromosome 21 duplications. The top panel shows individual TETRA21MI (Daumer-Haas et al., 1994) who has four copies of the region and genes indicated, associated with developmental delay, hypotonia, and some facial features of DS. The middle panel shows an individual, DUP21KJ, who has three copies of the region and genes indicated, associated with mild developmental delay and mild DS facial features. The bottom panel shows individual DUP21BS, who has three copies of the region and genes indicated, associated with congenital heart disease, developmental delay, and DS facial features.

chromosome 21 gene *APP* (amyloid precursor protein) have been associated with the familial form of AD. Moreover, although not associated with severe decline, after the age of 40 years, 100% of persons with DS reveal the neuritic plaques and tangles characteristic of the brain in AD (Wisniewski et al., 1985; Rumble et al., 1989). Further support for linking APP with AD in DS comes from a 78-year-old individual with DS clinical features and a duplication that did *not* include APP, who did *not* develop the plaques and tangles, nor cognitive decline (Prasher et al., 1998). Nonetheless, there are many other chromosome 21 genes that may contribute to the risk. These include *BACE2* (a beta secretase that modifies the APP protein) (Solans et al., 2000), *SOD1* (involved in superoxide metabolism and oxygen radical damage) (Brooksbank and Balazs, 1983; Ackerman et al., 1988), *PEP19* (involved in modification of neuronal calcium flux) (Gerendasy and Sutcliffe 1997; Johanson et al., 2000), and others, and study of individuals with partial trisomy may provide insight into the causes of AD in DS as well as in the remainder of the population.

Smaller regions of chromosome 21 have been shown to contain genes linked to duodenal stenosis (DST) and congenital heart disease (CHD) (Korenberg et al., 1992). Although the region and number of gene candidates for DST have been limited to the region including the genes for NCAM2 (a neural cell adhesion molecule) (Paoloni-Giacobino et al., 1997) through DSCAM (a neural cell adhesion molecule expressed in brain and peripheral nervous system including the wall of the intestines) (Yamakawa et al., 1998), there are many genes between and the incidence of DST is low, which may limit further cases. Nonetheless, the gene candidates in this region may now be tested for their role in the development of the intestines.

In the past year, the role of chromosome 21 genes in causing congenital heart disease in DS has been further defined; in individuals with CHD, duplication of the region including genes from D21S3 through the region of PFKL appears to be a common link (Barlow et al., 2001a) and will be described below. However, the mechanisms, pathways, and genes underlying mental retardation in DS are less well understood, as will now be discussed.

## Causes of Mental Retardation in DS

Mental retardation and abnormalities of the central and peripheral nervous systems (CNS and PNS) are features of individuals with DS that are noted from early development throughout adult life (Epstein, 1986). Unlike many of the other features of DS, which affect only a certain number of individuals, some degree of mental retardation is seen in all DS individuals. Furthermore, as discussed above, data from individuals with partial trisomy 21 suggest that the general quality of impaired mental function seen in DS

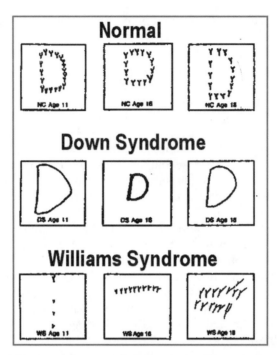

FIGURE 20.3. Cognitive abilities in DS. Individuals with DS have relative strengths in global processing but show impairments in local processing (Bihrle et al., 1989). Reprinted with permission by the Salk Institute.

cannot be mapped to any one region of chromosome 21 but rather that genes from many different parts of the chromosome are involved (Korenberg et al., 1994). How then can researchers begin to identify the genes responsible for mental retardation in DS?

To do this, we must first delineate a series of *measurable* cognitive features that *clearly* distinguish individuals with DS from the larger human population. Cognitive features include defects in auditory and visual spatial processing and in short-term memory, although there are relative strengths in visual-spatial short-term memory. One of the most specific cognitive features is the preservation of global versus the impairment of local processing (Bihrle et al., 1989; see Fig. 20.3), an example of the type of definable feature that may be amenable to mapping in partially trisomic individuals. Other DS cognitive features are less specific and thus would be difficult to map directly but may be related to mappable structural alterations in the brain. Thus it may be possible to map cognitive features indirectly, through understanding associated neurological, neuroanatomic, or functional changes in the brain. Structural abnormalities of the brain in DS include regression and distortion of the dendritic tree beginning after 4 months of age, a mean decrease in brain weight of 10–20% that begins after 6 months of age (Becker

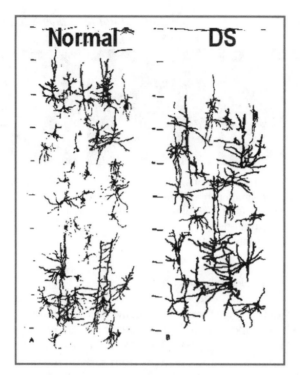

FIGURE 20.4. The development of the dendritic tree, part of the nervous system involved in sending and receiving signals, is impaired in individuals with DS, which may underlie some aspects of DS cognitive defects (Becker et al., 1993).

et al., 1993; see Fig. 20.4), abnormal formation of the sulci and gyri, and defective lamination of the cortex coupled with reduced cortical thickness (Golden and Hyman, 1994). Adults with DS also have substantially smaller cerebral and cerebellar hemispheres and hippocampal formations than the rest of the population (Pinter et al., 2001; see Fig. 20.5). Individuals with DS exhibit particular defects in speech and language that may involve regions of the prefrontal cortex, hippocampus and cerebellum and deficits in executive functions that may be associated with basal ganglia dysfunction (Pennington and Bennetto, 1996). Thus it may be possible, by uncovering the pathways that link these structural defects to cognitive function, to begin to map DS cognitive deficits to specific regions of chromosome 21. It is now important to understand the cognitive deficits seen in DS individuals in detail and to correlate these with detailed structural and functional studies employing new approaches to brain imaging [magnetic resonance imaging (MRI), functional MRI, and event-related potentials] variations in the brain. With this new level of information, it may be possible to correlate gene function with deficits in specific domains seen in persons with DS.

*The Hippocampus is smaller but not the amygdala in Down Syndrome*

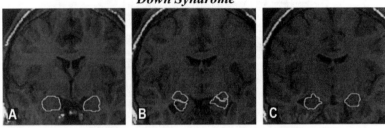

FIGURE 20.5. The hippocampus, a region of the brain central to learning and memory, tends to be smaller in individuals with DS (Pinter et al., 2001), which may contribute to the learning difficulties associated with DS. This was determined by measuring the boundaries of the amygdala (A and superior structures in B) and hippocampus (C and inferior structures in B).

Although none of the genes on chromosome 21 can as yet be related to these structural defects, genes expressed in the developing and adult brain are good candidates. These include *DSCAM* (Down syndrome cell adhesion molecule), which codes for a neural cell adhesion molecule mapping in 21q22 (Yamakawa et al., 1998). *DSCAM* is expressed in the developing central and peripheral nervous systems from early in the development of the fetal brain (Yamakawa et al., 1998) and continues to be expressed in the brain throughout adult life (Barlow et al., 2001b). Within the brain, *DSCAM* is expressed in the cerebral cortex, hippocampus, and cerebellum (Barlow et al., 2001b; see Fig. 20.6), all of which are affected in DS (Jernigan et al., 1993; Golden and Hyman 1994; Raz et al., 1995). In particular, the hippocampus is important for learning and memory as well as for retaining and possibly processing sensory inputs before transferring them to the cortex for long-term memory storage (Kandel et al., 1995), which are affected in individuals with DS (Pennington and Benetto, 1996). This pattern of *DSCAM* expression in the adult brain therefore suggests that *DSCAM* may play a role in the ongoing defects of learning and memory associated with DS.

## THE GENETIC ORIGIN OF CONGENITAL HEART DISEASE IN DOWN SYNDROME

Heart disease and defects of the cardiovascular system are responsible for the majority of premature deaths caused by congenital defects (Clark, 1987). Congenital heart disease (CHD) is particularly common in individuals with DS. It is detectable in 40–60% of individuals with DS and at autopsy in almost 70% of DS individuals. The schematic view of heart development shown in Figure 20.7 illustrates many of the regulatory molecules that play

## *DSCAM is Expressed in the Hippocampus*

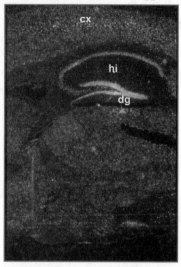

**3 months**

FIGURE 20.6. The chromosome 21 gene DSCAM is highly expressed in the hippocampus (hi), as indicated by the areas of white signals and has been proposed to contribute to DS cognitive defects (Barlow et al., 2001b). cx, cortex; dg, dentate gyrus.

## Cardiac Looping and Chamber Formation

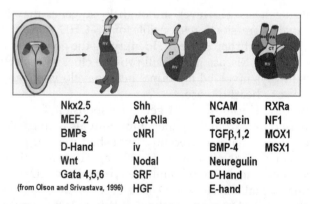

| Nkx2.5 | Shh | NCAM | RXRa |
|---|---|---|---|
| MEF-2 | Act-RIIa | Tenascin | NF1 |
| BMPs | cNRI | TGFβ,1,2 | MOX1 |
| D-Hand | iv | BMP-4 | MSX1 |
| Wnt | Nodal | Neuregulin | |
| Gata 4,5,6 | SRF | D-Hand | |
| (from Olson and Srivastava, 1996) | HGF | E-hand | |

FIGURE 20.7. Genes known to be involved in the different stages of the development of the heart (Olson and Srivastava, 1996). Although many genes have been identified, none of these is located on chromosome 21 and so cannot be directly responsible for the heart defects associated with DS.

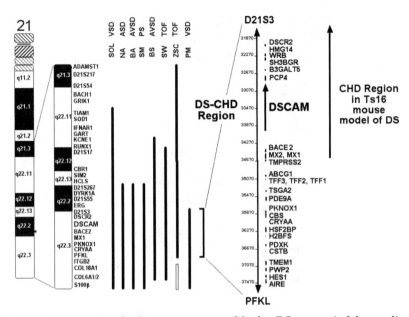

FIGURE 20.8. To identify the genes responsible for DS congenital heart disease (CHD), we compared the regions of chromosome 21 duplicated in eight different individuals with DS (represented by the black lines). The white box represents a single-copy region in individual DUP21ZSC. The region of overlap (candidate region) spans from D21S3 to at least PFKL and contains at least 35 known genes (shown on the right) (Hattori et al., 2000). Five of these genes are known to be expressed in the heart and may therefore contribute to heart disease in DS: *SH3BGR*, *DSCR2*, *WRB*, *DSCAM*, and *HES1* (Barlow et al., 2001a).

a role in cardiogenesis. However, although these genes may interact with those whose overexpression is responsible for DS-CHD, none of these known genes are located on chromosome 21. Identifying the genes and mechanisms responsible for heart disease in DS will provide clues to understanding the genes and pathways involved in normal heart development and the disturbances that lead to heart disease.

To identify the chromosome 21 gene(s) responsible for heart disease in DS, we have used data from the panel of individuals with partial trisomy 21 (Fig. 20.1) combined with the recently published map of chromosome 21 genes (Hattori et al., 2000; Barlow et al., 2001a). There are 19 individuals in the partial trisomy panel, 8 of whom have typical DS-CHD, which includes atrioventricular septal defects (AVSDs), atrial septal defects (ASDs), ventricular septal defects (VSDs), and tetralogy of Fallot (TOF). Figure 20.8 shows the regions of chromosome 21 triplicated in these eight individuals. All of their triplications overlap, and the total risk of CHD for individuals with this region (8/14 or 57%) is about the same as for full trisomy 21 (50–60%;

Korenberg et al., 1992), suggesting that a single gene or small group of genes is responsible for these types of CHD in DS. The region of overlap among the triplications defines the small region of chromosome 21 where these genes are located, between D21S3 and PFKL (Fig. 20.8). This "candidate" region is only 5.5 Mb in size, almost half the size of the previous candidate region (~10 Mb; Korenberg et al., 1994).

This narrowed candidate region excludes the region of D21S55, which was thought to contain genes responsible for many features of DS (Rahmani et al., 1989; Delabar et al., 1993; Korenberg et al., 1994). Also excluded is the region near the telomere (Fig. 20.8), which contains the genes encoding collagen VI. Collagen VI is expressed in the developing heart (Klewer et al., 1998) and has been considered a strong candidate for DS-CHD (Davies et al., 1995). It is important to stress that these data do not mean that collagen VI does not play a role in heart development, but rather that the overexpression of gene(s) in the region D21S3 through PFKL is sufficient to cause some forms of DS-CHD (discussed in Barlow et al., 2001a).

According to the recently published gene map of chromosome 21, the region from D21S3 through PFKL contains 39 known genes and a further 25 predicted genes (Hattori et al., 2000). Of these, we may reasonably assume

## DSCAM Expression in mouse embryonic heart

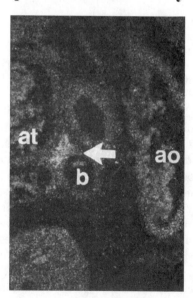

FIGURE 20.9. The chromosome 21 gene *DSCAM* is expressed in the cardiac ganglion (arrow), part of the nervous system controlling cardiac function, during the early heart development (Yamakawa et al., 1998).

## DSCR2 Expression in mouse embryo

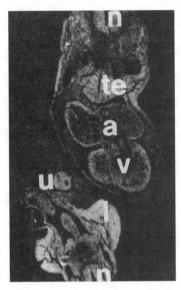

FIGURE 20.10. The chromosome 21 gene *DSCR2* is expressed in the muscular wall of the atria (a) and ventricles (v) of the heart during fetal development, as indicated by the area of white signals (Korenberg et al., manuscript in preparation).

that those responsible for DS-CHD are expressed at some time during development in the tissues that contribute to the fetal heart. However, the current map is new, many of these genes are recently identified, and their expression patterns are not yet known. At present, five are known to be expressed in the heart during development (Fig. 20.8). These include *DSCAM*, which encodes a cell adhesion molecule of the Ig superfamily (Yamakawa et al., 1998; Barlow et al., 2001; Fig. 20.9); *DSCR2*, which is thought to function in cell proliferation (Vidal-Taboada et al., 2000; Hubert et al., 1997; Fig. 20.10); *SH3BGR*, which encodes a glutamic acid-rich protein (Scartezzini et al., 1997; Fig. 20.11); *WRB*, which encodes a tryptophan-rich basic protein (Egeo et al., 1998); and *HES1*, which is thought to function in cellular metabolism (Scott et al., 1997). Thus combining data from DS individuals and the gene map of chromosome 21 has allowed the identification of five initial candidate genes for DS-CHD. Goals for future research include determining the effects of increased expression of these genes, using transgenic mice and other model systems to probe their functions, providing insight into the roles played by these genes in heart development and in heart disease both in DS and in the larger human population.

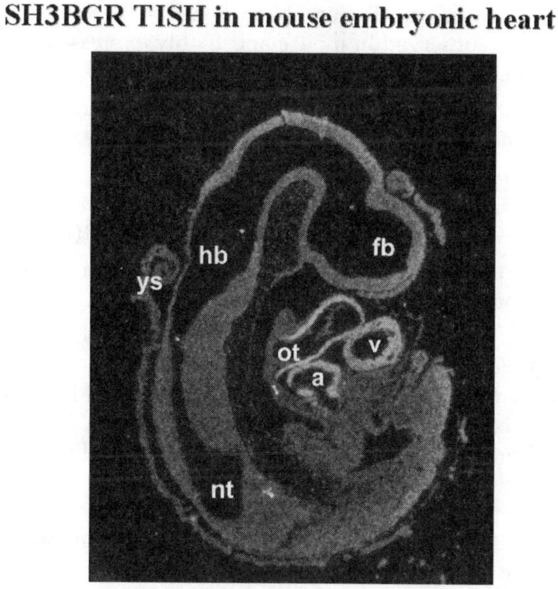

## SH3BGR TISH in mouse embryonic heart

FIGURE 20.11. The chromosome 21 gene *SH3BGR* is also expressed in the muscular wall of the atria and ventricles during fetal development (Korenberg et al., manuscript in preparation).

In summary, DS and its phenotypes are most accurately thought of as the result of the overexpression and subsequent interactions of a subset of genes on chromosome 21. All data together suggest that in the future we will be able to correlate the genetic basis of DS with phenotypes and associated defects. Ultimately, this knowledge will help to discover some of the causes of mental retardation and a cure for CHD, as well as a protocol of how to approach studies of other diseases associated with DS.

## REFERENCES

Ackerman AD, Fackler JC, Tuck-Muller CM, Tarpey MM, Freeman BA, Rogers MC (1988): Partial monosomy 21, diminished activity of superoxide dismutase, and pulmonary oxygen toxicity. New England Journal of Medicine 23; 318(25): 1666–1669.

Barlow GM, Chen X-N, Shi ZY, Celle L, Spinner N, Zackai E, Lyons GE, Mjaatvedt C, Pettenati MJ, Van Riper AJ, Vekemans M, Korenberg JR (2001): Down Syndrome Congenital Heart Disease: A narrowed region and a candidate gene. Genetics in Medicine, 3(2):91–101.

Barlow GM, Micales B, Lyons GE, Korenberg JR (2001): Down Syndrome Cell Adhesion Molecule is conserved in mouse and highly expressed in the adult mouse brain. Cytogenetics & Cell Genetics 94(3&4):155–162.

Becker LE, Mito T, Takashima S, Onodera K, Friend WC (1993): Association of phenotypic abnormalities of Down syndrome with an imbalance of genes on chromosome 21. APMIS Suppl 40:57–70.

Bihrle AM, Bellugi U, Delis D, Marks S (1989): Seeing either the forest or the trees: dissociation in visuospatial processing. Brain Cogniti 11(1):37–49.

Brooksbank BW, Balazs R (1983): Superoxide dismutase and lipoperoxidation in Down's syndrome fetal brain. Lancet 1(8329):881–882.

Cheung VG, Nowak N, Jang W, Kirsch I, Zhao S, Chen X-N, Kim UJ, Kuo WL, Oliver M, Conroy J, Furey T, Kasprzyk A, Massa H, Yonescu R, Sait S, Thoreen C, Snijders A, Lemyre E, Bruzel A, Burrill W, Clegg SM, Collins S, Dhami P, Friedman C, Lee J, Lowry S, Morley M, Narasimhan S, Peng Z, Plajzer-Frick I, Scott D, Sirotkin K, Thorpe AA, Eichler EE, Gray JW, Hudson J, Pinkel D, Ried T, Rowen L, Shen-Ong GL, Strausberg RL, Birney E, Cheng JF, Doggett N, Cox D, Carter NP, Haussler D, Korenberg JR, Morton CC, Albertson D, Schuler G, de Jong P, Trask BJ (2001): Integration of cytogenetic landmarks into the draft sequence of the human genome. Nature 409:953–958.

Clark EB (1987): Mechanisms in the pathogenesis of congenital heart defects. In: Pierpoint MEM, Moller JH (eds.), The genetics of cardiovascular disease. Martinus-Nijoff, Boston 3–11.

Cox AD, Goodall AH (1991) Activation-specific neo-antigens on platelets detected by monoclonal antibodies. Curr Stud Hematol Blood Transfus 58:194–199.

Cox DR (1992): Radiation hybrid mapping. Cytogenetics & Cell Genetics 59(3): 80–81.

Daumer-Haas C, Schuffenhauer S, Schipper RD, Portsmann T, Korenberg JR (1994): Tetrasomy 21 pter→q22.1 and Down syndrome: molecular definition of the region. American Journal of Medical Genetics 53(4):359–365.

Davies GE, Howard CM, Farrer MJ, Coleman MM, Bennett LB, Cullen LM, Wyse RK, Burn J, Williamson R, Kessling AM (1995): Genetic variation in the COL6A1 region is associated with congenital heart defects in trisomy 21 (Down's syndrome). Ann Hum Genet 59:253–269.

Delabar JM, Theophile D, Rahmani Z, Chettouh Z, Blouin JL, Preiur M, Noel B, Sinet PM (1993): Molecular mapping of 24 features of Down syndrome on chromosome 21. European Journal of Human Genetics 1:114–124.

Egeo A, Mazzocco M, Arrigo P, Vidal-Taboada JM, Oliva R, Pirola B, Giglio S, Rasore-Quartino A, Scartezzini P (1998): Identification and characterization of a new human cDNA from chromosome 21q22.3 encoding a basic nuclear protein. Hum Genet 102:289–293.

Epstein CJ, Korenberg JR, Anneren G, Antonarakis SE, Ayme S, Courchesne E, Epstein LB, Fowler A, Groner Y, Kemper TL, Lott IT, Lubin BH, Magenis E, Opitz JM, Patterson D, Priest JH, Pueschel SM, Rapoport SI, Sinet PM, de la Cruz, F (1991): Protocols to establish genotype/phenotype correlations in Down syndrome. American Journal of Human Genetics, 49:207–235.

Epstein CJ (1986): The consequences of chromosomal imbalance. Cambridge University Press, Cambridge.

Florea L, Hartzell G, Zhang Z, Rubin GM, Miller W (1998): A computer program for aligning a cDNA sequence with a genomic DNA sequence. Genome Research 8(9):967–974.

Gardiner K, Horisberger M, Kraus J, Tantravahi U, Korenberg JR, Rao V, Reddy S, Patterson D (1990): Analysis of human chromosome 21: Correlation of physical and cytogenetic maps: Gene and CpG island distribution. EMBO Journal 9:25–34.

Gerendasy DD, Sutcliffe JG (1997): RC3/neurogranin, a postsynaptic calpacitin for getting the response threshold to calcium influxes. Molecular Neurobiology 15(2):131–163.

Golden JA, Hyman BT (1994): Development of the superior temporal neocortex is anomalous in trisomy 21. J Neuropath Exp Neurol 53(5):513–520.

Hattori M, Fujiyama A, Taylor TD, Watanabe D, Yada T, Park HS, Toyoda A, Ishii K, Totoki Y, Choi DK, Soeda E, Ohki M, Takagi T, Sakaki Y, Taudien S, Blechschmidt K, Polley A, Menzei U, Delabar J, Kumpf K, Lehmann R, Patterson D, Reichwald K, Rump A, Schillhabel M, Schudy A, Zimmermann W, Rosenthal A, Kudoh J, Shibuya K, Kawasaki K, Asakawa S, Shintani A, Sasaki T, Nagamine K, Mitsuyama S, Antonarakis SE, Minoshima S, Shimizu N, Nordsiek G, Hornischer K, Brandt P, Scharfe M, Schon O, Desario A, Reichelt J, Kauer G, Blocker H, Ramser J, Beck A, Klages S, Henning S, Riesselmann L, Dagand E, Haaf T, Wehrmeyer S, Borzym K, Gardiner K, Nizetic D, Francis F, Lehrach H, Reinhardt R, Yaspo ML (2000): The DNA sequence of human chromosome 21. Nature 405:311–319.

Hubert RS, Mitchell S, Chen X-N, Ekmekji K, Gadomski C, Sun Z, Noya D, Kim U-J, Chen C, Shizuya H, Simon M, de Jong PJ, Korenberg JR (1997): BAC and PAC contigs covering 3.5 Mb of the Down Syndrome congenital heart disease region between D21S55 and MX1 on chromosome 21. Genomics 41:218–226.

Jacobs P, Baikie A, Court-Brown W, Strong J (1959): The somatic chromosomes in mongolism. Lancet I 710–711.

Jernigan TL, Bellugi U, Sowell E, Doherty S, Hesselink JR (1993) Cerebral morphologic distinctions between Williams and Down syndromes. Arch Neurol 50:186–191.

Kandel ER, Schwartz JH, Jessel TM (eds.) (1995) Essentials of neural science and behaviour. Appelton and Lange, Stanford, CT.

Klewer SE, Krob SL, Kolker SJ, Kitten GT (1998): Expression of type VI collagen in the developing mouse heart. Dev Dyn 211(3):248–255.

Johanson RA, Sarau HM, Foley JJ, Slemmon JR (2000): Calmodulin-binding peptide PEP-19 modulates activation of calmodulin kinase II in situ. Journal of Neuroscience 20(8):2860–2866.

Kimura M, Hirota H, Nishikawa T, Ishiyama S, Imamura S, Korenberg JR, Mizuno K, Nakayama T, Akagawa K, Shimizu N, Joh-o K, Diaz C, Tatsuguchi M, Komatsu K, Ando M, Takao A, Momma K, Matsuoka R (2000): Chromosomal Deletion and Phenotype Correlation in Patients with Williams Syndrome, Etiology & Morphogenesis of Congenital Heart Disease: Twenty Years of Progress in

Genetics and Developmental Biology. Futura Publishing, Armonk NY, pp. 381–338.

Korenberg JR, Barlow G, Chen X-N, Lyons G, Mjaatvedt C, Vekemens M (2000): Down Syndrome Congenital Heart Disease: Narrowed Region and DSCAM as a Candidate Gene. Etiology & Morphogenesis of Congenital Heart Disease: Twenty Years Of Progress In Genetics and Developmental Biology. Futura Publishing, Armonk NY, pp. 365–370.

Korenberg JR, Chen XN, Schipper R, Sun Z, Gonsky R, Gerwehr S, Berry K, Carpenter N, Daumer C, Dignan P, Disteche C, Graham J, Hudgins L, Lewin S, McGillivray B, Miyasaki K, Ogasawara N, Pagon R, Pueschel S, Sack G, Say B, Schuffenhauer S, Soukup S, Yamanaka T (1994): Down syndrome phenotypes: The consequences of chromosomal imbalance. Proceedings of the National Academy of Science USA, 91(11):4997–5001.

Korenberg JR, Shreck R, Yang-Feng T, Chen X-N (1992): Using fluorescence in situ hybridization (FISH) in genome mapping. Trends in Biotechnology, 10(1,2): 27–32.

Korenberg JR, Kawashima H, Pulst SM, Ikeuchi T, Ogasawara N, Yamamoto K, Schonberg SA, Kojis T, Allen L, Magenis E, Ikawa H, Taniguchi N, Epstein CJ (1990): Molecular definition of a region of chromosome 21 that causes features of the down syndrome phenotype. American Journal of Human Genetics 47:236–246.

Korenberg JR, Pulst SM, Neve RL, West R (1989): The Alzheimer amyloid precursor protein maps to human chromosome 21 bands q21.105–q21.05. Genomics 5:124–127.

Lejeune J, Gauthier M, Turpin R (1959): Etudes des chromosomes somatiques de neuf enfants mongoliens. C R Acad Sci (Paris)248:1721–1722.

McCormick MK, Schinzel A, Petersen MB, Stetten G, Driscoll DJ, Cantu ES, Tranebjacrg Mikkelsen M, Watkins PC, Antonarakis SE (1989): Molecular genetic approach to the characterization of the "Down syndrome region" of chromosome 21. Genomics 5(2):325–331.

McPherson JD, Marra M, Hillier L, Waterston RH, Chinwalla A, Wallis J, Sekhon M, Wylie K, Mardis ER, Wilson RK, Fulton R, Kucaba TA, Wagner-McPherson C, Barbazuk WB, Gregory SG, Humphray SJ, French L, Evans RS, Bethel G, Whittaker A, Holden JL, McCann OT, Dunham A, Soderlund C, Scott CE, Bentley DR, Schuler G, Chen HC, Jang W, Green ED, Idol JR, Maduro VV, Montgomery KT, Lee E, Miller A, Emerling S, Kucherlapati, Gibbs R, Scherer S, Gorrell JH, Sodergren E, Clerc-Blankenburg K, Tabor P, Naylor S, Garcia D, de Jong PJ, Catanese JJ, Nowak N, Osoegawa K, Qin S, Rowen L, Madan A, Dors M, Hood L, Trask B, Friedman C, Massa H, Cheung VG, Kirsch IR, Reid T, Yonescu R, Weissenbach J, Bruls T, Heilig R, Branscomb E, Olsen A, Doggett N, Cheng JF, Hawkins T, Myers RM, Shang J, Ramirez L, Schmutz J, Velasquez O, Dixon K, Stone NE, Cox DR, Haussler D, Kent WJ, Furey T, Rogic S, Kennedy S, Jones S, Rosenthal A, Wen G, Schilhabel M, Gloeckner G, Nyakatura G, Siebert R, Schlegelberger B, Korenberg JR, Chen X-N, Fujiyama A, Hattori M, Toyoda A, Yada T, Park HS, Sakaki Y, Shimizu N, Asakawa S, Kawasaki K, Sasaki T, Shintani A, Shimizu A, Shibuya K, Kudoh J, Minoshima S, Ramser J, Seranski P,

Hoff C, Poustka A, Reinhardt R, Lehrach H (2001): The International Human Genome Mapping Consortium. A physical map of the human genome. Nature 409:934–941.

Olson EN, Srivastava D (1996): Molecular pathyways controlling heart development. Science 272(5262):671–676.

Owen MJ, James LA, Hardy JA, Williamson R, Goate AM (1990): Physical mapping around the Alzheimer disease locus on the proximal long arm of chromosome 21. American Journal of Human Genetics 46(2):316–322.

Paoloni-Giacobino A, Chen H, Antonarakis SE (1997): Related Articles, Nucleotide, OMIM, Protein Cloning of a novel human neural cell adhesion molecule gene (NCAM2) that maps to chromosome region 21q21 and is potentially involved in Down syndrome. Genomics 43(1):43–51.

Pennington BF, Bennetto L (1996): Towards a neuropsychology of mental retardation. In: Burack JA, Hodapp RM, Zigler E (eds.), Handbook of mental retardation and development. Cambridge University Press, Cambridge.

Pinter JD, Brown WE, Eliez S, Schmitt JE, Capone GT, Reiss AL (2001): Amygdala and hippocampal volumes in children with Down syndrome: a high-resolution MRI study. Neurology 56(7):972–974.

Prasher VP, Farrer MJ, Kessling AM, Fisher EM, West RJ, Barber PC, Butler AC (1998): Molecular mapping of Alzheimer-type dementia in Down's syndrome. Annual Neurology 43(3):380–383.

Rahmani Z, Blouin JL, Creau-Goldberg N, Watkins PC, Mattei JF, Poissonnier M, Prieur M, Chettouh Z, Nicole A, Aurias A et al. (1990): Down syndrome critical region around D21S55 on proximal 21q22.3. American Journal of Medical Genetics Supplement 7:98–103.

Rahmani Z, Blouin JL, Creau-Goldberg N, Watkins PC, Mattei JF, Poissonnier M, Prieur M, Chettouh Z, Nicole A, Aurias A et al. (1989): Critical role of the D21S55 region on chromosome 21 in the pathogenesis of Down syndrome. Proc Natl Acad Sci USA 86(15):5958–5962.

Raz N, Torres IJ, Briggs SD, Spencer WD, Thomton AE, Loken WJ, Gunning FM et al. (1995) Selective neuroanatomic abnormalities in Down's syndrome and their cognitive correlates: evidence from MRI morphometry. Neurology 45: 356–366.

Rumble B, Retallack R, Hilbich C, Simms G, Multhaup G, Martins R, Hockey A, Montgomery P, Beyreuther K, Masters CL (1989): Amyloid A4 protein and its precursor in Down's syndrome and Alzheimer's disease. New England Journal of Medicine 320(22):1446–1452.

Scartezzini P, Egeo A, Colella S, Fumagalli P, Arrigo P, Nizetic D, Taramelli R (1997): Cloning a new human gene from chromosome 21q22.3 encoding a glutamic acid-rich protein expressed in and skeletal muscle. Hum Genet 99:387–392.

Scott HS, Chen H, Rossier C, Lalioti MD, Antonarakis SE (1997): Isolation of a human gene (HES1) with homology to an Escherichia coli and a zebrafish protein that maps to chromosome 21q22.3. Hum Genet 99:616–623.

Slavotinek AM, Chen XN, Jackson A, Gaunt L, Campbell A, Clayton-Smith J, Korenberg JR (2000): Partial tetrasomy 21 in a male infant. J Med Genet 37(10):E30.

Solans A, Estivill X, de La Luna S (2000): A new aspartyl protease on 21q22.3, BACE2, is highly similar to Alzheimer's amyloid precursor protein beta-secretase. Cytogenetics and Cell Genetics, 89(3–4):177–184.

Vidal-Taboada JM, Lu A, Pique M, Pons G, Gil J, Oliva R (2000): Down syndrome critical region gene 2: expression during mouse development and in human cell lines indicates a function related to cell proliferation. Biochem Biophys Res Commun 272:156–163.

Wisniewski KE, Wisniewski HM, Wen GY (1985): Occurrence of neuropathological changes and dementia of Alzheimer's disease in Down's syndrome. Annual Neurology 17(3):278–282.

Yamakawa K, Huo YK, Haendelt MA, Hubert R, Chen X-N, Lyons GE, Korenberg JR (1998): DSCAM: a novel member of the immunoglobulin superfamily maps in a Down syndrome region and is involved in the development of the nervous system. Hum Mol Genet 7:227–237.

## ABSTRACTS

Barlow GM, Chen X-N, Lyons GE, Mjaatvedt C, Kurnit D, Spinner N, Zackai E, Pettenati MJ, Van Riper AJ, Vekemans M, Korenberg JR (2000): Down syndrome congenital heart disease: Further delineation of the candidate region suggests components of the cardiac phenotype may be due to different candidate genes. Weinstein Cardiovascular Conference 2000, St. Louis, MO, June 2000.

Barlow GM, Chen X-N, Korenberg JR (2000): Down syndrome cell adhesion molecule: An endogenous promoter element drives the expression of a candidate gene for DS congenital heart disease in the developing mouse embryo. Weinstein Cardiovascular Conference 2000, St. Louis, MO, June 2000.

Barlow GM, Chen X-N, Lyons GE, Korenberg JR (2000): Down syndrome cell adhesion molecule: An endogenous promoter element drives the expression of a candidate gene for DS congenital heart disease in the developing mouse embryo. ASHG 50th Annual Meeting, Philadelphia, PA, October 2000.

Barlow GM, Chen X-N, Lyons GE, Korenberg JR (2001): Significance of specific chromosome 21 genes for the phenotypes of Down syndrome. International Conference on Chromosome 21 and Down Syndrome, Barcelona, Spain, April 6–7, 2001.

# THE ORIGIN AND ETIOLOGY OF TRISOMY 21

TERRY HASSOLD, PH.D., AND
STEPHANIE SHERMAN

## THE ORIGIN OF TRISOMY 21

Over the past decade, DNA polymorphisms have been used to investigate the parent and meiotic stage of origin of over 1000 trisomic fetuses and liveborns (Table 21.1). Trisomy 21 has been the most extensively studied condition, with over 700 informative cases. Chromosome segregation errors in the egg (i.e., maternal nondisjunction) predominate, accounting for approximately 90% of cases. Of these, over 75% are due to nondisjunction at maternal meiosis I (MI), with a smaller contribution from maternal meiosis II (MII) errors. A small proportion of cases of trisomy 21, about 10%, are apparently due to paternal meiotic errors or to postzygotic mitotic nondisjunction.

The other human trisomies that have been studied display remarkable variability in origin (Table 21.1). Nevertheless, the available evidence suggests that—like trisomy 21—errors at maternal MI are responsible for most human trisomies. It seems likely that factors associated with the origin of trisomy 21 pertain to other trisomies as well; thus studies of chromosome 21 nondisjunction likely serve as a paradigm for human nondisjunction in general.

*Down Syndrome*, Edited by William I. Cohen, Lynn Nadel, and Myra E. Madnick.
ISBN 0-471-41815-3   Copyright © 2002 by Wiley-Liss, Inc.

TABLE 21.1. STUDIES OF THE PARENT AND MEIOTIC/MITOTIC STAGE OF
ORIGIN OF HUMAN TRISOMIES (ADAPTED FROM HASSOLD AND HUNT, 2001)

| | | Origin (in %) | | | | |
| | | Paternal | | Maternal | | |
| Trisomy | No. of Cases | I | II | I | II | Mitotic |
| --- | --- | --- | --- | --- | --- | --- |
| 2 | 18 | 28 | – | 54 | 13 | 6 |
| 7 | 14 | – | – | 17 | 26 | 57 |
| 15 | 34 | – | 15 | 76 | 9 | – |
| 16 | 104 | – | – | 100 | – | – |
| 18 | 143 | – | – | 33 | 56 | 11 |
| 21 | 724 | 3 | 5 | 67 | 22 | 2 |
| 22 | 38 | 3 | – | 94 | 3 | – |
| XXY | 142 | 46 | – | 38 | 14 | 3 |
| XXX | 50 | – | 6 | 60 | 16 | 18 |

## THE ETIOLOGY OF TRISOMY 21

Despite years of study, we still know relatively little about risk factors that
influence the frequency of trisomy 21 in humans. However, recent studies
have identified an important correlate of human trisomy 21, namely, aberrant meiotic recombination, and have shed light on the only etiological factor
incontrovertibly linked to trisomy 21, namely, increasing age of the mother.

## RECOMBINATION AND NONDISJUNCTION OF CHROMOSOME 21

In virtually all organisms, the first meiotic division is a carefully orchestrated
process, consisting of three crucial steps: First, each of the homologous chromosomes find their partners and pair with one another (in humans, there
are 46 individual chromosomes, or 23 homologous pairs); second, each
pair of homologs exchanges genetic material, in a process known as genetic
recombination; and third, each of the homologous chromosomes separate
from their partners at metaphase to yield two daughter cells, each now containing 23 chromosomes.

Although errors in this final step (chromosome segregation) are ultimately responsible for generating trisomies, there is now considerable evidence that errors in the previous step (recombination) "set up" the cell for
nondisjunction. For example, in yeast and fruit flies, mutants that reduce
meiotic recombination invariably have increased frequencies of nondisjunction. In humans, the first evidence of an association between aberrant re-

combination and trisomy came over 10 years ago, when Warren et al. (1987) reported reduced levels of chromosome 21 recombination in meioses leading to trisomy 21. Subsequently, several laboratories have extended these observations, and it is now clear that most—if not all—human trisomies are associated with alterations in recombination; that is, significant reductions in recombination have been reported for paternally and maternally derived sex chromosome trisomies and for maternal trisomies 15, 16, 18, and 21 (for review, see Hassold et al., 2000).

In the Hassold and Sherman laboratories, we have focused on a relatively small number of trisomies, and especially on trisomy 21. We have found that the relationship between recombination and chromosome 21 nondisjunction is complex. Nondisjunction at maternal MI is linked to reduced recombination , with some cases involving outright failure of recombination between the homologous chromosomes 21 and others associated with distally placed exchange events (Lamb et al., 1997). Surprisingly— because recombination occurs at MI—maternal MII errors are also linked to altered recombination, but in this instance the effect involves increased, not decreased, recombination, especially in the proximal portion of the chromosome (Lamb et al., 1996). Presumably, this means that errors scored as arising at MII are, in fact, precipitated by events occurring at MI.

In general, the relationships we have observed for maternal trisomy 21 appear to apply to paternal MI and MII errors as well, although this conclusion is based on a limited sample (Savage et al., 1998). If confirmed, these observations would mean that alterations in recombination are important in virtually all chromosome 21 nondisjunction—in both paternal and maternal nondisjunction and in nondisjunction scored as arising at MII, as well as errors occurring at MI.

## MATERNAL AGE AND TRISOMY 21

The association between increasing maternal age and trisomy is probably the most important risk factor in any human genetic disease. Nevertheless, we know very little about the basis of the age effect. It is thought to originate in maternal MI, because in human females, oocytes enter meiosis during the fetal period and remain arrested in an early stage of MI until ovulation, many years later. The duration of this meiotic division suggests that any of four time periods may be important in maternal-age dependent nondisjunction. These include 1) the premeiotic fetal stage, when rapid mitotic divisions occur; 2) early fetal MI, when homologous chromosomes pair and recombine; 3) the arrested stage, which lasts from the fetal period until the time of ovulation, and thus may involve a span of 40–45 years; and 4) the periovulatory stage, when meiosis resumes and proceeds to metaphase of MII. Current data do not allow us to distinguish between factors acting at the four different stages of oogenesis. However, our data (Lamb et al., 1997) indicate that alterations in genetic recombination are an important contributor to age-dependent nondisjunction. Specifically, we have observed that, in comparison with normal genetic "maps" (which measure the amount and location of meiotic recombination events), the chromosome 21 genetic maps associated with maternal MI-derived trisomy 21 are similarly reduced in younger and older women, and the maps associated with so-called "MII" errors are similarly increased in younger and older women. We take this to mean that there are likely at least two steps or "hits" to maternal age-related nondisjunction. The first hit, which would be age independent, involves the establishment of a "vulnerable" pair of homologs (e.g., chromosomes 21 that are held together only by a single, distally placed meiotic exchange) in the fetal oocyte. The second hit, which would be age dependent, involves abnormal processing of the vulnerable homologous pair at metaphase of meiosis I (i.e., the time at which the homologs separate from one another). If this model is correct, it means that the nondisjunctional process is similar in younger and older women; it simply happens more frequently with age, possibly due to age-dependent degradation of cell cycle proteins or meiotic proteins responsible for segregating homologs.

## ARE THERE OTHER FACTORS THAT INCREASE THE RISK OF TRISOMY 21?

In addition to the well-characterized effect of maternal age, many other risk factors have been proposed to play a role in the genesis of trisomy 21. These include a variety of trisomy-inducing agents: environmental or occupational exposures (e.g., naturally-occurring DNA-damaging agents, medical irradiation, pesticides, and industrial chemicals), habituating agents (e.g., coffee, alcohol, tobacco, and drugs), and intrinsic risk factors (e.g., certain types of chromosome variants and defects in specific genes). However, despite intensive investigations, none of these, or other factors, has been convincingly linked to trisomies. Possibly, this means that, other than maternal age, no such factors exist or, if they do, their impact is so small by comparison with the age effect that they escape detection. However, it may also be that they exist, but we have simply failed to identify the correct ones to study. As described below, one recent set of studies has addressed this possibility by suggesting a link between nutritional status and nondisjunction of chromosome 21.

FOLIC ACID AND TRISOMY 21.   In 1999, considerable excitement was generated by a report that linked Down syndrome to a common "variant" for an enzyme involved in folic acid metabolism. Specifically, James et al. (1999) studied the frequency of a specific DNA change (i.e., at nucleotide 677, a C to T base pair substitution) in mehylenetetrahydrofolate reductase (MTHFR) in mothers of individuals with Down syndrome and in age-matched controls. This mutation occurs commonly in humans and typically has little, if any clinical importance; however, it leads to reduced enzyme activity in heterozygous and homozygous carriers and is known to be a risk factor for neural tube defects. James et al. (1999) hypothesized that aberrant cellular methylation reactions caused by the mutation might increase the likelihood of meiotic nondisjunction, thus making it a risk factor for Down syndrome as well as for neural tube defects. Their initial observations fit this idea because, among the mothers of individuals with Down syndrome, they found a highly significant increase in the proportion of women carrying one or two copies of the mutation. Subsequently, James and co-workers analyzed a commonly occurring mutation at a second gene in the folate pathway, namely, methionine synthase reductase (MTRR; the mutation involves a change from A to G at nucleotide 66) and—again—identified a significant increase in mutations among mothers of individuals with Down syndrome (Hobbs et al., 2000). Furthermore, an independent study of MTRR (O'Leary et al., in press) replicated the findings of James and colleagues. Thus results of three studies of two different folate pathway genes suggest an association between specific maternal folate variants and the risk of conceiving a trisomy 21 fetus.

These observations are remarkable for two reasons. First, the strength of the association is striking, given the relatively small number of cases and controls yet studied; indeed, they imply a major role of MTHFR and MTRR variants in the origin of Down syndrome. Second, the results suggest the possibility of relatively simple preventative strategies, because dietary folate and vitamin $B_{12}$ supplementation might overcome the risk of nondisjunction associated with the mutations.

Thus the confirmation of a link between folate pathway mutations and Down syndrome would represent an important advance in Down syndrome research. Unfortunately, however, recent studies suggest that this link may be less important than originally thought. That is, in two new studies of MTHFR and Down syndrome the mutation frequencies were similar between case (mothers of individuals with Down syndrome) and control individuals (Petersen et al., 2000; Chadefaux-Vekemans et al., in press). Furthermore, in recent studies of maternally derived trisomies involving other chromosomes (i.e., cases of trisomies 2, 7, 10, 13, 14, 15, 16, 18, 22, and sex chromosome trisomies), there were few differences in MTHFR or MTRR mutations in case mothers in comparison with controls (Hassold et al., in press). Thus there is little evidence that maternal folate variants alter the risk of nondisjunction for chromosomes other than 21, and the evidence for trisomy 21 is now equivocal. Nevertheless, the importance of the effect, if confirmed, and the considerable interest that the observations have drawn make it essential that additional analyses be conducted to clarify the situation.

## SUMMARY

The past decade has witnessed remarkable advances in our understanding of the way in which Down syndrome originates—we now have considerable information on the parental and meiotic sources of the additional chromosome 21 and we are beginning to unravel the molecular "mistakes" that occur in nondisjunctional meioses. However, despite intensive efforts, we remain woefully ignorant of risk factors that influence the frequency of meiotic nondisjunction. Identification and characterization of these factors remain two of the most important challenges facing human geneticists.

## ACKNOWLEDGMENTS

Research in the Hassold and Sherman laboratories discussed in this review was supported by NIH grants HD-21341 and HD-24605.

## REFERENCES

Chadefaux-Vekemans B, Coude M, Muller F, Oury J, Chali A, Kamoun P. Methylenetetrahydrofolate reductase polymorphisms in the etiology of Down syndrome. Pediatr Res. In press.

Hassold T, Sherman S, Hunt P (2000): Counting cross-overs: characterizing meiotic recombination in mammals. Hum Mol Genet 9:2409–2419.

Hassold T, Hunt P (2001): To err (meiotically) is human: studies of the genesis of human aneuploidy. Nat Rev Genet 2: 280–291.

Hassold T, Burrage L, Chan E, Judis L Schwartz S, James S, Jacobs P, Thomas N. Maternal folate polymorphisms and the etiology of human nondisjunction Am J Hum Genet. In press.

Hobbs CA, Sherman SL, Yi P, Hopkins SE, Torfs CP, Hine RJ, Pogribna M, Rozen R, James SJ (2000): Polymorphisms in genes involved in folate metabolism as maternal risk factors for Down syndrome. Am J Hum Genet 67:623–630.

James SJ, Pogribna M, Pogribny I, Melnyk S, Hine R, Gibson J, Yi P, Tafoya D, Swenson D, Wilson V, Gaylor D (1999): Abnormal folate metabolism and mutation in the methylenetetrahydrofolate reductase gene may be maternal risk factors for Down syndrome. Am J Clin Nutr 70:495–501.

Lamb N, Feingold E, Savage-Austin A, Avramopoulos D, Freeman S, Gu Y, Hallberg A, Hersey J, Pettay D, Saker D, Shen J, Taft L, Mikkelsen M, Petersen M, Hassold T, Sherman S (1997): Characterization of susceptible chiasma configurations that increase the risk for maternal nondisjunction of chromosome 21. Hum Mol Genet 6:1391–1399.

Lamb N, Freeman S, Savage-Austin A, Petay D, Taft L, Herset J, Gu Y, Shen J, Saker D, May K, Avramopoulos D, Petersen M, Hallberg A, Mikkelsen M, Hassold T, Sherman S (1996): Susceptible chiasmate configurations of chromosome 21 predispose to non-disjunction in both maternal MI and MII. Nat Genet 14: 400–405.

O'Leary VB, Parle-McDermott AP, Molloy AM, Kirke PN, Johnson Z, Conley M, Scott JM, Mills JL. MTRR and MTHFR polymorphisms: link to Down syndrome? Am J Med Genet. In press.

Petersen M, Grigoriadou M, Mikkelsen M (2000): A common mutation in the methylenetetrahydrofolate reductase gene is not a risk factor for Down syndrome. Am J Hum Genet 67(Suppl 2):141.

Savage A, Petersen M, Pettay D, Taft L, Allran K, Freeman S, Karadima G, Avramopolous D, Torfs C, Mikkelsen M, Hassold T, Sherman S (1998): Elucidating the mechanisms of paternal nondisjunction of chromosome 21 in humans. Hum Mol Genet 7: 1221–1227.

Warren AC, Chakravarti A, Wong C, Slaugenhaupt SA, Halloran SL, Watkins PC, Metaxotou C et al. (1987): Evidence for reduced recombination on the nondisjoined chromosomes 21 in Down syndrome. Science 237:652–654.

# PSYCHO-SOCIAL ISSUES

# Building Relationships/Social and Sexual Development

## Leslie Walker-Hirsch, M.Ed.

It is a wonderful, exciting time for people with disabilities, their families, and the professionals who support them. Many medical advances, educational techniques, and cultural changes have arisen in the last few years. These changes support the hopes and dreams for a satisfying and happy life for individuals with Down syndrome (DS) and their families. People of all ages with DS can and do enjoy an array of relationships with family members, friends, acquaintances, community members, and even sweethearts and spouses. Social development education and sexuality education lay the groundwork for the relationship opportunities that enrich lives and for the choices that maintain personal safety.

Having a disability such as DS can make the process of healthy sexual development confusing for families and for their children.

Different individuals define sexuality differently. For our purposes here, sexuality is best viewed as the lens through which a male or female sees and responds to the world. It includes biological, physiological, anatomic, cultural, social, spiritual, and even political aspects of our being.

Many forces influence a person's sexual role and the behavior that expresses that role; the hopes and dreams of that person, the values that his or her family conveys to that person, and the expectations that the person's culture has for him or her interact with the person's biological, intellectual, and emotional attributes as a boy or girl and as a man or woman.

*Down Syndrome*, Edited by William I. Cohen, Lynn Nadel, and Myra E. Madnick.
ISBN 0-471-41815-3   Copyright © 2002 by Wiley-Liss, Inc.

Sexuality is so much more than sexual intercourse or reproduction. It is an aspect of our very personality!

Sexuality starts that very moment when that sperm and that egg get together and continues throughout our lives into old age. Some very significant elements of sexual development are decided at the moment of conception. It has been decided at that moment whether those cells will grow to be a man or a woman. Even before a baby is born, its sexual systems are activated periodically. And so sexual development is begun even in utero.

When a child is born, many things have already been decided about sexual development over which a parent has had very little control. Each parent has provided half of the genes (the raw material) and has created a prenatal environment for the child to begin life as a sexual being.

After birth, environmental, cultural, and social influences come into play to influence sexuality:

- the way that the child is carried, nurtured, and cared for;
- the way the child is dressed, groomed, and toileted;
- the way the child expects to be touched and handled;
- how long the child is allowed to cry, or not cry;
- the kinds of toys and stimulation that the child enjoys and receives; and
- how the whole rest of the universe interacts with the child as either a baby boy or a baby girl

Environmental events and cultural practices influence the interpretation of maleness or femaleness in a particular culture at a particular time in history.

And as the child's awareness grows, family social practices interact with the personal characteristics of the child:

- the way that family members give and receive affection to the child and to each other;
- the way that privacy and modesty are expressed at home;
- the way that family members demonstrate being happy, sad, angry, or afraid;
- the way that family members make up from arguments; and
- the way that family members interact with friends and social contacts outside the family

Many factors that influence social and sexual expectation that are in action long before a child enters school and way, way before puberty appears on the horizon. The presence of DS and the experiences of a child with that condition may affect a child's self-perception and the family's perception of that child as a being without sexuality. These early experiences color the child's view as he or she continues to mature.

Long before puberty education is in order; many important elements of your child's sexuality education have been enacted. And YOU, parents and family members, are the first sex educators of your child. How you regard your children, how you teach them to regard their bodies, is all part of sexuality education. And the expectations and interactions you and your child have with the men and women in your social world all contribute.

Certainly, at the time of puberty there are more dramatic events that draw attention to sexual development. The good news is that most adolescents with DS show the biological signs of maturity within the typical age range of their peers without disabilities. That is, somewhere between the ages of 11 and 16, physical maturity becomes evident: body hair, voice change, breast enlargement, and an intensity of mood that signals adult hormones. However, the gap between physical maturity and social, intellectual, and emotional maturity begins to widen at this time. For this reason, additional attention and time may need to be devoted to managing the new behaviors and expectations that are now necessary.

Many youngsters are mainstreamed in their schools for health education, the class in which sexuality education is generally provided. Often the pace of instruction and the emphasis of the discussions are not effectively oriented to meet the needs of students with DS. The particular learning style and special educational techniques that support understanding for teenagers with DS may not be used because of time constraints or because the rest of the class is ready to cover new material rather than more repetition. And yet comprehensive, age- and ability-appropriate social/sexual education is very important to teens with a disability as well as all other teens. It is often advisable to create smaller groups of adolescents with a similar learning pace to be certain that the sexuality educational content is meaningful and conveyed in an effective manner.

There are six key components in sexuality education that support the development of sexually healthy teens and, eventually, responsible adults. If education is limited only to some of these components, misunderstanding and mistakes can occur and the person with DS may be more vulnerable to criticism or being taken advantage of.

The first component focuses on adult self-care. This is a standard and concrete area of sexuality education. Behavioral psychology has given us great insights into how to accomplish these tasks with task analysis, repetition, behavior shaping, and reward. Everybody needs to learn how to take a shower, use the toilet, learn the related social skills, distinguish the men's room from the women's room, and remember to wash his or her hands afterward.

The next area in which people need information and education related to sexuality has to do with anatomy and physiology. It is very important to know— and everyone is entitled to know—how his or her own body works, what parts he or she has and how to name them... not just eyes, nose, and mouth and then skip down to knees, ankles, and toes! There are important body parts in between. These private body parts, mostly sexual anatomy, have names and functions that should be learned as well: penis, vulva, scrotum, vagina, anus, and breasts. These parts of the body are worthwhile, too. Most people are really glad to have them!

It is true that these are not words to toss around lightly, and we do not use these words very often. However, it is very important to know them or their adult slang equivalent to talk about our bodies, find out whether they are healthy or not, and communicate if there is sexual encroachment or abuse.

It is important to know that sexual parts have other functions besides reproduction. Biology teachers in high school teach about the respiratory system, the digestive system, and the reproductive system. For most people, reproduction is not the main purpose of their sexual system. Often, more important sexual goals are intimacy derived from physical closeness, personal enjoyment of one's own body, or the enjoyment of pleasing another person.

It is sometimes hard or even embarrassing to put those sexual functions into words or to give a teen or adult both permission and rules for that physical pleasure.

According to Jane Brody, *The New York Times* health expert, puberty starts at age 6—slowly, of course! Children do not show the external changes of puberty at that age, but it does mean that there are significant hormonal changes at that age. There is evidence that puberty happens earlier than it has ever happened before, more than a year earlier than a generation ago on the average. As a child with DS approaches puberty, there will be many of the same maturity-related changes in that child's anatomy and physiology as in children without DS. If a child is not well prepared in anticipation of these exciting changes, they can be frightening. Imagine a girl who knows little about menstruation. One day, blood comes from a place that may not even have a name! She may assume that she is injured or ill. Or imagine a boy, who has had success with toilet training, who has a wet dream for the first time. He may be worried or ashamed that he has regressed in his toileting accomplishment.

Youngsters with DS are not usually significantly delayed in the age of onset for puberty, but there may be less social and emotional maturity and that may require some additional attention. Many schools have begun to educate students with intellectual disabilities about sexual anatomy in preparation for some of the physical changes of puberty. It is still important for parents and family members to corroborate this information and to support the behavior training that is involved in menstrual care and hygiene for ejaculation. It is also important to give a child permission to enjoy or be annoyed by these events as well as guidelines related to these very adult experiences.

The physical enjoyment of masturbation for teenagers and adults of both sexes is not something that is discussed in many schools. Jocelyn Elders, a U.S. Surgeon General, was criticized for talking about the "M" word. Most sex experts believe that masturbation that is done in private and that does not interfere with the other important social and intellectual activities of life is a harmless sexual outlet. For many people with developmental disabilities, it is the only available genital sexual outlet. Each family needs to decide what guidelines are appropriate and how to support both the individual's needs and the family's values. Parents can communicate values and preferences about masturbation and can insist on appropriate behavior in public, but whether a teenager will follow that value when in private is up to the teen.

Youngsters with DS need to discriminate between private and public places. Physically mature bodies are not acceptable to be displayed in public. The behaviors that relate to personal body parts must now be performed only in private. It is important to institute routines of privacy for the child and for other family members long before puberty is an issue. It will take some time to make the changes from childhood exuberance to modesty that is more adult; so do not wait until the last minute. Anatomy and physiology, especially around the time of puberty, is an important aspect of sexuality.

The third area of sexuality focuses on self-esteem and autonomy. This relates to decision making and taking control of the direction of one's life. People who have some control over their life choices are said to exhibit self-esteem. Sharing decision making with a teen with DS is an important step into adulthood. Begin to negotiate decisions and teach compromise. Help the teenager or child to see what choices and alternatives are available and what is likely to happen as a result of each choice. Young people need to understand that what they do today has a consequence tomorrow; it can be a wonderful consequence or something they don't like. Opportunity to practice making small decisions with little risk is an important step toward maturity. First decisions should be about what to have for lunch or what TV shows to watch. The slow process of taking responsibility for decisions begins early in life. Even if a person cannot envision all of the alternatives or their consequences, support can be offered without taking away the person's autonomy, as long as reasonable safety is maintained.

Too often, children with disabilities have their self-esteem assaulted. And the teasing is often related to their disability or sexuality. A 15-year-old girl with DS refused to go to school or speak anymore, after having loved school and after having charmed all of her teachers. As I got to know her, she told me that three girls in her gym class told her that because she had

DS and had one breast larger than the other, she was not a girl! They told her that because she was not a girl, she could not go into the girls' locker room or the girls' bathroom anymore. After spending some time talking about what it means to be a girl or a woman and what breasts are in all their different shapes and sizes, she was reassured that she was a girl. And that it was a good thing to be a girl. Sexuality can be a source of self-esteem or of fear and self-hatred.

The fourth component of sexuality has to do with relationships. It's my opinion that finding, cultivating, and maintaining good relationships are the single most difficult human task. It is also a task that affects overall happiness. We cannot live well without relationships. There is little joy without friends, family, acquaintances, schoolmates—all are different kinds of relationships. Many of the most important elements of our happiness generate from our relationships: family, spouse, children, parents, friends, colleagues, and others. This is what makes humans tick! Children, teens, and adults with DS can usually enjoy the benefits of these relationships. Friendships in younger years and learning about close relationships with siblings and other family members set the stage for the development of adult friendships and romances, too. Many people with DS want to have intimate relationships when they are adults. When adults with DS are able to learn and reason about important sexual information they will be able to meet the standards necessary to become consenting adults. That means that the person can participate in sexual relationships as full citizens. Some adults with DS marry and are partners in sexual relationships. The effort needed to enjoy this aspect of relationships can be considerable. But even if a person cannot manage an all-encompassing relationship such as a marriage, almost everyone enjoys being chosen as a boyfriend or girlfriend. Relationships that are mutual, that are not abusive, and that are within the person's ability to process and understand add great joy and excitement to life.

The most successful romantic couples that I have known are partners who enjoy each other's company, are of similar intellectual ability, and have a similar worldview, some common experiences, and lifestyles that are similar or overlapping. The "even playing field" minimizes the likelihood of sexual advantage taking and grossly unequal power in the relationship. It is important for children and teenagers to have friendships both with typical friends and with other friends with disabilities.

Often at puberty the nature of childhood friendships change. Sometimes the typical friend is no longer in the same school or class. Or the friends find they no longer have very much in common. Or the typical teen is less able to tolerate diversity in relationships. Or the friendship becomes a helping friendship instead of the peer friendship it used to be. Often, typical teens have more independence than teens with DS. This may mean that the teen with DS is not allowed by his or her parents to do the same activities that the typical friend is permitted to do. Teens and young adults, and even adults, may require a combination of included and specialized social events.

It is important to value the child's or teen's friendship with both typical and disabled friends. This will help to avoid a situation in which a child with a disability is prejudiced against others with disabilities or places a greater value on friendship with nondisabled peers. When it is time for romance, teens and adults are much more likely to find a satisfying partner with intellectual ability similar to their own. Most of the time being with a diverse network of people is advantageous, but it is also important to stay connected to others who have had experiences similar to your own and who share that culture.

The two final components focus on the social skills of sexuality and sexual rights and opportunities. These are still quite underdeveloped.

Social skills, such as saying please and thank you, using a tissue to catch a runny nose, saying hello and goodbye, and knowing how to set the table are every day social skills that parents and teachers want their children to learn so they will be accepted. Most typical children learn those skills as if by magic. In fact, they watch family members, select the specific action, and omit extraneous material. Copying is then an easy task. Everyday social skills often need to be taught directly to children with intellectual disabilities, often with repeated trials and frequently with hand-over-hand instruction.

TV and movies often show inappropriate, silly, or dangerous social skills related to romance and sexuality. Children and teens with DS need help from parents or older siblings to decipher which parts are unrealistic or funny and which are illegal and dangerous. When crushes, dances, and parties are part of a teenager's life, direct instruction about social skills is crucial to the teen's safety and well-being. Parents, counselors, and teachers can create a safe, welcoming environment to discuss and develop the social skills pertaining to sexuality that are required at a specific age.

Sometimes teenagers with and without disabilities use sexual terms that they do not understand. Being an "askable" teacher or parent can avoid many sexual misunderstandings if you clarify and explain the term to the child in a way that is useful and that reflects his or her age and social maturity. An enjoyable "teachable moment" instead of a reprimand should be your goal.

And, last but not least, the final key component focuses on social and sexual opportunities. What kinds and quantity of social opportunities are available, both included and specialized? How much sexual opportunity is appropriate to balance the right to personal freedom and the right to be protected from harm? What are your values? How do you balance the scale or tip it? What are the laws in your state that apply to a person's ability to give consent to participate in sexual activity with another person? By him or herself? These are just some of the questions that are asked and unanswered at the moment.

I have had the opportunity to help adults with DS date, explore their sexual interests in safe and responsible ways, and even to marry. This is best accomplished with supportive parents and a climate of teamwork and open discussion. Without parental support for romance and appropriate sexual development, there is a needlessly sad ending to many a romance.

This is not to say that every relationship that is romantic leads directly to sexual intercourse. Sometimes simply being chosen as a boyfriend or girlfriend and holding hands is a satisfying limit to sexual expression. Other times, passionate hugging and deep kissing reflect the emotion of the relationship. Or even a chance to go to a family holiday event with a date fulfills a need to be recognized as adult and desirable to the opposite sex. These are opportunities that are not as available to many teens and adults with DS. And the opportunities that are available are not always sufficiently diverse or frequent enough to satisfy every need.

Laws related to a person's ability to give consent to sexual interaction are an attempt to balance a person's right to sexual expression with the person's need for protection from harm that may result from that activity. The American Association on Mental Retardation recently published a book called *A Guide to Consent* (Dinerstein et al., 1999). The chapter concerning sexual consent represents state-of-the-art minimal guidelines for achieving this balance. Because each state has different laws governing consent, there is no single document that clarifies the issue. However, all state laws agree that the need to have knowledge, capacity, and voluntariness is basic to decision making about sexual interactions.

Picture yourself with your friends, and they all want to play Monopoly. You play a couple of times even though you've never played and you don't really know what the rules are and you lose every game. They are building hotels and houses and getting monopolies on properties, and you're going bankrupt every time. After a while you don't feel like playing anymore, and they do not want to play with you either because it's not so much fun. You are not a good player because you do not know the rules of the game.

That is the kind of experience many teens with DS have when it comes to making and keeping friends and having and enjoying a boyfriend or girlfriend.

*CIRCLES: Intimacy and Relationships*, also known as the CIRCLES Program (Walker-Hirsch and Champagne, 1993) is a very successful technique to introduce your child to the rules of the social world in a way that is fun to learn. The CIRCLES paradigm can be used in many settings.

Walker-Hirsch and Champagne, the creators of CIRCLES, theorized that they could use some of the same strategies successful in teaching other subjects to people with intellectual disabilities and apply them to social development and relationship issues. The CIRCLES floor mat is a life-size color graphic used to describe different degrees of relationships.

# Circles I®
## Intimacy
## & Relationships

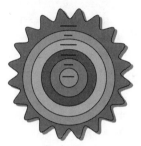

The CIRCLES schematic takes the abstraction of personal space and relationship boundaries and makes it concrete and specific. Each person is the center of all the circles, not unlike the sun and all the planets. The most important center circle embodies the self, self-esteem, autonomy, and empowerment; it is the place that is just for you. You are the most important person of your world of circles, and consequently you are the center of all the circles. The center circle is color-coded purple because that is the color for royalty. You deserve to be treated like a king or queen. This circle is around you at all times, even if you cannot see it. An iconic sign is paired with the purple color. The message is that your body is your own and private. You decide who will come close and who will stay away. There is a domain of privacy each person has and can learn to access, as well as possessions that are important and private to you. Thoughts, emotions, and experiences can be private, too. Be able to recognize that each person has a part of himself or herself that others will never know.

Around that circle, and touching it, is another circle. It is not very big, but it surrounds the purple private circle. It is the Blue Hug Circle. It is the size of a hug. The iconic sign looks like a hug. There are just a very few people that have this kind of closeness with us. For most people, the blue hug circle is filled with loving family members. When we are adults, and if we are fortunate, a sweetheart might enter that circle and fill the sweetheart spot. A person should be able to name all of the people with that kind of closeness to him or her. Although each of us has blue hug relationships, the actual individuals who fill that circle will be different for each of us.

Part of learning the CIRCLES concept involves creating an individual set of circles that specifies who is actually filling that relationship circle in real life. The boundary of a blue hug relationship and the other relationships we value are illustrated in high-interest, low-complexity video dramas across the parameters of touch, talk, and trust.

Around that circle is another one, a little bit less intimate, a little further away, and inclusive of more people. Usually, extended family members, or people who act like family members, and close friends populate this circle. This is the Green Far Away Hug Circle. Creating expectations for friends and family for touch, talk ,and trust assists the person to recognize encroachment and potential abuse at a time before harm is done.

Sometimes, when it is time to fill in the names of friends, it will become apparent a person has no one to fill in. Although it is sad to hear that someone has no friends, it may be the first step toward discovering the obstacle to friendships and addressing it.

Around that circle is another circle, the Yellow Handshake Circle. It represents the social distance for acquaintances. A person whose name you know and who knows your name qualifies for that circle. We can shake hands but limit our touch to hands only. Similarly, there is more remote conversation and less trust. There are usually many people in this circle. They are people who you only know slightly.

Around that is another circle, the Orange Wave Circle. There is no body contact or touch in this more distant circle. You can see a familiar face across the street and just wave. It is best to wave to children you do not know well. It is up to their parents to decide who touches their children.

Around that circle is the Red Stranger Space. Most of the people in the world are in this space. Most people are strangers: we do not touch them; we do not talk to them; we do not trust them. And they do not touch, talk to, or trust us, either. The exception in this group is the Community Helper. This person can be recognized because he or she wears a badge or a uniform and works in a specialized work-type setting. You can talk to community helpers about business. It is important to recognize what the limits are in business touch, business talk, and business trust for various community helpers.

The CIRCLES Program can be personalized according to the age and ability of the individual. The CIRCLES Guide Book gives suggestions for activities that support the large array of concepts that can be addressed through the use of CIRCLES at a variety of developmental stages and abilities.

As with typical teenagers, educating people with developmental disabilities about relationships is difficult. It is important to always keep the lines of communication open and to understand that mistakes in judgment may be made. However, if a person with DS is fully informed, those mistakes can be lessened. It is important to also recognize how relationships enhance the quality of life for people with DS throughout the life span, and, at the same time understand the need for education to minimize potential abuses and resolve other relationship issues.

## REFERENCES

Stavis P, Walker-Hirsch L (Chapter 4), Dinerstein, RD, Herr, S & O'Sullivan, Jr, eds. (1999): A Guide to Consent, AAMR, Washington, DC.

Walker-Hirsch L, Champagne M (1981): The CIRCLES Program, James Stanfield Co., Santa Barbara, CA.

Walker-Hirsch L, Champagne M (1981): CIRCLES: Stop Abuse, James Stanfield Co., Santa Barbara, CA.

Walker-Hirsch L, Champagne M (1985): CIRCLES: Safer Ways, James Stanfield Co., Santa Barbara, CA.

Walker-Hirsch L, Champagne M (1991): "CIRCLES Revisited—Ten Years Later," Sexuality and Disability, Vol. 9, No. 2, James Stanfield Co., Santa Barbara, CA.

Walker-Hirsch L, Champagne M. (1993): CIRCLES: Intimacy and Relationships, James Stanfield Co., Santa Barbara, CA.

Walker-Hirsch L, Acton, G., "Sexuality and Young Adults with Developmental Disabilities" (Fall 1994) Pursuing Healthy Lives for The Transition Years, IMPACT, University of Minnesota, Volume 7(2).

Walker-Hirsch L, Special Education Meets Sexuality Education, SIECUS Report, April/May 1995.

# FOOD, FEEDING, AND FAMILY: ON THE ROAD TO HEALTHY LIFESTYLES

JOAN E. MEDLEN, R.D., L.D.

Our dreams for our children begin when we learn of their existence. When a child has Down syndrome, the dreams change a bit, but we still dream. We dream about happy, healthy, fulfilling lives for our child with Down syndrome, his or her siblings, and ourselves. As we begin to live out those dreams, it's the little things that matter most: playing in the snow, cruising the pumpkin patch for the best pumpkin in town, riding a horse, being accomplished in a sport, learning to play the violin, and more. And yet, we are haunted by what Down syndrome means to our child's health over the course of his or her life. There are so many extra things to watch for, what if we miss one?

I remember my first images of our son's adult life as I held him in those early months. Although I had some experiences with children with multiple disabilities as a child, I knew little about Down syndrome. My thoughts were as limited as they come: I saw him sitting on a bench waiting for the bus. In my vision he was what is considered morbidly obese, not a comforting thought for a dietitian. Having waged a battle with my weight since my first pregnancy, the thought of my child having to endure the struggles I was currently facing was not acceptable. Not without a fight. My husband and I spoke about making some lifestyle changes to shape a healthy, active lifestyle in our son.

---

*Down Syndrome,* Edited by William I. Cohen, Lynn Nadel, and Myra E. Madnick.
ISBN 0-471-41815-3   Copyright © 2002 by Wiley-Liss, Inc.

Although some people argue that this is my own skewed view of life resulting from being a dietitian, I don't think so. I believe my concerns are not unlike many parents of children with Down syndrome. In fact, parents want the same thing for all children: the best, healthiest, most fulfilling life possible. I look for opportunities to learn how to encourage healthy lifestyles for children and adults with Down syndrome. I look for ways our children can teach me what is important in their lives. The following is a summary of some of the more striking concerns and lessons shared by parents and children and adults with Down syndrome.

In general, parents seem to have some consistent overall concerns that fall into age-related categories:

- Parents of younger children with Down syndrome are focused on texture progression and food choices (otherwise known as picky eating).
- Parents of teens and adults with Down syndrome are concerned about weight management and healthy living, which includes eating well.

Some answers to the first category have come through hindsight, reading, and research by others. An overview is provided in the following section. In response to the second category, weight management and healthy living, I sought to find answers from the people who matter most: teens and adults with Down syndrome. To gather this information, Mia Peterson, a young woman with Down syndrome, and I conducted a survey of 183 teens and adults with Down syndrome, asking about their habits and thoughts about healthy lifestyles. Some of what we learned is included in this article.

## THE TROUBLE WITH TEXTURES

Generally, children with Down syndrome are born with lower muscle tone than children without Down syndrome. This lower muscle tone, along with differences in the physical structure of the mouth or tongue and medical complications at birth, contributes to a general delay in the introduction of solid foods (Hopman et al., 1998). Not only are children beginning their experiences with solid food a bit later, they seem to take longer to progress through the stages of chewing development (Gisel, 1984). This may be due to low muscle tone, the need to adapt typical chewing styles for their tongue or mouth, or fatigue during the feeding process.

When parents express concern about "picky eating," the first thing to evaluate is where the child is in the texture progression and chewing development process. For instance, a 5-year-old child with Down syndrome may appear to eat a variety of foods. However, by listing the foods he readily accepts and eats well, you may find they are all "soft" in texture: mashed potatoes, french fries, cereal after it sits in milk a while, applesauce, ice cream, pasta, bread, eggs, yogurt, chicken nuggets, ground meat (although often meat is not a favorite), and so on. In this situation, the concern may be related to oral motor tone and chewing development rather than picky eating. (Medlen, 1999).

In a different situation, a 5-year-old with Down syndrome may eat foods such as mashed potatoes, taffy, jerky, celery with peanut butter (but not celery alone), a particular brand of macaroni and cheese (and no other), and a particular brand of breakfast cereal. This combination of chewy and crunchy textures along with the specific brands of otherwise available foods raises a different set of questions than oral motor development. In this situation, the issue is more likely related to sensory issues or the dynamics of the feeding environment.

Many times all that is needed is some coaching in methods to encourage children to develop oral motor skills by increasing the textures of foods slowly and playing different oral motor games. For children who struggle with sensory issues and environmental issues, parents may need some coaching on the art of introducing new foods. Even though most children with Down syndrome will eventually move on to a varied diet on their own, it is important to thoroughly investigate, educate, and coach parents through this mine field. Without this coaching, it is possible a child will be 7, 8, 9, or even 10 years old before the food battles end. The intervention involved is rarely intensive or extensive. However, with help from a speech pathologist, occupational therapist, or dietitian trained in the area of feeding, or a feeding team, success is expedient and mealtime is no longer something to dread. A feeding team is a group of professionals (physician, occupational therapist, speech-language pathologist, psychologist or behaviorist, and dietitian) who specialize in working with children who have difficulty learning to eat.

Why is this important? There are number of reasons that an assertive approach to texture progression and food acceptance is important.

- A delayed introduction to foods may have an impact on speech development (Hopman et al., 1998). Appropriate intervention for oral motor skills assists not only with texture progression but also with development of needed muscles and skills for speech.

- A child who begins school unable to manage crunchy or chewy textures may need to be watched more carefully for choking than his peers. Although on the surface this does not seem detrimental, it can lead to differences in seating arrangements in the lunch room or other situations that separate him from his same-age, nondisabled peers.

- If a child begins school with a need for texture modifications, it impedes his ability to participate in the regular lunchtime routine. Foods provided by the school will need to be modified separately, or the student will need to bring food from home.

Struggling with "picky eating" is common, if not a rite of passage for all children. Yet if it persists for a long period of time, it may be more than a food jag. When it is, parents must receive the support and coaching needed to overcome issues related to sensory, oral motor, and mealtime dynamics to build the foundation of a healthy adulthood. There are a few ways to determine whether you can benefit from a referral to a feeding specialist (speech pathologist, occupational therapist, dietitian or feeding team). Consider the following questions:

- Am I talking to more than one or two professionals about feeding (for instance, what foods my child eats, oral motor skills and exercises, or other medical conditions that affect feeding)?
- Am I getting advice from more than one or two professionals about feeding that is difficult to blend together or is conflicting?
- Is my child's eating or feeding taking a lot of time and therefore taking time away from my family because of stress and worry?
- Do I feel frustrated because I do not have one concise plan for helping my child learn to eat different textures and participate in family meals?

If you answered yes to two or more of these questions, it's probably a good idea to seek a referral to someone who can help. If your physician is hesitant about making the referral, suggest he obtain a PEACH (Parent Eating and Nutrition Assessment for Children with Special Health Needs) Survey to document the need for the referral. (Campbell and Kelsey, 1994)

## ENCOURAGING HEALTHY LIFESTYLES

Once children with Down syndrome get past texture progression, the focus is on more traditional aspects of a healthy lifestyle: weight management, activity, and food choices. To understand the complexity of these topics, it is helpful to have an understanding of some basic physiological differences between people with and without Down syndrome.

## METABOLISM

Studies suggest that people with Down syndrome have a lower basal metabolic rate (BMR) than those who do not have Down syndrome. One study found the difference in BMR in children to be up to 15% less for children with Down syndrome (Luke et al., 1994). Mia Peterson, my co-researcher, is also a young woman with Down syndrome. She explains the difference in metabolism to people with this story:

> *If you have a cookie and I have a cookie that is exactly like yours, it will do different things in our body when we eat it. When you eat the cookie, you will burn the calories from the cookie faster than I do. The reason is my metabolism is slower than the metabolism of people who do not have Down syndrome.*

Therefore, beginning in early childhood (1–12 years of age), the 1999 version of the *Health Care Guidelines for Individuals with Down Syndrome* (see Part V) suggests taking measures to correct for this difference. However, this reduction in overall calories for children requires parents to diligently encourage a variety of food choices to meet vitamin needs. If caloric reductions are followed, an over-the-counter multiple vitamin is a good idea, especially for picky eaters and peace of mind. (Luke et al., 1996)

## WEIGHT MANAGEMENT

Knowing that people with Down syndrome have a lower BMR makes the idea of weight management seem daunting. Add to that the statistic that 70% of Americans are overweight, with the numbers growing each year. And more: surveys show Americans claim to understand the importance of healthful choices regarding food and exercise, but less than 40% exercise on a regular basis. Is this also true for adults with Down syndrome? I don't know.

Mia and I began distributing our survey on healthy lifestyles in 1999. We asked teens and adults with Down syndrome questions about what they eat, how often they exercise, and how they feel about exercise. (Medlen and Peterson, 2000) It was an eye-opening experience both in the administration of the survey and in what we learned about eating and activity from the participants. The conclusions we found the most poignant were in the areas of:

- frequency of eating,
- nutritional balance of meals and snacks, and
- activity

## FREQUENCY OF EATING AND FOOD CHOICES

In our survey, Mia and I asked people to tell us when they were eating. We wanted to know whether adults with Down syndrome were skipping meals. When the surveys were complete, we counted the number of times out of six opportunities (breakfast, A.M. snack, lunch, P.M. snack, dinner, bedtime snack) adults with Down syndrome said they were eating. We learned that 97% ate three or more times each day, with most eating four to six times in a day. That means meals are not being skipped, which is good. In fact, not skipping meals is a good thing for weight management techniques. What matters next is what is being eaten.

According to the surveys, almost everyone ate breakfast, lunch, and dinner. Over 50% of those meals included foods from three of the five bottom food groups from the food guide pyramid. Next we looked at snacks. We found that over 50% had between-meal snacks, with 67% having a snack in the evening. Of those snacks, only 20–32% include just two of the bottom five food groups from the food guide pyramid. This means that most of the snacks had one or fewer servings from the bottom five food groups (bread, fruit, vegetable, meat, and milk) and most included a serving from the more calorie-rich group.

What does all this mean in practical terms? The information suggests that adults with Down syndrome are eating often. They are usually eating meals that are balanced in a general fashion, but snacks are often less nutritious. As a dietitian, it means when I work with families of children and adults with Down syndrome I want to look at the routines and habits related to snacks—such as breaks at work and evening snacks-as an opportunity to make meaningful changes. And yet any changes suggested must be absolutely respectful of the lifestyle and values of the person with Down syndrome. For some, an evening snack is something they have eaten as long as they can remember. It is part of the nightly routine that leads to falling asleep. Asking them to change that routine might mean changes in sleep patterns, which lead to other problems. It's important to agree on lifestyle changes together rather than to dictate them.

To do this, it is important to draw from the survey and experience. In the last 5 years I've had the opportunity to work with a number of teens and adults with Down syndrome in a workshop environment. As a group we've experimented with a variety of topics, but the best example of the current outcome of nutrition education and experiences goes something like this:

*The room is charged with excitement of being together with friends, new and old, and curiosity about what we'll be doing together. As I introduce the topic of nutrition, I can feel a handful of very sharp gazes directed at me. Rhetorically I ask the group, "You all know what the Food Guide Pyramid is, right?" while holding one in the air. They either say "yes!" or they groan aloud. Immediately, there are some comments from those who were giving me those sharp, guarded looks. One woman says, "I know what you're going to talk about.*

*"What?"*

*"Calories," she says with a moan.*

*"Nope," I reply.*

*She sits up a little straighter. Another participant, an older man who lives in his own apartment chimes in. "Well, I know. It's F-A-T."*

*"Nope," I reply again.*

*"Really?" they ask together looking quizzical.*

*"Yep," I answer while addressing them along with the rest of the group. "Today, we're going to talk about how to be healthy by eating a variety of foods—including desserts, french fries, and ice cream. We'll figure out how to decide if a meal is balanced, and if you want, we can create menus for you to take home and try."*

Of course it doesn't happen like this every time, but the idea is always the same. As soon as they hear we're going to discuss being healthy and food, those who have struggled with their weight or are meticulously managed with regard to food begin to build walls. Those who have not had those experiences expect to hear the mantra they've been hearing for years: no pizza, no french fries, no ice cream, no goodies . . . no, no, NO. I'm always happy to get past this point without getting covered in rotten tomatoes.

The survey confirms these personal experiences and adds depth to them as well. In fact, on the basis of my experiences, the survey data, and previous research, (Golden and Hatcher, 1997) I believe the outcome of nutrition education for many adults with Down syndrome today is an understanding

- of food groups,
- of the food pyramid,
- that too many calories cause you to be fat, and
- that never eating foods in the "sometimes" group of the pyramid prevents weight problems.

What they seem unsure of is what they *can* do with food to be healthy. We need to include what is possible in a manner that is as dynamic and memorable as possible to compete with all the restrictions. Otherwise, they do not have the tools to be able to enjoy eating and all that goes with it: friends, family, and the camaraderie of mealtime. Without that, like everyone else, our children will gravitate toward the restricted foods.

## ACTIVITY

The survey included a few questions that gave us an idea of how often adults with Down syndrome exercise and how they feel about exercise in general. It is presumed by many that adults with Down syndrome avoid physical activity or exercise. This might be because of the stocky build or low muscle tone of many adults and children with Down syndrome. It isn't always a sign of dislike for activity or even poor physical condition, as parents of children and adults with Down syndrome know. I will always remember the physician who included, "people with Down syndrome don't like to jog" in his description of what we could expect from our newborn child.

Among other things we asked our participants what their three favorite activities are. If you have ever attended a convention that includes people with Down syndrome of all ages, you already know the most talked-about events of the weekend are the dances. Everyone has fun, and *everyone* dances until they can barely stand. There is dancing of all kinds: ballroom dancing, swing dancing, rock-and-roll type dancing, and even the bunny hop. Partners are not required. It is a great workout. Knowing this, we were not surprised that the favorite activity chosen in the survey was dancing, closely followed by swimming and walking.

We asked our participants what they found the most difficult about exercise. The clear answer was "finding someone to do something with." This is consistent with a study investigating body mass index (BMI) in adults with Down syndrome. That study found that adults with Down syndrome have a lower BMI, which is a sign of lower risk for weight-related health problems, when they have friends to do things with. The lower BMI was not directly related to the total amount of exercise each week. Those who did not have friends to do things with had a higher BMI. In other words, friendships had a greater impact on BMI for the adults with Down syndrome in this study than how long or how often they exercised (Fujiura et al., 1997) This means that for any activity or exercise program to be effective for your child of any age, it helps to have a friend who is also involved in the activity. The friendships discussed in the above study may not be limited to those involved in activities, though. It may be just as effective to have a full circle of friends outside of physical activity.

It has been 12 years since I first pondered my son's adult life and what it might be like for him. I no longer imagine him as a morbidly obese man waiting for the bus. I do see a young man who is confident about how food and activity fit into his life. Unfortunately he, and many adults with Down syndrome, will struggle with weight management throughout his life. But then, so will most Americans.

## References

Campbell MK, Kelsey K (1994): The PEACH Survey: A nutrition screening tool for use in early intervention programs. J Am Diet Assoc 94(10):1156–1158.

Cohen WI (1999): Healthcare Guidelines for Persons with Down Syndrome: 1999 Revision (Down Syndrome Preventive Medical Check List) is published in Down Syndrome Quarterly (Volume 4, Number 3, September, 1999, pp. 1–16), and these excerpts are reprinted with permission of the Editor. Information concerning publication policy or subscriptions may be obtained by contacting Dr. Samuel J. Thios, Editor, Denison University, Granville, OH 43023.

Fujiura GT, Fitzsimons N, Marks B, Chicoine B (1997): Predictors of BMI among adults with Down syndrome: The social context of health promotion. Res Dev Disabil 18(4):261–274.

Gisel E, Lange L, Niman C (1984). Chewing cycles in 4- and 5-year-old Down's syndrome children: A comparison of eating efficacy with normals. Am J Occup Ther 38(10):666–670.

Golden E, Hatcher J (1997): Nutrition knowledge and obesity of adults in community residences. Ment Retard 35:177–184.

Hopman E, Csizmadia CG, Bastiani WF, Engels QM, de Graaf EA, le Cessie S, Mearin ML (1998): Eating habits of young children with Down syndrome in The Netherlands: Adequate nutrient intakes but delayed introduction of solid food. J Am Diet Assoc 98(7): 790–794.

Luke A, Rozien NJ, Sutton M, Schoeller DA (1994): Energy expenditure in children with Down syndrome: Correcting metabolic rate for movement. J Pediatr 125: 829–838.

Luke A, Sutton M, Schoeller DA, Roizen NJ (1996): Nutrient intake and obesity in prepubescent children with Down syndrome. J Am Diet Assoc 96(12):1262–1267.

Medlen JE (1999): From milk to table foods: A parent's guide to introducing food textures. Disability Solutions 3(3):1–9.

Medlen JE, Peterson M (2000): Food, activity, and lifestyles: A survey of adults with Down syndrome. Down Syndrome Q 5(4): 6–12.

# DOWN SYNDROME AND AUTISTIC SPECTRUM DISORDERS

GEORGE T. CAPONE, M.D.

## BACKGROUND

Autism and autistic spectrum disorders (ASD) are best defined as a neu-robehavioral symptom complex involving qualitative impairments in social interaction and communication and a restricted or stereotyped pattern of behavioral interests and activity (First, 1994). As a neurobehavioral symptom complex, autism is a classification based on observed behaviors and not eti-ology. For the purpose of this discussion ASD is meant to include infantile autism, pervasive developmental disorder (PDD), and late-onset autism (childhood disintegrative disorder). Approximately 75% of autistic persons also have mental retardation (Rapin, 1997), and cognitive level is signifi-cantly associated with the severity of autistic symptoms. The prevalence of ASD in persons with Down syndrome (DS) is estimated to be between 5% and 7% (Kent et al., 1999).

The prevalence of ASD appears to be substantially higher in the DS population than in the general population (0.1–0.2%) and higher than the predicted prevalence based upon the cooccurrence of either DS (1:1000 births) or autism (est. 1:1000 births). When conceptualized as biologically discrete and mutually exclusive diagnostic entities, the predicted preva-lence would be 1:1,000,000. We speculate that the presence of an extra copy of chromosome 21 lowers the threshold for the emergence of autistic behaviors in some DS children because of direct genetic and epigenetic

*Down Syndrome*, Edited by William I. Cohen, Lynn Nadel, and Myra E. Madnick.
ISBN 0-471-41815-3   Copyright © 2002 by Wiley-Liss, Inc.

influences on brain development during the prenatal and early postnatal period.

An epidemiological survey of autism in association with rare diseases conducted in the state of Utah revealed that trisomy 21 was the most common "rare disease" associated with autism (Ritvo et al., 1990). This study reported on six male DS subjects with severe or profound mental retardation. A subsequent review (conducted by this author) of epidemiological surveys and case reports published between 1979 and 1999 reveal 40 published cases of DS and autism (Wakabayashi, 1979; Coleman, 1986; Gath and Gumley, 1986; Gillberg et al., 1986; Bregman and Volkmar, 1988; Lund, 1988; Ritvo et al., 1990; Collacott and Cooper, 1992; Ghaziuddin et al., 1992; Howlin et al., 1995; Ghaziuddin, 1997; Kent et al., 1999). Thirty of the subjects were male, and five were female (ratio 6:1); the gender of five subjects was not provided. Karyotype data were given for only 14 subjects; 13 were trisomy 21, and 1 had a translocation. Other than these case reports virtually nothing is known regarding the causes, natural history, outcome, or treatment for this condition. What biological factors associated with trisomy 21 increase the risk for comorbid ASD? Are there distinctive features about the ASD symptomatology observed in DS that permit it to be distinguished from ASD seen in association with other medical-genetic conditions? Do children with DS/ASD respond to pharmacological treatments as described in non-DS persons with ASD?

Howlin and colleagues have recently called attention to the failure of health care providers and school personnel to appreciate the comorbid diagnosis of autism in children with DS/ASD (Howlin et al., 1995). They also speculate on the pathology of autistic disorder in DS, commenting on its association with lower IQ and apparent association with medical conditions (congenital heart disease, visual impairment, and seizures) in their subjects.

It has been noted previously that ASD may occur with increased frequency in certain medical conditions (Gillberg and Coleman, 1996) and that some variation in symptoms is frequently observed among different medical conditions. Thus Gillberg has urged greater emphasis on studying different subgroups of autism to explore the issue of behavioral phenotype as associated with specific medical-genetic conditions(Gillberg, 1992). In DS individuals, most of whom have trisomy 21, and with varying degrees of medical and neurodevelopmental involvement, this task may prove to be particularly daunting.

There is no consensus regarding the specific evaluations necessary to identify the syndrome or the degree to which certain "core features" must be present to establish the diagnosis. Unfortunately, the lack of specific diagnostic tests creates considerable confusion for professionals, parents, and others trying to understand the child and provide for his or her optimal education and care.

There is general agreement that:

- Autism is a spectrum disorder; it may be mild or severe. Many of the symptoms overlap with other conditions such as obsessive-compulsive disorder or stereotypic movement disorder.
- Autism is a developmental diagnosis; expression of the syndrome varies with age and the developmental level of the child.
- Autism can coexist with other conditions such as mental retardation, seizure disorder, fragile X syndrome , or Down syndrome.
- Autism is a life-long condition for which there is no known cure.

The most commonly agreed-upon "core features" of ASD include:

- Impairment in relating to people and social circumstances (disinterest, poor eye contact)
- Communication impairment (using and understanding spoken words, signs, or gestures)
- Repetitive body movements and/or persistent ritualistic behavior patterns

Children who do not manifest all three of these core features at levels considered significant, but who have many of these essential qualities, may be given a diagnosis of PDD. Aversion to certain sensory stimuli, which is frequently observed in ASD, is presently not considered to be one of the core features of the disorder.

## PSYCHIATRIC CONDITIONS

Compared with other groups of children (<21 years) with cognitive impairment, those with DS are less likely to have a psychiatric disorder. Having this additional label is sometimes referred to as having a "dual diagnosis" (mental retardation and psychiatric disorder). As any parent who has such a child knows, severe behavior problems may not be easily fixed. Concerns about a child's behavior are a common reason for referral to physicians and behavior specialists. It is important that the possibility of a comorbid psychiatric disorder be considered, in part because 1) it may be responsive to medication and/or behavioral treatment and 2) having such a diagnosis may entitle the child to more specialized educational or intervention services.

## CLINICAL EXPERIENCE

During the past 10 years we have had the opportunity to evaluate in excess of 70 children with suspected ASD through our Down Syndrome Clinic at

Kennedy Krieger Institute. Many of these children received their initial diagnosis as a result of their clinical evaluation by our DS team. In other cases, children were being seen for a confirmatory diagnosis, consultation, and participation in our research protocol. It has been our experience that children with DS and ASD often present in one of two ways.

## Group One

Children in this group may display atypical behaviors during infancy or toddler years. Behaviors often seen before 3 years of age include:

- Repetitive motor behaviors (mouthing fingers, waving hands, finger play)
- Fascination with and staring at lights, ceiling fans, or fingers
- Episodic eye movements (seizures may be suspected)
- Extreme food refusal (especially high-textured foods)
- Unusual play with toys and other objects (spinning, banging, waving)
- Receptive language impairment (limited understanding or may act as though deaf)
- Little or no meaningful spoken language, gestures, or signs

## Group Two

Another group of children are older when initially identified and often present with neurodevelopmental regression (loss of previously acquired skills, usually between the ages of 3 and 6 years), repetitive motor behaviors, sensory aversions, and/or disruptive behaviors. Some children are reported to have had subtle manifestation of inattention and repetitive behaviors before their regression, whereas others are said to have experienced typical development for DS. The behaviors commonly seen in this group include:

- History of developmental regression (esp. language and social skills)
- Hyper- or hypoactivity, short attention, impulsivity, and poor organization
- Unusual vocalizations (grunting, humming, or other throaty noises)
- Unusual sensory responsiveness (esp. sounds, lights, touch, or pain)
- Difficulty with changes in routine or familiar surroundings (or extreme noncompliance)
- Extreme anxiety, fearfulness, or agitation

- Sleep disturbance (frequent awakenings, decreased need for sleep)
- Disruptive behaviors (physical aggression or throwing objects)
- Self-injurious behavior (skin picking, biting, head hitting, or banging)

Because many of these same behaviors may be seen in other childhood disorders, the diagnosis of ASD may be overlooked or thought to be inappropriate in a child with DS and cognitive impairment. For instance, if a child has a high degree of hyperactivity and impulsivity only a diagnosis of attention deficit hyperactivity disorder, may be considered. Similarly, children with repetitive motor behaviors may only be regarded as having stereotypic movement disorder, which is common in individuals with more severe cognitive impairment. In older children with DS, obsessive-compulsive disorder may present with some of the same features as ASD.

## IMPLICATIONS

Although some of these same behaviors may be seen in other children with DS, neurodevelopmental regression is not normally seen and indicates the need for further investigation. In our experience the search for a concomitant medical cause for regression almost always proves unrewarding. In some children regression may be associated with abnormal EEG findings (Dr. Bonnie Patterson, personal communication). Most often, it is the presence of one or more of the associated behaviors (listed above) that motivate parents and other caregivers to seek out proper diagnosis and treatment. This is an important first step in coming to terms with the child's condition because many of these behaviors can be targeted for management using a combination of medications, behavior management, and augmentive communication techniques.

When deciding whether or not to attempt a medication trial, parents should consider a constellation of factors such as severity and chronicity of behaviors, the degree to which behaviors interfere with developmental or academic progress, and their impact on family or social relationships. In addition it is important to consider the potential impact of behaviors on the health and safety of the individual and caregivers. Even when medications are used a formal behavior management plan and establishing a functional communication strategy are also essential to ensure the greatest chance for success. This often requires establishing a team of teachers, therapists, and interventionists around the child in the school, home, and community. A diagnosis of ASD or PDD should entitle your child to more specialized and effective educational and intervention services. In many communities such services will be extremely difficult to establish and implement with any sense of cohesion. But it is an effort well worth undertaking as earnestly and early as possible once a diagnosis of ASD is established (Rogers, 1998).

## NEUROCHEMISTRY

The neurochemistry of autism is far from clear and most likely involves dysfunction in several different neurochemical systems of the brain that normally function to mediate communication among defined groups of neurons in discrete brain regions. Such information provides the basis for medication trials designed to modulate these neurotransmitter systems. Analysis of brain neurochemistry in autistic children without DS has consistently identified involvement of at least two and possibly three neurotransmitter systems:

- dopamine, which regulates attention, cognition, and reward behaviors
- serotonin, which regulates mood, aggression, sleep cycle, and sexual and feeding behaviors
- opiates, which regulate mood, reward, response to stress, and pain perception, may also be implicated

Detailed studies of brain neurochemistry in DS/ASD have not yet been done. However, our clinical experience in using medications that modulate the dopamine and/or serotonin systems has been favorable in some children with DS/ASD. This is in concordance with what has been reported in the literature (McDougle et al., 1997; Stein et al., 1997; Nicholson et al., 1998).

Newer neuroleptic medications such as risperidone (Risperdal), olanzapine (Zyprexa), and quetiapine (Seroquel), which block the action of dopamine and serotonin, may be helpful in promoting sleep, reducing hyperactivity, self-injurious, or disruptive behavior, and improving attention and organizational skills. Use of such medications must be medically monitored on a regular basis to avoid unwanted side effects that can include sedation, increased appetite, weight gain, or involuntary movements. For this reason, neuroleptic medications are usually started at very low doses and increased only as needed to achieve some improvement in target behaviors.

Newer antidepressant/antianxiety medications referred to as SSRIs (serotonin reuptake inhibitors) have also been helpful adjuncts in treating certain aspects of this condition. The medications fluoxetine (Prozac), paroxetine (Paxil), and fluvoxamine (Luvox), when used alone or in combination with a neuroleptic, may help to promote a normal sleep pattern, reduce anxiety or mood instability, and lessen the intensity of obsessional or perseverative behaviors. Likewise, SSRIs must be medically monitored to avoid unwanted side effects that may include headache, nausea, loose stools, or behavioral activation. Thus "starting low and going slow" is a mantra worth adhering to when using the SSRIs in young children.

Despite obvious concerns about unwanted medication effects it is helpful to know that side effects almost always abate when the medication is reduced or withdrawn, with no lingering or permanent problems as a result. Many families have reported an improved quality of life for themselves and their child once certain behaviors come under control.

It is unclear whether early diagnosis and treatment with medication results in an improved functional outcome for children with DS/ASD. One impediment to early treatment is that a proper diagnosis is often delayed until later in childhood; another is that some professionals are not comfortable using medications in preschoolers or the parents simply may not be interested, opting to choose from the wide variety of other therapies that they inevitably learn about (Campbell et al., 1996).

## GENERAL RECOMMENDATIONS FOR INTERVENTION IN MANAGING A CHILD WITH ASD

### PRESCHOOL CHILD (2–5 YEARS)

Because young children may show variability in their mood, attention, and interest in "therapies," it is best to try and incorporate these into daily routines as much as possible.

1. Emphasize pragmatic aspects of communication (eye contact, turn taking).
2. Utilize a visual communication strategy early on (picture symbols, photographs, or object board) in addition to spoken language.
3. Although repetitive or self-stimulatory behaviors may not be easily stopped, they can often be redirected so as to avoid harm or self-injury. Try distracting your child with a pleasurable game or activity instead of a verbal reprimand. Repeating "No" or "Stop" quickly loses effectiveness.
4. Promote and reward desirable behaviors early and often. Beware of new or unfamiliar environments or transitioning your child too abruptly, because this may precipitate noncompliance or tantruming. Seek out behavior management as needed.
5. Be mindful of the sensory environment; avoid sounds that may be disturbing (noisy crowds, vacuum cleaners, loud arguments, etc.).
6. Try to educate and enlighten medical and early intervention personnel about your child and his condition. Try not to become adversarial, especially when requesting services. It is not known what techniques work best for any given child—that will need to be discovered by you in cooperation with the intervention team. Having

more services may not be as beneficial as finding a specific therapeutic approach that your child accepts. The personality and style of the therapist are also important.

7. Try to have realistic goals for therapy. Of course, you would probably be happy just to have the usual hurdles experienced by parents of typical DS children, but you have more than that now. Target specific behaviors or developmental tasks when deciding goals, you cannot change everything or address all issues at the same time.

8. Accept your child for the person that he or she is and have fun together!

9. Seek out other parents of children with ASD and educate yourself about this condition. You are not alone; it only feels that way.

## School-Age Child (>5 years)

1. Most children will do best in a small, structured classroom where they can get a high degree of supervision and where the program is consistent and predictable. Continue to educate school personnel about your child and what does and does not work. If educational progress is slow, be open to a trial period of some new or different technique; try to use the same techniques at home that are used in school so that learning can be generalized.

2. Seek help with behavior management if and when behavior becomes an issue. Maladaptive behaviors can interfere with learning, socialization, and adaptive abilities. Problem behavior can dominate a person's perception of any child; you do not want this to be the predominant view that others have of your child. Input from behavior personnel helps the child, teachers, and parents to manage behaviors effectively.

3. Don't feel compelled to try every new idea that you hear or read about. Be very skeptical of treatments that sound too good to be true. Although they may be safe and therefore "worth a try," some can consume your emotional and financial resources. Find out as much as you can about any proposed treatment, its cost in time and money, and the specific goals for your child. Ultimately, the decision regarding treatment modality is yours. Remember that many treatments have never been clinically tested for safety and efficacy in large numbers of children with ASD, and there are no studies that focus on children with DS/ASD specifically.

4. Puberty may mark a more difficult time for your child in terms of mood and behavior. Don't be surprised.

5. Take care of yourself and your family. You have a life and a family to consider. Recognize that there is only so much time, energy, and

resources that you can put into this "project." Of course there will be cycles of good times and bad, but if you can't find some way to renew your emotional spirit, then "burn out" is inevitable. There is a higher rate of anxiety, sleep problems, lack of energy, depression, and failed or struggling marriages under these circumstances. Learn to recognize your own difficulties and be honest with yourself and your spouse about the need for help. Counseling and medication may go a long way in helping you to be at your best, for everyone's sake.

## SUMMARY

Clearly there is a great deal yet to be learned about children with DS who are also dually diagnosed with ASD. In the meantime, parents can educate themselves and others about this condition and work on building a team of health care professionals, therapists, and educators who are interested in working with their child to promote the best possible outcome. Research efforts must move beyond mere description to address causation, natural history, and early identification . Specific neurobiological markers that can distinguish DS/ASD from typical DS and typical autism should be sought because they may provide important clues about causation. Finally, the possible benefits of various treatment modalities must be carefully studied and documented. Realization of these goals will take a very long time to accomplish and must be approached with a spirit of support, cooperation, and caring both for individual children and the larger community of children with DS and autism.

## REFERENCES

APA (1994): Diagnostic and Statistical Manual of Mental Disorders. Washington, DC: American Psychiatric Association.

Bregman J, Volkmar F (1988): Autistic social dysfunction and Down syndrome. J Am Acad Child Adol Psychiatry 27(4):440–441.

Campbell M, Schopler E et al. (1996): Treatment of autistic disorder. J Am Acad Child Adolesc Psychiatry 35(2):134–143.

Coleman M. (1986). Down's syndrome children with autistic features. Down Syndrome Papers and Abstracts for Professionals 9(3): 1–2.

Collacott R, Cooper S (1992): Adaptive behavior after depressive illness in Down's syndrome. J Nerv Ment Dis 180:468–470.

Gath A, Gumley D (1986): Behaviour problems in retarded children with special reference to Down's syndrome. Br J Psychiatry 149:156–161.

Ghaziuddin M, Tsai L et al. (1992): Autism in Down's syndrome: Presentation and diagnosis. J Intellect Disabil Res 36:449–456.

Ghaziuddin M (1997): Autism in Down syndrome: Family history correlates. J Intellect Disabil Res 41(1):87–91.

Gillberg C (1992): Subgroups in autism: Are their behavioral phenotypes typical of underlying medical conditions? J Intellect Disabil Res 36:201–214.

Gillberg C, Coleman M (1996): Autism and medical disorders: A review of the literature. Dev Med Child Neurol 38:191–202.

Gillberg C, Persson E et al. (1986): Psychiatric disorders in mildly and severely mentally retarded urban children and adolescents: Epidemiological aspects. Br J Psychiatry 149:68–74.

Howlin P, Wing L et al. (1995): The recognition of autism in children with Down syndrome—Implications for intervention and some speculations about pathology. Dev Med Child Nerol 37:398–414.

Kent L, Evans J et al. (1999): Comorbidity of autistic spectrum disorders in children with Down syndrome. Dev Med Child Neurol 41:153–158.

Lund J (1988): Psychiatric aspects of Down's syndrome. Acta Psychiatr Scand 78: 369–374.

McDougle C, Holmes J et al. (1997): Risperidone treatment of children and adolescents with pervasive developmental disorders: A prospective, open-label study. J Am Acad Child Adolesc Psychiatry 36(5):685–693.

Nicholson R, Awad G et al. (1998): An open trial of Risperidone in young autistic children. J Am Acad Child Adolesc Psychiatry 37(4):372–376.

Rapin I. (1997): Autism. N Engl J Med 337(2):97–104.

Ritvo E, Mason-Brothers A et al. (1990): The UCLA-University of Utah epidemiologic survey of autism: The etiologic role of rare diseases. Am J Psychiatry 147(12): 1614–1621.

Rogers S (1998): Neuropsychology of autism in young children and its implications for early intervention. Ment Retard Dev Disabil Res Rev 4:104–112.

Stein D, Bouwer C et al. (1997): Risperidone augmentation of SSRI in obsessive-compulsive and related disorders. J Clin Psychiatry 58:119–122.

Wakabayashi S. (1979): A case of infantile autism associated with Down's syndrome. J Autism Dev Disord 9(1):31–36.

# EDUCATION/INCLUSION

# INCLUSION: WELCOMING, VALUING, AND SUPPORTING THE DIVERSE LEARNING NEEDS OF ALL STUDENTS IN SHARED GENERAL EDUCATION ENVIRONMENTS

RICHARD A. VILLA, ED.D., AND
JACQUELINE THOUSAND, PH.D.

In a growing number of schools in the United States, it now is possible to walk into elementary, middle, and secondary classrooms and observe students who could be identified as having mild, moderate, and severe cognitive, physical ,and emotional disabilities successfully receiving their education together with similar-aged classmates who have no identified special education needs (Falvey, 1995; Lipsky and Gartner, 1997; Villa and Thousand, 1995). This practice of welcoming, valuing, and supporting the diverse academic and social learning of all students in shared general education environments and experiences is referred to as inclusive education. This article examines inclusive education along a number of dimensions. First, the evolution of the inclusion movement is briefly examined. Second, the construct of "severe disability" is considered in the context of inclusive

*Down Syndrome,* Edited by William I. Cohen, Lynn Nadel, and Myra E. Madnick.
ISBN 0-471-41815-3   Copyright © 2002 by Wiley-Liss, Inc.

education. Third, various rationales for inclusion are examined along with outcome data, legislation, and legal and U.S. Department of Education decisions that forward inclusive policy. Finally, eight factors most frequently associated with successful inclusive education are described.

## HISTORICAL TREND TOWARD INCLUSIVE EDUCATION

For over a decade, researchers, policy makers, parents, consumers, and educators have discussed changing the predominant delivery of special education services, using such terms as "mainstreaming," "integration," "regular education initiative," and "inclusion." These discussions have highlighted some of the perceived requirements for these new types of service delivery to be successful, including restructuring, merging general and special education, creating a unified educational system, and developing shared responsibility for students (Gartner and Lipsky, 1987; Lipsky and Gartner, 1997; Reynolds et al., 1987; Villa et al., 1992).

The "regular education initiative" (REI), first proposed under that name by then U.S. Assistant Secretary for Education Madeline Will (1985), was the term originally used to convey the notion that students with mild disabilities could be served within the regular education setting. It was not long before advocacy efforts expanded the REI concept to incorporate serving all students, including those with severe and profound disabilities, in general education classrooms in neighborhood schools (Biklen, 1988; Thousand et al., 1986; Villa and Thousand, 1988). By the 1990s, the concept had grown to one in which the focus was on "heterogeneous" schooling (frequently called "inclusionary schooling"), in which all children are educated with necessary supports in general education environments in their local neighborhood schools (Villa and Thousand, 1988). In these schools, the traditional schooling paradigm was altered, with curriculum and instruction modified for *all* students (Falvey, 1995; Lipsky and Gartner, 1997; Neary et al., 1992; Stainback and Stainback, 1990, 1992; Villa et al., 1992).

During the past several years the movement toward inclusion has gained unparalleled momentum. By 1993, almost every state was implementing inclusion at some level (Webb, 1994).

## INCLUSION AS PART AND PARCEL OF EDUCATIONAL REFORM

Tremendous attention at the federal, state, and local level is focused on educational reform. Policy makers are emphasizing the establishment of national and state standards, greater flexibility in the use of funds used to support categorical programs, and new, more authentic forms of assessment. Until recently, the inclusive education movement was viewed as a separate initiative running parallel or even counter to concomitant general education reform efforts (Block and Haring, 1992). In contrast, as Udvari-Solner and Thousand (1995) illustrated, established and emerging general education theories in education actually emulate the principles and practices under-pinning inclusionary education. General education school reform initiatives they identify as offering great promise for facilitating inclusive education include multicultural education, outcome-based education, multiple intelli-gence theory, interdisciplinary curriculum, constructivist learning, authentic assessment of student learning, multiage groupings, use of technology in the classroom, forms of peer-mediated instruction such as cooperative group learning, teaching responsibility, and peacemaking and collaborative team-ing among adults and students.

Today the inclusion debate has expanded beyond special education and become part of the total school reform movement. Reports like *Winners All: A Call for Inclusive Schools* by the National Association of State Boards of Education (NASBE) (1992) support the concept of inclusionary schools and urge states to create a new belief system of inclusion and to retrain teachers and revise funding formulas to support inclusive practice. Major educa-tional organizations (e.g., Association for Supervision and Curriculum Development, 1992) have passed resolutions supporting the same notions.

In 1995, 10 of the most prominent national educational associations acknowledged schools successfully implementing inclusive schooling practices and identified their characteristics (Council for Exceptional Children, 1995):

- Diversity is valued and celebrated.
- The principal plays an active and supportive leadership role.
- All students work toward the same educational outcomes based on high standards.
- There is a sense of community in which everyone belongs, is accepted, and is supported by his or her peers and other members of the school community.
- There is an array of services.
- Flexible groupings, authentic and meaningful learning experiences, and developmentally appropriate curricula are accessible to all students.
- Research-based instructional strategies are used, and natural support networks are fostered across students and staff.
- Staff have changed roles that are more collaborative.
- There are new forms of accountability.
- There is access to necessary technology and physical modifications and accommodations.
- Parents are embraced as equal partners.

## Who are Students with "Severe Disabilities?" Why are They Considered so Challenging to Educate?

Whether or not a student is considered as having a severe disability often depends on the idiosyncratic definition adopted by the state and community in which the student resides. The U.S. federal definition identifies students with severe disabilities as those who:

> because of the intensity of their physical, mental or emotional problems need highly specialized education, social, psychological and medical services in order to maximize their full potential for useful and meaningful participation in society and for self-fulfillment. The term includes those children with disabilities with severe emotional disturbance (including schizophrenia), autism, severe and profound mental retardation and those who have two or more serious disabilities such as deaf-blindness, mental retardation and blindness and cerebral palsy and deafness.
>
> (CFR chapter III, Sec. 315.4, 7-1-95, p.176)

At the local school level, such formal definitions oftentimes have little functional meaning or use. What is considered a "severe disability" varies from one school to the next and is contingent on each school community's beliefs about and experience with students whose educational needs go beyond the school's standard curriculum or instructional practices (Thousand and Villa, 1992). For example, a school community with little experience in accommodating for individual students may think of a new student with Rett syndrome as "severely disabled." A second school, with extensive experience accommodating for individual students who have a broad range of needs, may view a much more challenged student as "just another student" with unique needs that must be met. Given this phenomenon of "relativity," the term "students with severe disabilities" will be used throughout this chapter to represent those students with moderate and severe cognitive, physical, health, and emotional/social disabilities described in the previous paragraphs as well as other students who, for whatever reason, are perceived by school personnel as "most challenging" to the current school culture or ecosystem.

There has been and continues to be disagreement as to whether students with severe disabilities belong in general education classrooms, despite the fact that entire texts have been devoted to describing strategies that have been successful for including these and all students, regardless of their perceived exceptionalities, within general education and community environments (e.g., Falvey, 1995; Lipsky and Gartner, 1989, 1997; Stainback and Stainback, 1996; Thousand et al., in press; Villa and Thousand, 1995, 2000). Years ago, Williams, Villa, Thousand, and Fox (1993) suggested that the special versus regular class placement debate was inappropriate for a number of reasons. The successful placement and education of students with intensive educational challenges in regular classes have been occurring for years in schools throughout the United States (e.g., Thousand et al., 1986). Furthermore, the Individuals with Disabilities Education Act (IDEA) clearly specifies that placement of any student must be based on the individual's identified needs, not the student's handicapping condition or categorical label. To even raise the question of whether regular class placement is appropriate for a category of learners (i.e., students with intensive educational needs) "assumes that placement can be made based upon handicapping condition without documentation, of an individual student's identified needs and examination of whether the needs could be met in a regular class-based placement" (Williams et al., 1993, p. 333). Finally, learning and social benefits in inclusive settings for students with and without disabilities have been documented (National Study of Inclusive Education, 1994, 1995; Stainback and Stainback, 1996; Villa, Thousand, Meyers, and Nevin, 1996), as have benefits for teachers, when educators collaborate to invent individualized responsive educational programs (Villa, Thousand, Nevin, and Malgeri, 1996).

The "Who belongs in general education?" placement question for students with severe disabilities may be inappropriate for all of the above reasons. Yet the norm within most schools is still for intensively challenged students to be educated in separate schools and classrooms for all or most of their day. Why? Gartner and Lipsky (2000) identify potential perceptual, cultural, and emotional barriers, which cause people to balk at idea of the inclusion of students with severe disabilities:

- Attitudes of disdain and prejudice;
- The belief that only those closer to "normal" can be/should be included;
- The belief that the needs of students with severe disabilities are unique and beyond the capacity of general educators;
- The "severity" of the disability;
- The need for more extensive related services to enable these students to benefit from instruction;
- The need for access to particularized expertise to support the student's academic and social learning;
- The relationship of educational goals for students with severe disabilities to the general education curriculum;
- Concern that the behavior of students with severe disabilities might be disruptive to the learning of other students in the general education classroom;

- Unfamiliarity with students with severe disabilities because the vast majority of them are served in settings apart from the district's general education population of teachers and students;
- The cost of providing special education and related services to students with severe disabilities; and
- The belief that functional life skills cannot be addressed in general education settings.

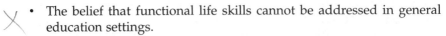

Nevertheless, despite these potential barriers, models of inclusive education for students with severe disabilities do exist and, in some places, have existed for some time. These living demonstrations have taught us much about how to facilitate systems change in the structure of the school and the school day, the everyday operation of the classroom, and the roles of educators, students, and community members, so that students with severe disabilities have equal educational opportunities, meaningful access to the general education curriculum, and effective educational and related services in neighborhood schools. Before sharing the "hows" of inclusive education learned in these schools, let us first examine the "whys" of inclusion—the data and related rationale for including students with disabilities in general education. Adults and students alike are more likely to learn *how* to do something (i.e., inclusive education) if they understand *why* doing so is important.

## RATIONALE AND DATA IN SUPPORT OF INCLUSIVE EDUCATION

What leads people to get beyond their perceptual, cultural, and emotional barriers and to shift their beliefs, attitudes, values, practices, and policy making toward more inclusive educational opportunities for students with identified learning differences? This section presents some of the rationale associated with the growing advocacy for inclusive schools where all students are welcomed, valued, supported, and learning in shared environments

## EFFICACY DATA: HOW GOOD IS SEPARATE SPECIAL EDUCATION?

Over a decade ago, research reviews and meta-analyses known as the special education "efficacy studies" already showed that placement outside of general education had few or no positive effects for students regardless of the intensity or type of their disabilities (Lipsky and Gartner, 1989). Reviewing the findings, Lipsky and Gartner (1989) observed the basic premise of special education was that students with deficits will benefit from a unique body of knowledge and from smaller classes staffed by specially trained teachers using special materials. But there is no compelling body of evidence demonstrating that segregated special education programs have significant benefits for students.

(p. 19)

A 1994 review of three meta-analyses concerned with the most effective settings for educating students with special needs concluded that regardless of the type of disability or grade level of the student, "special-needs students educated in regular classes do better academically and socially than comparable students in non-inclusive settings" (Baker et al., 1994, p. 34). Hunt, Farron-Davis, Beckstead, Curtis, and Goetz (1994) found that students with disabilities in inclusive settings had higher-quality individualized education programs (IEPs) and higher levels of engaged time compared with students with disabilities who were educated in separate classes.

Specifically, for students with severe disabilities, Keefe and Van Etten (1994) found higher levels of "active academic responding" and lower levels of competing behavior in general education settings compared with segregated classes and schools. Hollowood, Salisbury, Rainforth, and Palombaro (1994) found the inclusion of students with severe disabilities not to be detrimental to classmates. Others found inclusion to enhance classmates' (Costello, 1991; Kaskinen-Chapman, 1992) as well as their own learning (e.g., Cole and Meyer, 1991; Hollowood et al., 1994; Strain 1983; Staub and Peck, 1994) and to yield social and emotional benefits for all students, with self-esteem and attendance improving for some students considered "at risk" (Kelly, 1992). Burchard and Clark (1990) noted that for a child with severely maladjusted behavior it is considerably more cost effective to individualize services in the community than to place the child in a segregated residential program and that services provided in local schools and community are considered to be better.

In response to the fear that students with disabilities would have a detrimental effect on nondisabled classmates, Staub and Peck (1994) found in an analysis of studies using quasi-experimental designs "no deceleration of academic behavior for nondisabled children" (p. 36) when children with mild, moderate, or severe disabilities were placed full-time in general education. Sharpe, York, and Knight (1994) found no decline in the academic and behavioral performance on standardized tests and report card measures of the classmates of students with disabilities.

As for postschool employment data for graduates of separate special education programs, Wagner and colleagues (1991) found high levels of unemployment (over 50% 1 year after graduation) and underemployment. In contrast, Ferguson and Ash (1989) found that the more time children with disabilities spent in regular classes, the more they achieved as adults in employment and continuing education. This held true regardless of the gender, race, socioeconomic status, or type of disability of the child or the age when the child was afforded access to general education. In 1995, the U. S. Department of Education reported that "across a number of analyses of post-school results, the message was the same: those who spent more time in regular education experienced better results after high school [p. 87]."

## FEDERAL LEGISLATION AND CASE LAW

Since 1975, federal court cases have clarified and continue to clarify the intent of the law in favor of the inclusion of students with disabilities in general education. For example, in 1983, the *Roncker v. Walter* case addressed the issue of "bringing educational services to the child" versus "bringing the child to the services." The case resolved in favor of integrated versus segregated placement and established a *principle of portability*, that is, "if a desirable service currently provided in a segregated setting can feasibly be delivered in an integrated setting, it would be inappropriate under P.L. 94-142 to provide the service in a segregated environment" (700 F. 2d at 1063). The 1988 U.S. Court of Appeals ruling in favor of Timothy W., a student with severe disabilities whose school district contended he was "too disabled" to be entitled to an education, clarified school districts' responsibility to educate all children and specified that the term "all" included in IDEA meant *all* children with disabilities, without exception. In 1993, the U.S. Court of Appeals for the Third Circuit upheld the right of Rafael Oberti, a boy with Down syndrome, to receive his education in his neighborhood regular school with adequate and necessary supports, placing the *burden of proof* for compliance with the IDEA's mainstreaming requirements squarely on the school district and the state rather than the family. In 1994, the U.S. Court of Appeals for the Ninth Circuit upheld the district court decision in the *Holland v. Sacramento Unified School District* case in which Judge Levi indicated that when school districts place students with disabilities, the presumption and *starting point is the mainstream.*

## PHILOSOPHICAL RATIONALE

A third compelling rationale for inclusive education is moral, philosophical, and ethical in nature and compliments the data-based and legal rationales discussed above. This rationale is that categorical segregation of any subgroup of people is simply a violation of civil rights and the principle of *equal citizenship*. Many believe what Chief Justice Earl Warren clarified in the landmark *Brown v. Board of Education* decision over four decades ago, that is, that separateness in education can generate a feeling of inferiority as to [children's] status in the community that may affect their hearts and minds in a way unlikely ever to be undone. This sense of inferiority . . . affects the motivation of a child to learn . . . [and] has a tendency to retard . . . educational and mental development.

(Warren, 1954, p. 493)

Many advocates of inclusive education see the parallels to other struggles for human and civil rights and recall images of school personnel of the 1950s and 1960s blocking "white" schoolhouse doors to keep out African-American children. In far too many communities, administrators, teachers, and other school personnel (e.g., social workers, school psychologists) figuratively still block the doors, but this time to keep out children with disabilities. The number one determinant of whether or not a child with disabilities has access to regular education is *where* that child's family happens to live.

## EIGHT FACTORS FOR SUCCESSFUL INCLUSIVE PRACTICE:

What have nearly 25 years of the implementation of P.L. 94-142/IDEA taught us about what facilitates successful inclusive education? Analysis of the reports from some 1000 school districts on their inclusive education efforts in the National Center on Educational Restructuring and Inclusion's *National Study* (1994, 1995) identifies at least eight factors for success: visionary leadership, collaboration, refocused use of assessment, support for staff and students, effective parental involvement, implementation of effective program models, effective classroom practices, and funding. What follows is a description of the eight factors and specific National Center findings as well as suggestions for the role of special educators' and related services personnel in promoting each of the factors.

### FACTOR 1: VISIONARY LEADERSHIP

Villa, Thousand, Meyers, and Nevin (1996), in a study of 32 inclusive school sites in five states and one Canadian province, found the degree of administrative support and vision to be the most powerful predictor of general educators' attitude toward full inclusion. Although traditionally leadership is viewed as emanating from the school superintendent or principal, in districts across the country the initial impetus for inclusive education has come from many sources. Visionaries may be educators, related services personnel (e.g., psychologists, occupational therapists), parents, students, and, on occasion, from a university or state-level project. The issue is less the initiator but more recognition that for inclusive education to be successful the vision must be articulated and ultimately all stakeholders must become involved.

## FACTOR 2: COLLABORATION

Reports from school districts across the nation clearly indicate that the achievement of inclusive education presumes that no one person can or ought to be expected to have all the expertise required to meet the educational needs of all the students in a classroom. Having the *opportunity* to collaborate and to learn about and develop the *skills* to be effective and efficient collaborative team members (Thousand and Villa, 1992; 2000) is a minimum requirement for inclusive education to work. In a study of over 600 educators, collaboration emerged as the only variable across general and special education teachers and administrators that predicted positive attitudes toward inclusion (Villa, Thousand, Nevin, & Meyers, 1996). Building planning teams, scheduling time for teachers to work together, recognizing teachers as problem solvers, conceptualizing teachers as front-line researchers—these means were all reported to the National Center on Educational Restructuring and Inclusion (1994, 1995) as critical for successful collaboration.

## FACTOR 3: REFOCUSED USE OF ASSESSMENT

Historically, the practice of special education has led to an overwhelming amount of special educators' and school psychologists' time being spent in assessment activities related to the determination of special education eligibility of a student. Up to 50% of the special educator's time, and even more of the psychologist's time, has been spent in noninstructional assessment and paperwork activities. This left little time for the special services personnel to offer other types of services that fall within their purview.

As a screening device for special education determination and classification, many studies have documented the inadequacy of the present system of assessment. According to assessment leader James Ysseldyke, given one or another state's definition of learning disabilities, a substantial majority of all students would be so classified; indeed, he says, the determination is "little better than a flip of the coin." With regard to assessment as a measure of student progress, inclusive education schools and districts are reporting moving toward more "authentic assessment" designs, including the use of portfolios of students' work and performances, and generally working to refocus assessment to determine how a child is smart rather than how smart a child is.

FAMILY-FRIENDLY ASSESSMENT.    Making Action Plans (MAPs) (Falvey et al., 1994) is example of an authentic assessment process particularly useful with students with severe disabilities whose needs and lives may be so complex that it is not always clear which directions are the "correct" ones to take. The MAPs process is initiated by gathering a team that includes the student, peers, family members, friends, and anyone else the student wants to attend, including school staff. With the help of a "neutral" facilitator, the team addresses a sequence of key questions to visualize a desired future and develop an action plan.

Vehicles for translating long-term dreams into specific goals and objectives, daily schedules, and individualized accommodations are based on three fundamental assumptions: 1) the student has a *caring support team* that meets regularly, communicates often and effectively with one another using MAPs and other strategies, and holds the long-range dreams and nightmares in mind when making more short-term decisions with and on behalf of the student; 2) the *student* as well as peers and family members are *included as team members* at every step of the way (Villa and Thousand, 1996) and their voices are heard and are as valued as the voices of the professionals; and 3) the process used for futures planning (e.g., MAPs) is dynamic, meaning that *priorities*—dreams and nightmares—are *reexamined regularly.*

## FACTOR 4: SUPPORT FOR STUDENTS AND STAFF

From the student's vantage point, support for inclusion may mean integrating needed therapy services into the general school program; peer support such as "buddy systems" or "Circles of Friends" (Falvey et al., 1995); communication support (e.g., facilitated communication); supplementary aids and services (including short- or long-term, part- or full-time paraprofessional support); and effective use of computer-aided technology and other assistive devices as classroom tools rather than fancy gadgets in a special room. Best practices in providing support are based on an "only as much as needed" principle, to avoid inflicting "disabling help" on students who do not need or necessarily want the human or material support that could be provided. Thus paraprofessionals are assigned to a class as a member of a teaching team, rather than "velcroed" to an individual child. The "only as much as needed" principle recognizes that related services are supposed to be educationally *necessary* (not all that might be required to meet a child's other-than-educational needs) to enable the student to interact with the curriculum. It goes without saying that related services need to be coordinated, so that supports don't pull in opposite directions and actually pull the student away from the general education classroom and curriculum.

## FACTOR 5: EFFECTIVE PARENTAL INVOLVEMENT

Successful inclusive schools report the critical importance of parental participation. They encourage parental involvement by providing family support services and effective collaboration and communication opportunities.

Programs that bring a wide array of services to children in the school set-tings report at least two sets of benefits—direct benefits to the children and the opportunities for parents and other family members to become involved in school-based activities. As the child in an inclusive school becomes a part of the fabric of the school along with her/his nondisabled peers, so, too, the parents of children with disabilities become less isolated.

The 1997 IDEA renewal also enhances parental participation. It does so by requiring their participation in all eligibility and placement decisions involving their child(ren) and by requiring that they be informed about their child(ren)'s progress no less frequently than is the district's practice for nondisabled children.

## FACTOR 6: IMPLEMENTATION OF EFFECTIVE PROGRAM MODELS

There are many partnership and shared responsibility models of inclusion that have been successful (National Study of Inclusive Education, 1994, 1995). They include:

- a co-teaching model, in which the special educator (and other support personnel such as the psychologist) co-teaches alongside the general education teacher;
- parallel teaching, in which the special educator (and other support personnel such as the psychologist) works with a small group of students from a selected special education population in a section of the general education classroom;
- a co-teaching consultant model, in which the special educator (and other support personnel such as the psychologist) provides assistance to the general educator, enabling her or him to teach all the students in the inclusive class;
- a team model, in which the special educator (and other support personnel such as the psychologist) joins with one or more general education teachers to form a team, sharing responsibility for all the children in the inclusive classroom;
- a methods and resource teacher model, in which the special educa-tor (and other support personnel such as the psychologist), whose students have been distributed in general education classes, works with the general education teachers, providing direct instruction, modeling of lessons, and consultation; and
- a dually licensed teacher, who holds both general and special educa-tion certification and thus is equipped to teach all of the students in an inclusive classroom (with the support of other support personnel such as the psychologist).

Schools have had success with each of these designs or variations of the designs. Factors in adopting a particular model are local decision making and educators' preferences. Basic to any design is a strong professional development component that includes formal training and ongoing technical assistance both before and during the initiation of the model.

## FACTOR 7: EFFECTIVE CLASSROOM PRACTICES

Effective classroom practices, as reported by districts implementing inclusive education, have two overarching characteristics. The first is that the adaptations appropriate for students with disabilities benefit all students. The second is that the instructional strategies used in inclusive classrooms oftentimes are practices recommended by educational reformers and researchers for general education students. Cooperative learning is the most important instructional strategy supporting inclusive education. Well over half of the districts implementing inclusive education included in the National Center on Educational Restructuring and Inclusion's National Study of Inclusive Education (1994, 1995) reported using cooperative learning. Additional instructional strategies cited by a quarter or more of the districts include curricular adaptations, students supporting other students, paraprofessional support, and use of instructional technology.

ADDITIONAL EFFECTIVE PRACTICES FOR STUDENTS WITH SEVERE COG-NITIVE, PHYSICAL, AND HEALTH CHALLENGES.   Students with severe cognitive, physical, and health challenges are students for whom many teachers question the value of general education classroom experiences. A frequently asked question is why students who have learning objectives very different from those of the majority of class members would be included in activities that, at first glance, do not seem to relate to the students' needs. Sometimes people do not realize just how rich the general education environment is, particularly for a student with intensive challenges. The variety of people, materials, and activities is endless and provides an ongoing flow of opportunities for communication and human relationship building, incidental learning in areas not yet targeted as priority objectives and direct instruction in a student's high-priority learning areas.

Key to ensuring a student's meaningful participation is the creative thinking of the members of the student's educational support team. The team always has at least four options for arranging a student's participation in general education activities (Giangreco et al., 1993). A student can do the *same* as everyone else (e.g., practice songs in music class). *Multilevel curriculum and instruction* can occur; that is, all students are involved in a lesson in the same curriculum area but are pursuing varying objectives at multiple levels based on their unique needs. For example, in math class students may be applying computation skills at varying levels—some with complex word problems, others with one-digit subtraction problems, and yet others with materials that illustrate counting with correspondence. *Curriculum overlapping* involves students working in the same lesson but pursuing objectives from different curricular areas. For example, Bob, a teenager with severe disabilities, was working in a cooperative group in science class with two other students, using the lap tray attached to his wheelchair as the team's work space. Most students were dissecting frogs for the purpose of identifying body parts. Bob's objectives came from the curriculum areas of communication and socialization. One communication program (e.g., discrimination of objects, including his blue drinking cup) was simple for Bob's teammates to carry out along with their dissection throughout the activity. Another communication objective of vocalizing in reaction to others and events was frequently and readily achieved as Bob giggled and vocalized to teammates' wiggling of frog parts in the air. *Alternative activities* may be needed in a child's schedule to allow for community-based or work options or to address management needs (e.g., catheterization in the nurse's office). Alternative activities also may be considered when a regular education activity cannot be adapted.

Extreme caution is advised in classifying an activity "impossible to adapt" or the general education classroom as inappropriate for a student with severe disabilities. Experience has taught the authors that general education (e.g., science class for Bob) can meet most needs of children with severe disabilities, given creative thinking and collaboration on the part of the adults and children of the school and greater community. Current theories of learning (e.g., multiple intelligences, constructivist learning), teaching practices that make subject matter including science more relevant and meaningful (e.g., cooperative group learning, project- or activity-based learning, community-referenced activities), and authentic alternatives to paper and pencil assessment (e.g., artifact collection for a portfolio, role playing, demonstration) are now available to empower and equip educators to adapt instruction for any student, including one with a severe disability.

Finally, to make assumptions about an individual based on a classification of disability is dangerous, because it can lead to tunnel vision. Specifically, it can blind others to an individual's strengths and abilities and cause them to see only the person's disability—a phenomenon Van der Klift and Kunc describe as "disability spread" (1994, p. 399). Without a students strengths and abilities in view, it is easy to limit expectations, "overaccommodate," or ignore ways in which strengths and abilities can be employed to motivate and support a student's learning.

## FACTOR 8: FUNDING

Historically, special education funding formulas favored restrictive placements for students in special education. The 1997 IDEA renewal required states to adopt policies that are "placement neutral," that is, ones that do not contravene the law's program mandate as to least restrictive environment placement. Funds must follow the student, regardless of placement, and must be sufficient to provide the services necessary. Districts report that, in general, inclusive education programs are no more costly than segregated models ("Does inclusion cost more?" 1994; McLaughlin and Warren, 1994; Parrish, 1997). However, districts must anticipate one-time "conversion" costs, especially for necessary planning and professional development.

## CONCLUSION

To expand inclusive or democratic schooling nationwide, we, who are in or who are interested in education, must push the limits of our abilities to learn new skills, ways of thinking, and ways of dealing with our own and our colleagues' struggles to make behavioral, cognitive, and attitudinal transformations. Pushing our limits to effect change in educational systems and to talk about that change in ways that make sense to educators, families, and community members will be a challenge. But, as Pierre Teilhard de Chardin observed, "our duty as [humans] is to proceed as if limits to our abilities do not exist."

## REFERENCES

Association for Supervision and Curriculum Development. (1992): Resolutions, 1991. Alexandria, VA: Association for Supervision and Curriculum Development.

Baker E, Wang M, Walberg H (1994): The effects of inclusion on learning. Educ Leadership 52(4):33–35.

Biklen D (Producer) (1988): Regular lives (video). Washington, DC: State of the Art.

Block J, Haring T (1992): On swamps, bogs, alligators, and special education reform. In Villa R, Thousand J, Stainback W, Stainback S (eds.), Restructuring for Caring and Effective Education: An Administrative Guide to Creating Heterogeneous Schools. Baltimore: Paul H. Brookes Publishing , pp. 7–24.

Burchard JD, Clark RT (1990): The role of individualized care in a service delivery system for children and adolescents with severely maladjusted behavior. J Ment Hlth Admin 17(1):48–60.

Cole D, Meyer L (1991): Social integration and severe disabilities. A longitudinal analysis of child outcomes. J Spec Ed 25, 340–351.

Costello C (1991): A comparison of student cognitive and social achievement for handicapped and regular education students who are educated in integrated versus a substantially separate classroom. Unpublished doctoral dissertation. Amherst: University of Massachusetts.

Council for Exceptional Children (1995): Inclusive Schools: Lessons from 10 Schools. Reston, VA: Council for Exceptional Children.

Falvey M (1995): Inclusive and Heterogeneous Schooling: Assessment, Curriculum, and Instruction. Baltimore: Paul H. Brookes Publishing.

Falvey M, Forest M, Pearpoint J, Rosenberg R (1994): Building connections. In; Thousand J, Villa R, Nevin A (eds.), Creativity and Collaborative Learning: A Practical Guide for Empowering Students and Teachers. Baltimore: Paul Brookes Publishing, pp 347–368.

Ferguson P, Ash A (1989): Lessons from life: Personal and parental perspectives on school, childhood, and disability. In: Biklen D, Ford A, Ferguson D (eds.), Disability and Society, Chicago: National Society for the Study of Education, pp 108–140.

Gartner A, Lipsky D (1987): Beyond special Education: Toward a quality education system for all students. Harvard Educ Rev 57:367–395.

Gartner A, Lipsky D. (2000): Inclusion and school restructuring: A new synergy. In Villa R, Thousand J (eds.), Restructuring for Caring and Effective Education: Putting the Pieces of the Puzzle Together (2nd. ed.). Baltimore: Paul H. Brookes Publishing.

Giangreco MF, Cloninger CJ, Iverson VS (1993): Choosing Options and Accommodations for Children (COACH): A Guide to Educational Planning for Students with Disabilities (2nd ed.). Baltimore: Paul H. Brookes Publishing.

Hollowood TM, Salisbury CL, Rainforth B. Palombaro MM (1994): Use of instructional time in classrooms serving students with and without severe disabilities. Exceptional Children 61(3):242–253.

Hunt P, Farro-Davis F, Beckstead S, Curtis D, Goetz L (1994): Evaluating the effects of placement of students with severe disabilities in general education versus special class. J Assoc Persons Severe Handicaps 19(4):290–301.

Kaskinen-Chapman A. (1992): Saline area schools and inclusive community concepts. In: Villa R, Thousand J, Stainback W, Stainback S (eds.), Restructuring for Caring and Effective Education. Baltimore: Paul H. Brookes Publishing, pp. 169–185.

Keefe E, VanEtten G (1994, December 8): Academic and social outcomes for students with moderate to profound disabilities in integrated settings. Paper presented at conference of The Association for Persons with Severe Handicaps, Atlanta, GA.

Lipsky D, Gartner A (1989): Beyond Separate Education: Quality Education for All. Baltimore: Paul H. Brookes Publishing.

Lipsky D, Gartner A (1997): Inclusion and School Reform: Transforming America's Classrooms. Baltimore: Paul H. Brookes Publishing.

McLauglin M, Warren S (1994): Resource implication of inclusion: Impressions of special educators. Palo Alto, CA, Center for Special Education Finance.

National Association of State Boards of Education Study Group on Special Education (1992): Winners All: A Call for Inclusive Schools. Alexandria, VA: Author.

National Study of Inclusive Education (1994): New York: City University of New York, National Center on Educational Restructuring and Inclusion.

National Study of Inclusive Education (1995): New York: City University of New York, National Center on Educational Restructuring and Inclusion.

Neary T, Halvorsen A, Kronberg R, Kelly D (1992, December): Curricular Adaptations for Inclusive Classrooms. California Research Institute for the Integration of Students With Severe Disabilities.

Oberti v. Board of Education, 995F. 2nd 1204 (3rd. Cir. 1993).

Parrish T (1997): Fiscal issues relating to special education inclusion. In: Lipsky DK, Gartner A (eds.), Inclusion and School Reform: Transforming America's Classrooms. Baltimore: Paul H. Brookes Publishing, pp 275–298.

Reynolds JC, Wang MC, Walberg HJ (1987): The necessary restructuring of special and regular education. Exceptional Children 53:391–398.

Roncker v. Walter (1983). 700F.2d 1058, 1063 (6th Cir.) cert. denied, 464 U.S. 864.

Sacramento City Unified School District v. Rachael H., 14 F 3d 1398 (9th Cir. 1994).

Sharpe MN, York JL, Knight J (1994): Effects of inclusion on the academic performance of classmates without disabilities. Remedial Spec Educ 15(5):281–287.

Stainback S, Stainback W (1996): Inclusion: A Guide for Educators. Baltimore: Paul H. Brookes Publishing.

Stainback S, Stainback W (1990): Inclusive schooling. In: Stainback W, Stainback S (eds.), Support Networks for Inclusive Schooling: Interdependent Integrated Education. Baltimore: Paul H. Brookes Publishing, pp 25–36.

Staub D, Peck CA (1994): What are the outcomes for nondisabled students? Educ Leadership 52(4):36–40.

Strain P (1983): Generalization of autistic children's social behavior change: Effects of developmentally integrated and segregated settings. Anal Intervention Dev Disabil 3(1):23–34.

Thousand J, Fox T, Reid R, Godek J, Williams W, Fox W (1986): The Homecoming Model: Educating Students Who Present Intensive Educational Challenges Within Regular Education Environments (Monograph No. 7-1). Burlington: University of Vermont, Center for Developmental Disabilities.

Thousand J, Villa R (1992): Collaborative teams: A powerful tool in school restructuring. In: Villa R, Thousand J, Stainback W, Stainback S (eds.), Restructuring for Caring and Effective Schools: An Administrative Guide to Creating Heterogeneous Schools. Baltimore: Paul H. Brookes Publishing, pp 73–108.

Thousand J, Villa R, Nevin A (in press): Creativity and Collaborative Learning: A Practical Guide to Empowering Students, Teachers, and Families. Baltimore: Paul K. Brooks Publishing.

Thousand J, Villa R, Nevin A (1994): Creativity and Collaborative Learning: A Powerful Guide to Empowering Students and Teachers. Baltimore: Paul H. Brookes Publishing.

Udvari-Solner A, Thousand J (1995): Exemplary and promising teaching practices that foster inclusive education. In: Villa R, Thousand J (eds.), Creating an Inclusive School. Alexandria, VA: Association for Supervision and Curriculum Development.

U.S. Department of Education (1995): Seventeenth Annual Report to Congress on the Implementation of the Individuals With Disabilities Education Act. Washington, DC: US Dept of Ed.

Van der Klift E, Kunc N (1994): Beyond benevolence: Friendship and the politics of help. In: Thousand J, Villa R, Nevin A (eds.), Creativity AND Collaborative Learning: A Powerful Guide to Empowering Students and Teachers. Baltimore: Paul H. Brookes Publishing, pp. 391–401.

Villa R, Thousand J (1988): Enhancing success in heterogeneous classrooms and schools: The powers of partnership. Teacher Educ Spec Educ 11:144–154.

Villa R, Thousand J (1995): Creating an Inclusive School. Alexandria, VA: Association for Supervision and Curriculum Development.

Villa R, Thousand J (1996): Student collaboration: An essential for curriculum delivery in the 21st century. In: Stainback S, Stainback W (eds.), Inclusion: A Guide for Educators. Baltimore: Paul H. Brookes Publishing, pp. 171–192.

Villa R, Thousand J (2000): Restructuring for Caring and Effective Education: Piecing the Puzzle Together. Baltimore: Paul Brooks Publishers.

Villa R, Thousand J, Nevin A, Malgeri C (1996): Instilling collaboration for inclusive schooling as a way of doing business in public schools. Remedial Spec Educ 7(3):182–192.

Villa R, Thousand J, Meyers H, Nevin A (1996): Teacher and administrator perceptions of heterogeneous education. Exceptional Children 63(1):29–45.

Villa R, Thousand J, Stainback W, Stainback S (1992): Restructuring for Caring and Effective Education: An Administrative Guide to Creating Heterogeneous Schools. Baltimore: Paul H. Brookes Publishing.

Wagner M, Newman L, D'Amico R, Jay ED, Butler-Nalin P, Marder C, Cox R (Eds.) (1991): Youth with Disabilities: How are they doing? The First Comprehensive Report from the National Longitudinal Transition Study of Special Education Students. Menlo Park, CA: SRI International.

Wang MC, Reynolds MC, Walberg HJ (1987): Handbook of Special Education Research and Practice. Oxford, UK: Pergamon Press.

Warren E (1954): Brown v. Board of Education of Topeka, 347 U.S. 483, 493.

Webb N (1994). Special education: With new court decisions behind them, advocates see inclusion as a question of values. Harvard Educ Lett 10(4):1–3.

Williams W, Villa R, Thousand J, Fox W (1993): Is regular class placement really the issue? A response to Brown, Long, Udvari-Solner, Schwarz, VanDeventer, Ahlgren, Johnson, Grunewald, and Jorgensen. J Assoc Persons Severe Disabil 14:333–334.

Will M (1985, December): Educating children with learning problems: A shared responsibility. Wingspread Conference on The Education of Special Needs Students: Research Findings and Implications for Practice, Racine, WI.

# POSITIVE BEHAVIORAL SUPPORTS: CREATING SUPPORTIVE ENVIRONMENTS AT HOME, IN SCHOOLS, AND IN THE COMMUNITY

HANK EDMONSON, M.ED., AND
ANN TURNBULL, ED.D

"I wasn't prepared in college for this . . . . I took classroom management. . . . I learned how to make cutesy bulletin boards and how to have parent/teacher conferences and how to get little Johnny to lunch, but . . . ," says a teacher in the urban middle school, as he expresses his sentiment, and the sentiments of many others, when discussing how to support individuals whose behaviors impede their learning. The purpose of this chapter is to provide insights into research being conducted on positive behavioral supports (PBS).

This paper addresses supporting students through a discussion of the following: a definition, PBS and the law, key components of PBS, and a blueprint of the four levels of support.

## WHAT IS PBS?

According to Turnbull et al. (in press), PBS involves both positive behavior and support. It is both a philosophy for supporting interventions and a framework for organizing supports. As a philosophy, behavioral interventions should focus on increasing skills. Simply focusing on the repression

*Down Syndrome*, Edited by William I. Cohen, Lynn Nadel, and Myra E. Madnick.
ISBN 0-471-41815-3   Copyright © 2002 by Wiley-Liss, Inc.

and punishment of undesired skills has several side effects (Sidman, 1989). These side effects include, but are not limited to, making the behavior harder to change in the future, increased escape and avoidance behaviors, and counter-coercion (e.g., revenge).

PBS focuses on teaching appropriate behaviors. It is related to discipline in that this term comes from the Latin root word *discipulus*, which literally means "to teach." To understand why certain behaviors occur, a process known as functional behavioral assessment is used (discussed in greater detail below). The purpose of this process is to increase the likelihood that interventions will be efficient, powerful, and effective. All decisions should be based on data regarding the student's behaviors, environment (within the school and without), and physiology. It is the flow of information between key stakeholders that brings about change at many different levels (Briggs and Peat, 1999; Wheatley, 1992).

Within PBS, there is a focus on the larger context within which the behavior occurs. As Dewey (1997/1938) explained, students have miseducative experiences when there is a mismatch between the student and the setting. PBS strategies attempt to focus on altering systems (e.g., whole school, classroom, communities, family settings) to improve the educational experiences for children, their families, and teachers.

Another factor is that data-based decisions should be made by teams of people concerned with the welfare of the individual. No one person can shoulder responsibilities of supporting people whose behavior significantly impedes their ability. The adage has been that, "It takes a village to raise a child." An extension of that would be that it is helpful to have access to the resources of the village to keep the child from burning it down!

As a structure, PBS provides a way of organizing resources to decrease the duplication of services, to track needs, to evaluate what succeeds, and to make ongoing adjustments. Although the unit of analysis does change (e.g., the whole school, class, community), the key principles still apply. The four levels of support (universal support, group support, individual school support, and individual comprehensive supports) discussed below provide teachers, parents, and community members with a way of self-organizing (Briggs and Peat, 1999), to ensure the success of all students. It is the assumption of researchers at Loyola University, Chicago, and the University of Kansas that each of these levels is critical and interrelated. Without any one of these levels of support, stakeholders in the child's life will find themselves without the necessary resources to provide appropriate experiences.

## WHAT IS THE LAW?

Meeting the needs of an individual with disabilities can be difficult when discipline problems are added to the equation. The person's support providers must ask themselves, "How can we set up situations in which individuals receive an appropriate education when behavior impedes their success?"

When schools are faced with problem behavior of students with disabilities, the federal government calls for the consideration of PBS. It requires that the individualized education plan (IEP) team consider, when appropriate, "... strategies, including positive behavioral interventions and supports: strategies, and supports to address that behavior" [IDEA, Section 1415(d)(3)(B), 1997].

The Individuals with Disabilities Education Act (IDEA) 1997 also (a) allows for students not receiving special education services to have incidental benefit from supports; (b) encourages the use of schoolwide approaches; (c) considers school improvement a method for creating supportive general education environment; and (d) encourages partnerships among schools, families, and service providers. The following section will provide a discussion of four components of PBS. These levels are an attempt to bring together these IDEA considerations when creating supportive environments.

## The Levels of PBS

### Universal Support

The term "universal" indicates that the whole school population receives this level of support. At this level, every student is universally exposed to the same behavioral instruction.

INTERVENTION.    Whether at work, at home, at school or during recreation, people want to know what is expected of them. Think how frustrating it would be to try to play any sport without an understanding of its rules and expectations. Take basketball, for instance; it would be considerably more effective if we could sit on the shoulders of a teammate and place the ball inside the rim. We are not, however, allowed to do this; it is against the rules. If a person is going to play that sport, we hope that someone will take the time to explain the behaviors that are expected before he or she actually plays the game. If not, people will find many of their efforts very frustrating.

In the previous example, and in other settings, people expect that individuals know what is expected of them. Inappropriate behaviors are often punished without the person being taught (disciplined) the correct responses.

As with any sport activity, it is best to start with the basics. Universal support involves:

- The identification of three to five positively stated expectations (e.g., be safe, be cooperative, be ready to learn);
- Directly teaching these expectations in multiple settings;
- Making sure these expected behaviors "work"; and
- Keeping track of the expected behaviors.

These expectations should be short, easy to memorize, stated positively, posted in frequently traveled (e.g., classrooms, hallways) areas, and developed and agreed upon by everyone in the setting. Teachers can develop their expectations by asking staff and students to describe the steps to being successful in their school. Teachers at one school identified the expectations: be safe, be cooperative, be ready to learn, be respectful and be responsible. These five expectations are the framework for their classroom codes of conduct and are posted in every classroom, cafeteria, office, and hallway.

One would not explain to a child the intricacies of a free-throw basketball shot and expect that would be enough. To teach that skill, one would probably explain what was to be taught and why it was important, describe the specific steps of the shot, model the shot, allow the person to practice, and provide feedback about the performance. These same steps are the components of teaching behavioral expectation. These steps (identify the skill, state the rationale, teach the skill, allow practice, provide feedback) are also components of good instruction. In schools in which this level of support is being provided, teachers use a combination of these steps to teach the expectations of their setting to their students.

These expectations should then become a part of the culture of the setting and be acknowledged; most importantly, these behaviors should work (e.g., desirable things happen for doing the right thing). In schools where this research is being conducted, teachers used their three to five expectations to provide the framework for their codes of conduct (classroom rule). Most schools require development of these codes. The teachers obtain input from the students about how expected behaviors appear during the myriad of activities throughout the school day. A benefit of incorporating the students in the development of the codes of conduct is that people own what they create (Fullan, 1998).

A school that implemented PBS reported that 81% of the students had at least one referral during the course of the baseline year (Warren et al., in press). This statistic illustrates the culture of the school: it was "cool" to be "bad." The teachers developed a system to change this culture of "badness." The five expectations for the school were placed on small slips of paper, along with a space for student and teacher names. For instance, when a student was cooperative, the teacher would provide the student with one of the slips with a check mark next to the "cooperative" behavior. The student would then take the slip to the office, where the slip would be placed into one of three boxes, depending on the student's grade level. At the beginning of each school day, the vice principal would select one student from each grade-level box and read the students' names, the teachers' names, and the engaged behaviors over the intercom system during class time. Next, the students were sent to the office, where they would have their picture taken, as a group, and select a single prize from a glass display case. Each student's picture was then mounted in the display case accompanied by the specific behavior exhibited to win the prize. This cabinet is located next to the cafeteria, where all students must pass on their way to lunch.

BENEFITS FOR SCHOOLS.    The teachers at this middle school suggested there were several benefits to this approach (Edmonson, 2000; Turnbull et al., in press). Teachers reinforcing the student "expected" behaviors improved student-to-teacher relationships. These behavior–reward systems helped the teachers to look for the positive behaviors of the students rather than to focus on the negative ones. When the expected behaviors were taught and rewarded, the students knew what they were doing right. Also, the staff suggested that the reward system gave the students something to look forward to; it provided motivation for being at school and for being successful. The staff also suggested that the system provided principles of IDEA: normalization and dual accommodations.

Normalization involves creating a situation in which people with disabilities are treated and feel like "normal" members of society. The teachers reported that because all students participated in the behavior–reward system, the students receiving special education services were part of the setting. Teachers reported a favorable effect when students were called over the loud speaker to come down to the office.

Dual accommodations involve creating supports that focus directly on the individual and simultaneously improving the individual's environment. By using the behavior–reward system, expected individual student behaviors (e.g., being safe, being cooperative) were rewarded, therefore increasing the likelihood they would use these behaviors to be successful in school. The entire school environment was "richer" in the amount of positive outcomes for students, because teachers had a reason to look for expected behaviors. The first year of data indicated that teachers provided twice as many positive reward slips as punitive office referrals. Although a ratio of three or four positive interactions for every one negative interaction is ideal, the teachers have taken a large step in the right direction.

Perhaps the strongest selling point of the universal support system is that it focuses on prevention. Without this type of system, the teachers would have to wait for the student to engage in the wrong behavior and then provide correction. This correction is typically punishing the problem behavior (e.g., "stop that") without telling the student what the behavior should be replaced with (e.g., "please use an inside voice"). With the universal system of support, the teachers do not have to wait for problem behaviors to teach (discipline) the expected behaviors. This saves time. In fact, the staff of this middle school increased their instructional time after implementing this level of support. Teaching and rewarding expected behaviors prevents negative interactions between students and teachers (e.g., power struggles), which set the tone for future problems (e.g., escape, avoidance, revenge).

Two factors must be considered with universal support. First, some students at this middle school needed to be taught how to accept praise and rewards. Many of the youths' experiences with adults had been negative, so they had not developed skills to accept positive praise (e.g., saying thank you, acknowledging their accomplishment). Accepting rewards was a skill that had to be taught like any other. Secondly, there was some concern about the novelty and consistency of the reward system. The teachers recommended ongoing adjustments for the reward system (e.g., fading the number of drawings, changing the prizes), based on data about the students' behaviors (e.g., office referrals). Some teachers simply did not use the reward system as much as others; further studies will need to be done to address "why" certain teachers do and do not use this system.

IMPLICATIONS FOR FAMILIES.    The translation of universal support to the home setting seem to be guided by several questions:

What are the behaviors that are expected in one's home? One might want to sit down, as a family, and discuss what behaviors are expected for both children and adults. One could have children write, draw, or dictate how these behaviors might appear. Shorten this list to three to five, short, positively stated expectations. These expectations could include, but are not limited to, being safe, cooperative, kind, and respectful. It would be most helpful to post these expectations in areas of high traffic or play. This will allow family members to refer to the expectations whenever necessary.

How do the family members know these behaviors? What do these expectations look like in different settings? Once one has agreed on these expectations, there should be discussion about how these behaviors appear in different settings. Think about all of the settings in which one would like his or her family to engage in these behaviors. Be specific! Once one has expectations and settings identified, one needs to teach how they work together. This will be discussed more thoroughly in the group support section.

What happens to people when they engage in these behaviors? One should ensure that these expected behaviors "work" for family members. Thus if a family member demonstrates one of these behaviors, such as being respectful during play with a brother, something desirable happens to the child who initiated the expected behavior. This could be a regular outcome (access to a game, food, praise, or activity) or a token system (reward ticket that a child can trade for a preferred reward). The trick to reward systems is that the reward should immediately follow the desired behavior. Typically, the reward is paired with a specific statement about the behavior. This includes a description of the behavior (e.g., you were respectful to your brother when you gave him back his toy), a rationale for the behavior (e.g., that is really good because we can all have time with the toys), checking to see whether the rationale makes sense (e.g., do you understand why being respectful is so good?), and a delivery of the reward (e.g., praise, presentation of object or activity). A general rule of thumb is that one wants to spend a lot of energy at first in rewarding desired behaviors. A good standard is to have four positive interactions for every one corrective interaction.

How does one know that people are engaging in the expected behaviors? The next consideration is program evaluation. This is going to look different at home than it will at school. The idea, however, is the same. First, monitor how well one is doing with implementation. Are the rules posted in the home, car, and other recreational locations? Does one have more positive interactions than negative (use a golf counter to keep track of these)? Do the family and close friends know your expectations? Periodically, ask members of family if they can remember what these expectations are. Providing this information to friends, family members, and baby sitters could prevent some potential problems. Also, it would be ideal if some of these expectations matched with the expectations of the child's classroom(s), school, and/or workplace.

Next, monitor the "so what" of the universal "housewide" plan. What difference has this made in the life of one's family? Are there fewer arguments? Do the children have more access to activities they really like? On the whole, do family members have more energy at the end of the day? Are parents in a better mood when spending time with their children? One way to track one's mood would be to write a number, from 1 to 10, on your calendar. A 1 would indicate a terrible day (e.g., considerable time spent in correcting behaviors), a 5 would indicate an average day (e.g., neither especially positive nor punitive), and a 10 would indicate an extremely positive day (e.g., most interactions with the children were positive, little time was spent in "correcting" behaviors). Another way to measure the outcomes of one's interventions would be the products left behind by those who live in your home. These outcomes could include:

- The number of toys left out at the end of the day;
- The condition of beds and bathrooms after use;
- The number of clothes left on the floor as opposed to a hamper;

There are two benefits for tracking the behaviors of children. First, the minute tracking a behavior begins, the behavior is impacted. Second, by tracking behaviors, it is easier to consider behaviors (even one's own) as data rather than personal interactions. Data collection gives the adults a behavior that interrupts their typical reactions to their child's problem behaviors (e.g., yelling, physical intervention). It also gives the parents a sense that they are doing something about the problem behavior. This will decrease one's frustration level when times get tough!

## GROUP SUPPORT

Although universal support does prevent problem behaviors, sometimes more specific strategies are needed. Group support involves identifying specific situations, settings, expectations, and behaviors that need more development.

INTERVENTION.    In the middle school where this research was being carried out, many of the sixth graders were having difficulty during hallway passing periods. These problems included hitting, pushing, running, and yelling. The staff were concerned that these behaviors were not safe, and perhaps created problems, as the students moved into their next class. Teachers and researchers took the PBS approach when dealing with these behaviors.

First, the researchers and teachers used interviews and observations to identify the students, times, and universal expectation that related to these behaviors (be safe). Next, the teachers used the teaching strategy identified in Table 26.1 (Taylor-Green et al., 1997).

A critical component to these "discipline" sessions was the use of behavioral momentum (Dunlap and Morelli-Robbins, 1990). The students were asked to engage in behaviors in which they were very likely to change (e.g., unsafe hall walking). Whether they realized it or not, the students were complying with teachers' instructions. The teachers were able to build momentum toward compliance. With only one exception, all of the students were able to demonstrate safe hall walking. The one exception involved the students walking on the wrong side of the hall on the first attempt at safe walking.

BENEFITS FOR SCHOOLS.    The teachers at the middle school where this research was conducted suggested that this level of support was effective (Edmonson, 2000). When asked whether a follow-up session was necessary, the teachers suggested that it was not. There was a suggestion that this level of support also changed some teachers' view of students' behaviors. Many of the teachers also suggested that it was very helpful to be able to redirect the students in the hallway. The students had enough prior knowledge to be able to take responsibility for their own behaviors. The staff did suggest that it would be very helpful to provide additional self-management strategies (e.g., tracking performance on a specific behavior) to sustain behaviors after the initial training. Some teachers combined the behaviors taught through group support with self-management systems in their classrooms.

TABLE 26.1. Steps for Group Instruction

| Teaching strategy | Implementation |
| --- | --- |
| State and identify the expectation and setting | Be safe in the hallway. The students were taken to a hallway near the auditorium. |
| Identify the reason this expected behavior is necessary | Students suggested: "So no one will be hurt." |
| Describe what the expected behavior *does not* look like (Be specific) | Students suggested: Hitting each other, running, pushing |
| Describe what the expected behaviors *do* look like (Be specific) | Students suggested: Walking with hands to self, walking on the right side of the hallway, using an inside voice |
| Practice: Students demonstrate the inappropriate behavior first, then end with the appropriate behaviors | Students were precorrected before demonstrating the inappropriate behaviors not to do anything that would be considered a major violation of school policy (e.g., punching, cursing). Students were also taught a signal that would indicate it was time to end the demonstration of unsafe hall walking |
| Provided feedback/recognition for expected behaviors | The students earned certificates that indicated they were "certified" safe hall walkers |
| Ongoing feedback about expected behaviors | Teachers were able to redirect students who were not walking safely by asking, "Are you being safe or unsafe in the hallway right now?" The students were able to evaluate and change their own behaviors without the use of punishment |

*Note.* Teaching strategies adapted from Taylor-Greene et al. (1997)

IMPLICATIONS FOR FAMILIES. The basis for this level of support is that problem behaviors provide insight into possible interventions. It is critical that one has established "housewide" expectations. For example, if a child yells when she or he asks for a toy, then the expectation might be respect. The location for this behavior is wherever it occurs. The replacement behaviors will typically be the opposite of the problem behavior. Table 26.2 provides a grid to help one plan group support lessons in the home.

Sometimes group supports are not enough. A more individualized approach is needed to prevent problem behaviors and improve the quality of life for everyone involved in the child's life.

TABLE 26.2. GRID FOR TEACHING EXPECTATIONS AT HOME

| Expectation | Setting 1: Kitchen | Setting 2: Living Room | Setting 3: Bedroom | Setting 4: Backyard |
|---|---|---|---|---|
| Be Safe | P: Touching hot stove<br>T: | P: Climbing on coffee table<br>T: Proper use of furniture | P:<br>T: | P: Hitting others with bat<br>T: Proper use of baseball bat |
| Be Responsible | P: Messy table manners<br>T: How to use utensils | P: Leaving toys out<br>T: Where to keep toys when done | P: Leaving clothing on the floor<br>T: Putting clothes in a hamper | P: Leaving bike in driveway behind car<br>T: Where to park bike when done |
| Be Respectful | P: Yelling, "Give me salt!"<br>T: How to say "please and thank you" | P: Talking when others talk<br>T: How to interrupt or waiting for turn | P: Playing radio too loud<br>T: Appropriate sound level inside the house | P: Not taking turns with friends during games<br>T: How to take turns/ share activities |
| Be Cooperative | P: Not coming to the table when called<br>T: How to follow directions the first time given | P:<br>T: | P:<br>T: | P:<br>T: |

Note. P = Problem Behavior, T = What to teach to replace problem behaviors.

## INDIVIDUAL SCHOOL SUPPORT

Positive behavioral supports involve several steps at the individual level: assessment, development of support team, interventions and ongoing adjustment/evaluation.

INTERVENTION.    Individual intervention begins with three levels of assessment: behavioral, personal, and environmental factors. Each of these factors should be addressed within a functional behavioral assessment (FBA). The FBA is a critical component of the PBS approach. At a minimum, an FBA involves interviews with people familiar with the student, observations in multiple settings and at different times, development of hypotheses about the behavior, and a description of behaviors targeted for improvement. An important addition is an understanding of the strengths of the student as well. The goal of the FBA process is to increase the likelihood that the behavioral intervention plan will be effective and efficient.

A simple way to remember the interview process is to remember one's first composition class. The teachers probably suggested that any story should have at least five components: who, what, where, when, and why. This is also an effective guide to developing a better understanding of the purpose of the behavior and developing interventions that meet that purpose in a more appropriate way. All five of these questions should be used, with both the occurrence and nonoccurrence of behaviors.

The following is an example of a student involved in a University of Kansas research study on PBS.

Ted was a 12-year-old boy who had received special education services. He lived with his mother but stayed nights with his grandmother, while his mother worked. His mother would pick him up around midnight, and they would go home.

Ted had several strengths. He seemed to enjoy using the computer, reading, doing arts and crafts, and working with students in an English as a second language program. He was also very good at evaluating his own behaviors. He knew when he was having a good day and when he was not. Ted also seemed to respond very well to individual attention.

According to Ted's mother, he had asthma. Also, since 1995, he had had sleeping problems. His mother suggested that Ted and his brothers would sneak out and watch television after she would put them to bed. She also reported that he and his brothers frequently would fight at home.

According to his teachers, Ted was failing in school. He did not keep up with basic hygiene (e.g., combing his hair, picking scars in class). But the behaviors of concern were being "off-task" and social isolation.

On the basis of teacher reports and his records, Ted had a 4-year history of not completing or of avoiding work. As one teacher described, Ted wasted time "playing with things." Being off-task involved two behaviors: sleeping

TABLE 26.3. TED'S FUNCTIONAL BEHAVIORAL ASSESSMENT TABLE

| Question | Occurred | Did not occur |
|---|---|---|
| Who | When working with one teacher and multiple students | When working one-on-one with an adult |
| What | When asked to do something he did not like to do (e.g., writing). He would draw instead. | Art class |
| Where | In math, science, and language arts; Class discussions; and smaller classes | Would participate in the activities listed below |
| When | When asked to awaken in class; When asked to read silently in class; On days when his personal hygiene was especially lacking | Group reading; During hands-on activities; Well groomed; Familiar with the content of the lesson |
| Why (hunch about the purpose of the behavior) | Escaping/avoiding frustrating or less preferred work; Adult attention received for sleeping in class | He is a kinesthetic learner; Adult attention is important to Ted; He is more likely to engage topics he is familiar with |

*Note.* Data Sources included teachers, parent, aunt, and Ted himself. Settings included his home and school.

and repetitive behaviors. Sleeping was described as head nodding or having his head on his desk. Repetitive behaviors involved playing with pencils or paper or picking at scars.

Social isolation for Ted involved a lack of positive peer interactions. Other students picked on Ted, typically as a result of his problem behaviors. He did not appear to have significant relations with any other students. This social isolation seemed to be related to the concerns about personal hygiene. He was described as typically having a "downtrodden" affect.

The tools used to collect additional information included interviews, direct observations, positive environment checklist, learning styles interviews, document reviews, and sleep checklists. The researchers used interviews and observations to document when problem behavior did and did not occur (see Table 26.3).

The hunch that Ted's ability to be on-task related to his preferred activities was tested as the only theory of "why" the problems were occurring. His social studies teacher allowed Ted to read a topic that he determined to be interesting. As a result, this teacher reported that Ted was on-task during this activity and that he was reading more in class.

The initial support team involved one of the vice principals of the school, two teachers, the school counselor, the parent liaison, his mother, and a researcher. One of Ted's teachers took the lead role and served as the single point of contact at the school for coordinating data, meetings, and interventions. The researcher served as the facilitator for data collection, initial team meetings, and intervention development.

The team determined that they would focus on replacing off-task behaviors with on-task (PBS has a focus on increasing rather than decreasing behaviors). Table 26.3 describes the initial hunches that were addressed during the development of the behavior intervention plan (BIP). The components of a BIP include, but are not limited to, a description of the behaviors to be increased, statements about the hunches for the problem behaviors, and strategies that address the hunches for the problem behaviors. Some of these strategies are included in Table 26.4.

As you will probably notice from Table 26.4, a greater emphasis is placed on interventions before problems occur. As stated above, a foundational principle of PBS is that prevention is typically the most powerful, effective, and efficient way to address problem behavior. Table 26.5 provides a description of interventions developed specifically for Ted.

The teachers reported that Ted began to do better at school. During a 3-month period, Ted had nine disciplinary office referrals. After the FBA and implementation of the behavioral intervention plan, Ted had no more referrals for the rest of the year. Although the plan continued to require adjustment, many of the teachers reported that Ted was doing much better.

BENEFITS FOR SCHOOLS.    Researchers reported several lessons from this process with Ted and other students (Edmonson, 2000). When one works with one student, one improves the quality of life of others in the setting. After these interventions, the teachers had more time to work with other students, thus increasing their ability to meet the other students' needs. The student's lead teacher reported that the BIP served as a tool for the implementations of supports. Without a plan, according to this veteran teacher, she never would have been able to provide this level of support to Ted. The use of a behavioral team also decreases the likelihood that a person will "burn out" from trying to meet one individual's every need. The team process divided the work, provided an opportunity to share responsibility, and provided access to resources no one person would know.

Several factors must be brought into account when implementing this level of support (Edmonson, 2000). Typically, one intervention will not last

## TABLE 26.4. Positive Behavioral Support Interventions

| Before the behavior occurs | When the behavior occurs | After the behavior occurs |
|---|---|---|
| **Task Interspersal:** Interchanging preferred and nonpreferred tasks for a person;<br><br>**Incorporating preferred activities/learning modalities:** Incorporate content that is interesting to the student, incorporate activities that address the person's learning style (problem behaviors provide insights into preferred interests and activities;<br><br>**Behavioral Momentum:** Asking the person to do something they are likely to comply with (e.g., "please take this piece of candy"), followed by something they are less likely to comply with (e.g., "please hand me your pencil");<br><br>**Choice Making:** Providing the person with options between several activities;<br><br>Teach Replacement Behaviors: Teach the person behaviors that serve the same purpose as the problem behaviors (e.g., teaching a signal that indicates a person need a break from a stressful activity);<br><br>**Pre-Teaching:** Similar to group instruction. Teach and/or remind the individual of the expected behaviors prior to the next activity or change of setting.<br><br>**Social Stories:** These are stories that the individual writes in their own language pictures that describe behaviors that are expected in certain settings (hint: this is useful for pre-correction)<br><br>**Scheduling:** Identifying and posting a schedule that provides structure for activities. Any major change in the schedule should be pre-corrected to increase the success of the transition; | **When expected behaviors:** Acknowledge behaviors that reflect the universal expectations of your setting (e.g., delivery of universal ticket);<br><br>**When problem behaviors occur:** Redirect the person to the expected behavior—if the person has been through group instruction for those behaviors, then ask whether or not the person is engaging in the expected behaviors. | **When expected behaviors occur:** Immediately following deliver praise, object and/or reward slip (e.g., universal ticket). If possible, check to see if the person understands why the reward was received;<br><br>There will be natural outcomes for appropriate behaviors (e.g., access to preferred activities, completed work, success);<br><br>**When problem behaviors occur:** Review the social story with the person and practice expected behaviors;<br><br>Acknowledge others who are demonstrating the appropriate behaviors;<br><br>Deliver a positive consequence the moment the desired behavior occurs |

TABLE 26.5. INTERVENTIONS FOR TED

| Before the problem behaviors occur | When the behavior occurs | After the behaviors occur |
|---|---|---|
| Practice handwriting skills; Teachers personally greet Ted on his way into class; Teac Ted a morning routine for personal hygiene; Provide Ted with his own alarm clock; Uncle will watch the boys at their home until their mother gets home from work; Enroll and his brothers in an after-school program; Allow Ted to work with students who receive English as a second language services; Include preferred activities (e.g., art), and topics in his lessons; Directly teach Ted introduction skills for making friends. | Ted will keep a behavioral tracking sheet that will allow he and his teachers to rate his on-task behaviors and personal hygiene. | **Following expected behaviors:** Ted and his teachers will discuss his performance on his behavioral tracking sheet. Ted will earn time on the computer for days with high ratings for his target behaviors; Computer time will be in the classroom of his favorite teacher; **Following problem behaviors:** When Ted sleeps in class, his teachers will walk up to him and ask him about a topic his interested in, rather than comment about his sleeping in class; Provide praise for on-task behaviors as soon as they occur. |

forever. People and settings change; therefore, supports need to change. For instance, during the first year of the research, one of the young men involved in the case studies was disrupting class for adult attention. He did not have many interactions with peers, hence, peer attention did not seem to be very important. During the second year, however, this young man began to spend more time interacting with peers. The intervention strategies that were in place were designed for someone whose disruptive behaviors were maintained by adult attention. Although the team considered it a plus that the young man was interacting with his peers, they had to adjust their strategies accordingly.

Two additional lessons have been learned from this research. It appears to take between 2 and 3 months from the time the FBA begins to when the team begins to have a firm handle on an intervention plan. The reasons for this delay seem to include the teams' lack of prior experience with the process, scheduling issues (e.g., absences, suspensions), the level or intensity of the behaviors, and the beliefs of the individual teams members about what "support" really means.

It also seems to take about 1 year before lasting and substantive change begins to occur. For most of the first year with the students involved in the case studies, it was one step forward and two steps backward. Throughout, students needing individual support, the team went through a process of identifying supports for supports. For instance, if a counselor were located for a student, there was a concern about transportation to get to the services. If reduced rate bus passes were located, the team had to find a way to bring the paperwork across town before the students and their families obtained resources.

IMPLICATIONS FOR FAMILIES.    It is hard to limit the number of implications of this research for families. Perhaps it would be best to think in terms of options. By asking the questions stated at the beginning of this section, family members can gain ideas about why problem behaviors are occurring. An individual data collection process makes it possible for family members to gain this information. This makes it easier for them to not view behavior personally but rather to understand that the child is providing them with information about quality of life. When families have a better understanding of the issues, they have a better idea about what to do. Parents move from having one option to a problem behavior (e.g., saying "stop that") to multiple responses (e.g., preteaching, reinforcing expected behaviors).

## INDIVIDUAL/COMPREHENSIVE SUPPORT

This fourth level of support involves working with setting events (Smith and Iwata, 1997). These setting events involve things that happen before the behavior that impact how a person responds to events and/or stimulus. For example, missing dinner can make food the next morning extremely desirable. If having gone for a long period of time without attention, behaviors that provide access to attention from others can provide desirable outcomes. According to Ferguson (1991, as cited in Kansas Commission on Teaching and America's Future, 2000), these family and home issues contribute the greatest percentage of variability for student success (49%), while having a qualified teacher and reduced class size contribute 42% and 8%, respectively. Some students need individual support across multiple settings (in addition to school) including home, neighborhood, and community.

INTERVENTION.    An understanding of how setting events impact behaviors brings us back to the discussion of the larger "why" behind behavior. For example, in Ted's situation, sleeping in class was a more preferred activity than reading aloud. Although there were certainly academic issues involved, they did not seem to address the entire issue. The team could have simply developed a reward system across every class in which Ted was sleeping to ensure on-task behavior. It was considerably more powerful and efficient to address "why" sleep was preferred. Although his mother's late working hours were a factor, there was something even more critical then that. Ted did not have a bed of his own in which to sleep. The beds that were available were too small and required that he share them with at least one of his brothers. He preferred sleeping on his grandmother's couch to his situation at home. The teachers, along with the support of researchers, located a bed and a truck to transport it. It is important to mention that it took at least two attempts to make arrangements to deliver the new bed. Scheduling problems required that multiple attempts be made, another example of supports needed for supports. The teachers reported that, after receiving his bed, Ted was able to stay awake for longer periods of time in class.

The larger community can, in certain circumstances, contribute to problem behaviors at school. For example, many of the mothers, including Ted's, suggested that they did not allow their children to play outside at night. Frequent drive-by shootings, drug usage, and gang activity kept their children indoors. While indoors, these students did not have the opportunity to develop social skills with other children through playing games and other recreational activities. When students are asked at school to participate in interactive activities, such as cooperative learning, they do not have the requisite skills to participate. This frustrates teachers and impedes the children's ability to learn.

The teachers, parents, students, and community members of Ted's middle school have been meeting on a regular basis to address these very issues. They use the site-based management plan (or school improvement plan) to organize their efforts and provide the structure for planning. Typically these plans: (a) require representative participation from the larger community, (b) are team driven, (c) are data driven, (d) provide a plan of operation for the school at large, and (e) require meetings on a regular basis to evaluate and adjust planning.

Currently this team is focusing on developing plans that will impact the children, teachers, and families of their school community and the entire county. This team has decided to pursue diagnostic tutoring programs, mentoring programs, and community school efforts (e.g., one-stop shopping for community resources through the school). These three supports will buttress the student improvement team and individual levels of supports by providing additional options and resources for interventions.

Benefits for school.    The staff of this middle school have mentioned several benefits for comprehensive levels of support (Edmonson, 2000). The staff mentioned that data about the child's quality of life created empathy for them. The teachers reported that empathy (instead of sympathy) for the student increased their willingness to try different interventions and supports. Also, sharing data (communicating) between the home and the school improved the teacher-student-parent relationships.

At the larger community level, the school improvement plan provided a way to organize data, resources, and interventions that reduced duplication of services. The meeting format necessary for the school improvement plans provided a mechanism to provide a common focus for the 52 different programs that were running at the school. These meetings also provided opportunities to share information about the school with the community and to receive input about improving supports.

IMPLICATIONS FOR FAMILIES.   To make a significant impact on problem behavior in home, neighborhood, and community settings, it's important to ask the following questions:

1. What supports does an individual child need?
2. Are there other children who need similar supports?
3. What resources does one's community/school have that could meet this need?
4. Who else in one's community would find meeting this need important? (e.g., How does everybody win by meeting this need?)
5. What is one's school or community doing (or need to be doing) that could be a natural place to house these additional supports? (e.g., school improvement plan, city planning commission)
6. How can one organize this information in a way that makes sense to one's community members?

Three principles of PBS will provide guiding light as one moves forward: efforts should be team driven, data driven, and focused on increasing skills and supports.

## SUMMARY

The purpose of this chapter has been to increase the reader's understanding of PBS and its application. It is hoped that the generalizations of structures, assessments, and interventions to the home setting will provide the reader with additional tools for support. Most importantly, it is hoped that the reader has been provided with different, and perhaps more effective, ways to think about problem behaviors.

## REFERENCES

Briggs J, Peat FD (1999): Seven Lessons of Chaos: Timeless Wisdom from the Science of Change. New York: Harper Collins.

Dewey J (1997/1938): Experience and Education. New York: Touchstone.

Dunlap D, Morelli-Robbins M (1990): A guide for reducing situation-specific behavior problems with task intersperse [Field Test Draft]. Florida Mental Health Institute, University of South Florida.

Edmonson H. (2000): A Study of the Process of the Implementation of School Reform in an Urban Middle School Using Positive Behavioral Supports: "Not One More Thing." Dissertation Abstracts International.

Fullan M (1998): Change Forces: Probing the Depths of Educational Reform. London: Falmer Press.

Individuals with Disabilities Education Act [Chapter 33]. (1997). 20, Parts A–C.

Kansas Commission on Teaching America's Future. (2000). Put Students First: A Competent, Caring and Qualified Teacher in Every Classroom. Lawrence, KS: Institute for Educational Research and Public Service.

Sidman M (1989): Coercion and its Fallout. Boston, MA: Authors Cooperative.

Smith R G, Iwata B (1997): Antecedent influences on behavior disorders. J Appl Behav Anal 30(2):343–375.

Taylor GS, Brown D, Nelson L, Longton J, Gassman T, Cohen J, Swartz J, Horner R, Sugai G, Hall S (1997): School-wide behavior support: Starting the year off right. J Behav Educ 7(1):99–112.

Turnbull A, Edmonson H, Griggs P, Wickham D, Sailor W, Beech S, Freeman R, Guess D, Hale N, Lassen S, McCart A, Riffel L, Smerchek D, Turnbull R, Warren J, Brennan W (in press). A Blueprint for Schoolwide Positive Behavior Support: Full Implementation of Three Components, Exceptional Children.

Warren J, Edmonson H, Turnbull A, Sailor W, Wickham D, Griggs P, Beech S. (in press): School-wide Application of Positive Behavior Support: Implementation and Preliminary Evaluation of PBS in an Urban Setting. Journal of Educational Psychology Review.

Wheatley M (1992): Leadership and the New Science. San Francisco: Berrett-Koehler Publishers.

# POSTSECONDARY EDUCATION

## PHYLLIS JACKS, ED.D.

If you subscribe to the theory that life's challenges are character-developing experiences, families of individuals with disabilities must have a wealth of "character" by the time their sons/daughters are exiting secondary school. Not surprisingly, and just when families and individuals with disabilities thought they had faced enough "character building experiences" for a life-time, a new set of challenging decisions relating to future planning for their child, now grown to adulthood, appear on the horizon in the student's final years with the school system. Not underestimating the difficulty of decid-ing among the choices available, or lack thereof, the planning process has improved considerably in the last decade as the result of transition planning mandates that are embodied in IDEA. That families do not leverage this mandate to its fullest, that schools do not attend to it with the vigilance that advocates had hoped they would, and that government agencies created to fund and/or provide services to disabled adults have not measured up to expectations in this area is unfortunate. However, it is incumbent on fami-lies, school personnel, and staff from adult provider agencies to employ this "statutory tool" to safeguard and enhance the special education investment that has already been made in the individual no longer under the school's auspices and now eligible for continued services.

Although all parties have a definite role, families can and must make the difference at this juncture in the life of their son/daughter. It is not possible to adequately describe the concern, sometimes fear, in the eyes of families searching for services that will ensure their sons/daughters the array of

*Down Syndrome*, Edited by William I. Cohen, Lynn Nadel, and Myra E. Madnick.
ISBN 0-471-41815-3   Copyright © 2002 by Wiley-Liss, Inc.

services that will allow their adult children to meet their potential—often the hope of an independent life, albeit with ongoing support services. Conversely, it is also hard to describe the immense pleasure one feels in seeing the relief in the eyes of family members who feel that they have found the right setting and program for their son/daughter.

Initially, the most important thing to remember about postsecondary services is that the eventual choices made are the result of sustained, careful planning during the individual's high school years. Under federal law, planning for life after a student exits the school system must begin when the student is 14 years old. The elements of the transition plan are delineated in IDEA and include addressing "instruction, community experiences, the development of employment and other post-school adult living objectives, and, when appropriate, acquisition of daily living skills . . ." [20 U.S.C. sect. 1401(a)(19)]. The forum for creating the plan is the annual meeting at which the student's IEP is reviewed and the next year's plan is created. In fact, the transition plan, including goals, objectives, and evaluative measures, is part of the IEP. Employing the areas indicated in the law, the plan should identify those skills that will be required for the student to reach his or her potential. Ideally, starting with the initial transition goals there will be a progression from an emphasis on skills learned in the classroom to specific plans for application of these skills in the real world, culminating with a student ready to graduate and benefit from further programming that addresses living arrangements, employment, and social needs and that can be realized in settings ranging from institutions of higher learning to specialized programs that teach advanced skills for successful independent living to permanent structured living arrangements with 24-hour supports.

A radical difference between program planning before the mandated age of 14 and after that age is the introduction of adult service providers as part of the team. Before the age of 14, services are delivered by educators or professionals who are providing a related service. Once transition planning begins, the federal statute requires the school system to identify those adult agencies in the state for whose services the student will be eligible. Furthermore, staff from these agencies should be contacted and invited to the official planning meetings. In the early years of transition planning, it may not be necessary for the adult agency staff to be at the meeting, but early identification of the adult state agency that will follow the school system is essential.

Although special education guidelines are derived from a federal statute (with companion state statutes), most adult services are mandated under state laws and regulations. Families should become familiar with the departments that oversee adult services and learn the departments' criteria for eligibility and the services that they provide (directly or through purchase from a private agency). Families should be aware that through federal legislation and funding each state does have a rehabilitation agency charged with assisting adults with disabilities to become employed (these agencies will go under different names in each state). Representatives of the state rehabilitation agency should be included in transition planning meetings along with staff from other relevant state agencies (the names and types of these agencies will vary from state to state.)

Understanding and negotiating the process of transition planning is a good start, but it does not answer the pivotal question of how one identifies programs that provide the services your son/daughter will need on exiting the school system. It is encouraging that new public and private programs have been developed over the last decade. However, the route to finding appropriate options can be difficult. Unlike the industry that has grown up around finding higher education services (various guides in print or on the Internet), there are no comparable publications or websites that have all the information centralized and categorized for the consumer. Essentially, families are in the position of researching the options that are available through whatever means are possible. School systems, in particular special education departments, may be aware of local programs, but as a rule, school districts do not have the breadth of knowledge regarding postsecondary programs that most families would consider adequate in attempting to identify all of their options.

Resources that can be utilized to identify programs include:

- State agencies for adult services—As noted above, representatives from these agencies should be included in the transition planning meetings mandated by IDEA. However, it is incumbent on families to research further the services for which their son/daughter is eligible and understand thoroughly the process for accessing these services. It is helpful to speak with other families who have navigated the process or professionals who are familiar with it. Even with the best of intentions, bureaucracies are not known for providing the most comprehensive information or for being easy to navigate. Therefore, the experience of a family who came before or a professional conversant with the services can be invaluable.

- There are frequently advocacy groups within a state that also have current information on available services and processes. If you do not know how to reach these associations, it is likely that state chapters can be identified through the national organizations. Most national organizations now have a presence on the Internet, and even if one does not know the organization title, it can be reached through a fairly easy web search using key descriptors. Again, do not overlook other families or professionals who would have this information.

- Families should investigate institutions of higher learning, particularly community colleges, in their search to identify the step that follow high school. These institutions have offices that can assist your son/daughter in discerning whether there is a program at the institution that meets their needs.

- NAPSEC—The National Association of Private Special Education Centers can provide referrals to postsecondary programs notwithstanding its emphasis on special education through the high school years. [They can be reached at 202-408-338; E-mail *napsec@aol.com*.]

- IECA—Independent Educational Consultants Association is an organization of professionals who work with families to identify appropriate programs for individuals. In recent years their familiarity with special education settings, both undergraduate and postsecondary has increased significantly, allowing them to narrow your search to specific programs. More information about IECA can be found at *IECAassoc@aol.com* or *www.IECAonline.com* or by calling 703-591-4850.

There is a significant amount of work involved in identifying the right program and set of services for an individual who is exiting the education system. Although it is fortunate that IDEA has mandates that identify the school's responsibilities in the transition process, it is critical for families to become familiar with all aspects of adult services, including what their son/daughter is eligible for and how to obtain the service. The responsibility of advocating for one's child is never really over, but finding the right setting and program for your son/daughter after they have graduated will allow families to have peace of mind and most importantly will allow the individual to become a contributing member to society and have the opportunity to meet his or her potential.

# ASSISTIVE TECHNOLOGY AND DEVELOPMENTAL DISABILITIES

JOSEPH F. WALLACE, PH.D.

Assistive technology represents an area of increasing importance in the lives of individuals with developmental disabilities. Simply put, assistive technology includes any device, piece of equipment, or service that provides an opportunity for increased independence, academic inclusion, community integration, or employment or just makes life easier. Assistive technology can be something very simple, inexpensive yet practical, such as a wooden backscratcher that allows people with limited reach and hand strength to press an elevator button or drag something on a table top toward them without asking for help. Examples also include more high-tech solutions, for example, a voice output device that assists a person with severe speech difficulties in communicating with others. For persons with developmental disabilities, an assistive technology application might be computer software to assist in visual learning. It could also include traditional pocket organizers that provide memory enhancement for work tasks, schedule reminders, etc. This section will provide an overview of assistive technology and the process for acquiring needed devices and services through the education system and will include examples of real-life solutions for persons with Down syndrome and other developmental disabilities.

*Down Syndrome,* Edited by William I. Cohen, Lynn Nadel, and Myra E. Madnick.
ISBN 0-471-41815-3   Copyright © 2002 by Wiley-Liss, Inc.

## CLARIFYING THE DEFINITION

Many of the legislative origins of assistive technology culminated in the Technology-Related Assistance for Individuals with Disabilities Act of 1988 (PL 100-407). Congress concluded that provision of assistive technology devices and assistive technology services enables some individuals with disabilities to:

1. have greater control over their lives;
2. participate in and contribute more fully to activities in their home, school, and work environments and in their communities;
3. interact to a greater extent with nondisabled individuals; and
4. otherwise benefit from opportunities that are taken for granted by individuals who do not have disabilities (Tech Act of 1988, p. 1044).

Of particular note is that this is the first law to specifically address the technology-related needs of persons with disabilities and, equally important, the charge to state agencies to develop consumer-responsive systems that are directed and influenced by the technology users themselves (Wallace et al., 1995).

In the current version, now formally known as the Assistive Technology Act (PL 105-394), assistive technology devices are defined as:

> any item, piece of equipment or product system, whether acquired commercially off the shelf, modified or customized, that is used to increase, maintain, or improve functional capabilities of an individual with a disability.
>
> [Section 4]

The legal definition of an assistive technology service as stated in the Act is:

> any service that directly assists an individual with a disability in the selection, acquisition or use of an assistive technology device.

Specifically these include:

- The evaluation of the technology needs of the individual, including a functional evaluation of the individual in his or her customary environment;
- Purchasing, leasing ,or otherwise providing for the acquisition of assistive technology devices;
- Selecting, designing, fitting, customizing, adapting, applying, maintaining, repairing, or replacing assistive technology devices;
- Coordinating and using other therapies, interventions, or services with assistive technology devices;

- Training or technical assistance for an individual with a disability or, if appropriate, the individual's family; and

- Training or technical assistance for professionals, employers, or other individuals who provide services to, employ, or otherwise are substantially involved in the major life functions of an individual with a disability [Section 5].

It is important to note that assistive technology devices and those services necessary for their successful acquisition and integration into the individual's life are equally important. A device without the appropriate service supports may lead to unnecessary technology abandonment. Assistive technology is similarly defined in the Developmental Disabilities Act of 2000, the Americans with Disabilities Act, and the amendments to the Individuals with Disabilities Education Act of 1997.

Many misconceptions exist about the nature and application of assistive technology that in some cases, lead to difficulties in acquisition or prevent it from being considered in the first place. The first of these misconceptions is that assistive technology is primarily applicable to individuals with physical and sensory disabilities. Although the benefits to individuals who may have vision, hearing, or mobility deficits may seem obvious, persons with developmental disabilities may also benefit from devices and applications that improve their community integration and approach to learning. These may include accommodations such as time aid devices to assist with time abstraction issues and alternative keyboards to provide support for persons who have fine motor or other mobility difficulties or those with visual issues. There are many other examples which will be discussed later.

Other misconceptions include the fallacy that most assistive technology is of a high-tech nature. The implication is that assistive technology typically is something electronic, such as a computer or specialized software requiring some degree of programming, and of course is expensive in nature. Very often, low-tech solutions can provide an effective technique for overcoming a presenting barrier facing an individual. Simple low-cost electronic organizers demonstrate an affordable approach to assist with scheduling, appointments, medication reminders, etc. These are widely used, fit unobtrusively in a shirt pocket or purse, and provide a dignified and professional alternative for persons to independently make it through their day.

## THE PROCESS FOR ASSISTIVE TECHNOLOGY ACQUISITION

The question is often asked, "How do I go about determining what assistive technology is right for me, and then successfully include it in my life?" The primary steps include evaluation, device and service identification, and funding. The process of acquiring needed assistive technology can be a challenging but necessary experience. As in all experiences no two will be alike, some will be quick and easy, whereas others may be confusing and frustrating. It requires an informed consumer to be resourceful, flexible, and most important, persistent. The following steps are intended to provide both guidance and helpful hints.

## STEP 1: DEFINE THE NEED

Start by being prepared; know what you need and why you need it. This may be initiated through speaking with other consumers with disabilities to see what has worked for them and what they learned from the process. The advice of therapists and other professionals can provide good introductory knowledge from which to proceed.

## STEP 2: DOCUMENT THE NEED

An assistive technology evaluation from a trained professional can be invaluable at this stage. It provides objective proof of the need and recommends devices within the evaluation. An evaluation can be initiated by obtaining a physician's order. Collect all past information that might be of benefit to the evaluation team or professionals to help in documenting the need. The documentation may include input from a combination of professionals, some or all of whom may be willing to provide assistance throughout the request process.

## STEP 3: IDENTIFY THE DEVICE OR SERVICE NEEDED

The evaluation will match your need with a specific device(s) and/or service. It is helpful to include all devices that were used in the evaluation and the benefits or weaknesses of each. Rarely is one device the perfect solution for an individual. Be sure to obtain written prescriptions or recommendations from professionals to substantiate the specific request. Find out prices of the device and service; and who can best provide it. Typically, the evaluator/therapist will provide this. As you look at prices and options, be aware of alternative devices and services that you could use. Knowledge of the alternatives can give you options regarding funding.

Remember, the right technology is crucial if it is to be used successfully after it is acquired.

## STEP 4: DETERMINE WHETHER NO- OR LOW-COST ALTERNATIVES ARE AVAILABLE

Before applying for funding, investigate alternatives and options. For example, would an adaptation suffice or could the device be borrowed from a loan closet or library? Could it be rented or leased first to ensure a successful trial before formal purchase?

Check to see whether the same device or service is available at a lower cost. Also, determine whether private insurance, the school system, rehabilitation agency, or another type of third-party provider will cover the cost.

If there are no alternatives, have the facts well documented to show all options have been explored before applying for funding.

## STEP 5: IDENTIFY APPROPRIATE FUNDING SOURCE(S)

Funding sources are often determined by the age of the individual consumer (school system), level of income, relationship to certain state agencies (aging, rehabilitation, deaf and hard of hearing, visual impairment, etc.). Private or public insurance are considerations but primarily for purchase of medically related equipment, which often excludes assistive technologies such as computers, software, memory devices, etc.

Do not limit your options; keep a list of possible funding sources and decide where to start first. Get as much support and guidance as possible to ensure that all funding options, both public and private, are identified.

## STEP 6: SUBMIT A REQUEST TO THE FUNDING SOURCE

Make contact with the funding source to determine what you need to do to submit a request. It is important to note that there is no single specific method to ensure success. Try to get as much information on the process and required paperwork before submitting the request. Seek out the assistance from a therapist or other professional who has had success in funding assistive technology from this source before.

It helps to find one person in the agency as a contact during the process. As you collect information and prepare the request, call your contact at the agency with questions and concerns. Making sure you have a current and accurate understanding will save time and energy later. Keep a written record of all contacts with the agency.

Complete the application and send in all the needed information with the request, keeping copies of everything that is sent. Do not be surprised if a funding source asks for resubmission with additions and/or changes, particularly on a request for expensive items. Once the request is submitted and has met all the required criteria, the only thing to do is wait.

If notification of approval or denial of a request is not received within the indicated time frame, a courtesy contact to the funding source may be advantageous.

## STEP 7: AUTHORIZATION IS RECEIVED

Hopefully, your request for funding has been approved. Be sure to understand the exact amount of the authorization, along with the terms and processes for obtaining the requested device or service. Know whether the funding source will purchase the device or provide the service directly or make arrangement with the vendor for the device or service.

If the full amount of funding is not approved, go to your list of other options to supplement the amount awarded. Other options to supplement the approved funding may include community civic groups or other philanthropic organizations.

## STEP 8: APPEAL

If your request is denied, make contact with the funding source and be sure why it was denied. If the denial was due to a lack of information or a misunderstanding, appeal the decision. Get information on the appeal process; also determine legal options and processes and know when they may be appropriate to use.

## STEP 9: GO TO YOUR NEXT FUNDING OPTION

Do not give up. If you agree with the denial of your request, go back to Step 4 and continue with the next funding source on your list. The search for funding is not often quick or easy. Investigate and exhaust all possible options for funding.

## ASSISTIVE TECHNOLOGY APPLICATIONS FOR INDIVIDUALS WITH DEVELOPMENTAL DISABILITIES

Assistive technology holds great potential for individuals with developmental disabilities, but all too often the choices and options are not generally familiar to parents, professionals, and the individual consumers themselves. When considering areas of need such as learning development, speech improvement, mobility enhancement, etc. it is important to consult with assistive technology providers who possess expertise in the particular area of concern. The Rehabilitation Engineering and Assistive Technology Society of North America (RESNA) serves as a technical assistance provider and clearinghouse for information at a state level for this very purpose (*www.resna.org*).

Table 28.1 provides a variety of examples of assistive technology solutions that may assist in initiating an individual with a developmental disability across a variety of performance areas. This is by no means a complete list and is intended to provide some basic direction from which to explore further.

TABLE 28.1. ASSISTIVE TECHNOLOGY DEVICES HELPFUL TO INDIVIDUALS WITH
DEVELOPMENTAL DISABILITIES

Writing
Adaptive pencil/pen grips
Electronic speller, dictionary, or thesaurus
(Franklin Speller, American Heritage Talking Dictionary)
Typewriter
Portable word processor        (AlphaSmart, Braille 'n Speak)
Software standard to the computer
      (Easy Access, Accessibility Options, Close View)
Word prediction/Abbreviation Expansion
      (Co:Writer, Abbreviate!)
Grammar checker
Mapping/Outlining       (Inspiration, Writer's Blocks)
Talking word processor       (Write OutLoud, IntelliTalk)

Reading
Books-on-Tape
Scanner
OCR       (OpenBook, TextHELP)

Math
Calculator
Software       (MathPad, Blocks-In-Motion, Big Calc)

Communication
Communication books
Communication boards
Communication vests
Communication indicators       (All-Turn-It, ScanLite)
Single-message output       (BigMack, Talking Frame)
Multi-message output       (CheapTalk, AlphaTalker, Dynavox)
Language software       (First Words, Teach Me To Talk)

Sports, Recreation, and Leisure
Modified crayons, brushes, or markers
Adapted TV remote control
Computer games

Specialized Computer Equipment
Keyguard
Moisture guard
Trackball/Trackpad
Expanded keyboard       (Flexiboard, IntelliKeys, BigKeys)
Touch Screen

Additional Equipment, Materials, and Software
Single-switch       (RadSounds, UKanDu series, MultiScan)
Special Needs Software       (Sentence Master, I Can Read)
Tactile cues       (texture labels, foam, sandpaper)

**Teacher/Parent Tools**
Productivity software       (BoardMaker, OverlayMaker)
Lesson makers       (IntelliPics, Clicker4)
Authoring tools       (HyperStudio, AuthorWare)
Prompting devices       (TimePad)

George, 2001

## FEDERAL AND STATE LEGISLATION THAT SUPPORTS ASSISTIVE TECHNOLOGY ACQUISITION

### THE INDIVIDUALS WITH DISABILITIES EDUCATION ACT

The Individuals with Disabilities Education Act (IDEA) (PL 105-17) is a federal law that requires states to ensure that children with disabilities between the ages of 3 and 21 receive a free and appropriate education (FAPE). The law mandates a free and appropriate public education for those children receiving special education. The law provides procedural safeguards that include mediation and due process protections to ensure that students with disabilities receive the special education and related services, including assistive technology devices and services they require to benefit from their special education program.

### EARLY INTERVENTION SERVICES: PART C OF THE IDEA

Part C, formerly Part H, was added to IDEA in 1986 to expand access to early intervention/family services for children with disabilities from birth to 3 years of age. Children 3 and older are served under Part B of IDEA. Part C was designed to provide coordinated service delivery to infants, toddlers, and their families and to fill gaps in existing services as needed.

Services available to children under Part C as "early intervention services" are varied and include, among others, special instruction, physical therapy, nutrition services, audiology, nursing services, physical therapy, speech-language pathology, family training, counseling and home visits, vision services, and assistive technology. However, Part C programs are payors of last resort—meaning that Part C will only fund devices and services if the family has exhausted all other possible sources of funding including Medicaid and private insurance. Service coordinators assist families in identifying and pursuing such funding sources.

Many infants and toddlers can benefit from assistive technology to develop communication, perceptual and fine motor skills, as well as improved mobility. Assessments are critical in selecting appropriate technology and should be conducted by qualified professionals as part of a developmental assessment team. It is particularly important to recognize that infants and young children are developing quickly and their needs may change rapidly. Assessments should be considered an ongoing process. The assistive technology assessment should consider the following:

- Developmental needs and functioning of the child
- Equipment and device options
- Needs of family and the child

- Use of equipment
- Proper prescription for a device
- Current needs
- Use of loan equipment

## Primary and Secondary Public Schools

Children who qualify for special education services under the Individuals with Disabilities Education Act (IDEA) are entitled to receive assistive technology as needed to ensure that they are receiving a "free and appropriate public education" (FAPE). Children with disabilities also have rights that are defined by Section 504 of the Rehabilitation Act of 1973, Title II, of the Americans with Disabilities Act (ADA). These nondiscrimination laws require schools to accommodate the needs of children with disabilities (including those who do not qualify for IDEA) to provide, to the extent possible, an equal opportunity to enjoy the educational benefits offered by their district.

Although both IDEA and the nondiscrimination laws require schools to provide this technology for children with disabilities, there is an important difference between them. Under IDEA, the state provides schools with extra funding for each child designated as receiving special education services. A small percentage of this funding comes from the federal government; the rest comes from the state general fund. Under the nondiscrimination laws, schools do not receive any special funding or reimbursement for expenses incurred in accommodating children with disabilities. Funding for such accommodations comes from the school's "general" fund. Although this funding difference does not impact a child's legal rights in any way, it may be easier for a child to obtain assistive technology if he or she is requesting it under IDEA rather than the civil rights statutes.

## The Americans with Disabilities Act

The Americans with Disabilities Act (ADA) of 1990 is a nondiscrimination statute. Under Title II of the Act, public entities must provide program access in an integrated setting (unless separate programs are necessary to ensure equal benefits or services). The ADA provides direct references to assistive technology within each of the four titles of the Act. The ADA extends federal civil rights to protect people with disabilities from discrimination in the workplace and to provide them with equal access in many other areas. This Act requires employers who receive federal funding to provide "reasonable accommodation" to people with disabilities to enable them to perform work for which they are qualified. In Titles I and III, the purchase and modification of equipment is included in the definition of "reasonable accommodation." The ADA is considered a civil rights bill rather than a funding bill that attempts to promote the integration of assistive technology as a civil right for all persons with disabilities.

In the context of public education, the ADA requires schools to make their programs and services accessible to children with disabilities within the context of the legal requirements relative to "reasonable accommodation" and "undue burden." The school may employ assistive technology or various other means to make the necessary accommodations, but there are limitations. School districts are not required, under the ADA, to take actions that would cause "fundamental alteration of the nature of the program or activity or undue financial or administrative burdens. However, public entities must [still] ensure that individuals with disabilities receive access to the same benefits and services offered to others without disabilities."

## SECTION 504 OF THE REHABILITATION ACT

Specifically, Section 504 of the Rehabilitation Act of 1973, as amended in 1992 (P.L. 102-569) states that,

> No otherwise qualified disabled individual shall, solely by reason of his disability, be excluded from the participation in, be denied the benefits of, or be subjected to discrimination under any program or activity receiving federal financial assistance.

This statute includes all entities that receive federal funds, and the protections in Section 504 can be used to support the legal right to assistive technology across all of those environments. It is appropriate in the school setting, for example, if the technology is needed to ensure equal access to the school program. For students with disabilities, this means that schools may need to make special arrangements so that these students have access to the full range of programs and activities offered. Other modifications that might be required under Section 504 include installing ramps into buildings and modifying bathrooms to provide access for individuals with physical disabilities. Section 504 does not provide individual funding. It is a civil rights statute that requires equal access and equal opportunity to persons with disabilities.

### REFERENCES

Americans with Disabilities Act (ADA) of 1990, PL 101-336. (July 26, 1990). Title 42, U.S.C. 12101 et seq: U.S. Statutes at Large, 104, 327–378.

Assistive Technology Act of 1998, PL 105-394. (October 9, 1998). Title 29, U.S.C. 2201 et seq: U.S. Statutes at Large, 102, 1044–1065.

George C (2001): Assistive Technology Devices Helpful to Individuals with Developmental Disabilities. Kellar Institute for Human disAbilities, George Mason University.

Rehabilitation Act Amendments of 1992 P.L. 102-569. (October 29, 1992). Title 29, U.S.C. 701 et seq: U.S. Statutes at Large, 100, 1807–1846.

Technology-Related Assistance for Individuals with Disabilities Act of 1998, PL 100-407. (August 19, 1988). Title 29, U.S.C. 2201 et seq: U.S. Statutes at Large, 102, 744–765.

Technology-Related Assistance for Individuals with Disabilities Act of 1988, PL 100-407. (August 19, 1988). Title 29, U.S.C. 2201 et seq: U.S. Statutes at Large, 108, 50–97.

Wallace J, Flippo K, Barcus M, Behrmann M (1995): Legislative foundations of assistive technology policy in the United States. In: Flippo K, Inge K, Barcus M (eds.), Assistive technology: A Resource for School, Work, and Community. Baltimore, MD: Brookes Publishing.

# COMMUNICATION, MATH, AND LANGUAGE SKILLS

# STARTING OUT: SPEECH AND LANGUAGE INTERVENTION FOR INFANTS AND TODDLERS WITH DOWN SYNDROME

## LIBBY KUMIN, PH.D., CCC-SLP

Infants with Down syndrome are ready to communicate, but they can't use speech yet. So they communicate first by crying, then by smiling and laughing. It's a long journey from crying to speaking, and there are many milestones and many skills to be mastered. Although some early intervention programs include speech and language services, many early intervention programs do not provide speech and language services until a specific age (1, 2, or 3 years) or until the child is speaking. There are communication, sensory, and motor developmental skills that contribute to readiness for language and speech that can be targeted in early intervention programs.

The broadest system for interaction between people is communication. When we think of adults communicating with each other, we generally think about speech. But adults also use many gestures, facial expressions, body postures, and emotions in their voice. In fact, researchers have found that in most daily interactions, the nonverbal (such as a scowl or a smile) and vocal (such as anger in the voice) carry the meaning of the message more than the words themselves.

Communication is holistic. It includes not only what is said, but also

*Down Syndrome,* Edited by William I. Cohen, Lynn Nadel, and Myra E. Madnick.
ISBN 0-471-41815-3   Copyright © 2002 by Wiley-Liss, Inc.

how it is said. Communication includes how close I stand to you, whether I shrug my shoulders, whether I look confident or defeated, how my voice sounds, whether I am smiling, smirking, or scowling. Communication may be unintentional, or it may be planned and intentional. On a day when you are about to come down with the flu, you may unintentionally communicate that you don't feel well by your demeanor. For a business interview, or at a major social event, people communicate intentionally. They think about the messages that they want to send and intentionally tailor clothes, shoes, hairstyles, accessories, speech (formal or informal), and presentation to send that message.

Language is less holistic and more specific than communication. Language is a structured system of symbols that catalogs the objects, relations, and events within a culture. It is a shared code that is understood by the members of a language community and that infants learn within that language community. Infants and toddlers learn language through social interaction, and we must *learn* language, because language is an arbitrary code. Why do we call a table a table and a desk a desk? There is no intrinsic "tableness" to a table. We call it a table, because that is what we have been taught and because everyone in our language community understands what we mean when we say "table." Americans use the term "pen," while the French use the term "plume." Words such as "sandwich" and color names such as "green" are arbitrary symbols. Because they represent a specific object or a specific color, we must use those words to be understood. Language may include various types of structured systems, including speech, signs, gestures, and pictures, computer-generated speech or symbols, or writing.

Speech is verbal language. Speech is the process of producing voice and making sounds and combining them into words to communicate. Speaking is an overlaid or secondary function of the same structures used for breathing, swallowing, and feeding. Speech involves strength, coordination, and timing of precise muscle movements. It is the most neurologically and physiologically complex of the communication systems.

When we compare speech, language, and communication, speech is by far the most difficult for children with Down syndrome to use. Children with Down syndrome understand the concepts of communication and language very well and have the desire to communicate at an early age. Most children with Down syndrome are capable of communicating and of using language many months before they are able to use speech. Most children with Down syndrome will, however, progress to using speech as their primary communication system. The basis for communication is the desire and the ability to communicate and to interact with other people. Infants with Down syndrome exhibit the desire and the capability to communicate at an early age. There are many communication skills that they can learn at an early age to prepare them to speak.

## COMMUNICATIVE INTENT

Communicative intent is the knowledge and understanding that you can influence your environment and get results by communicating, for example, if you cry, someone will come to help you; if you make sounds, you will attract attention from those around you. It is the most important single foundation skill for later language and speech. The primary way to help children develop communicative intent is by being responsive. Interpret the infant's behaviors as communicative. If the child kicks her feet, assume that it is a communication and respond by playing a game with her toes, or put a balloon near her feet so that she can kick. If the child points to a ball, give him the ball and label it as "ball." Interpret looking, kicking, making noises, and pointing as the child's desire to communicate with you and show the child by your actions not only that his communication is received, but also that his communication brings results. That's very powerful—that's why we all communicate!

## TURN-TAKING

All two-way communication depends on turn-taking; on the fact that there is a speaker and a listener and that they change roles. The way to foster development of this skill is to create and model turn-taking opportunities. When the baby makes sounds, imitate his sounds. These may be screeching or cooing sounds or any other sounds and probably won't be recognizable speech sounds or words until much later. Then wait and allow your child time to take his turn, that is, to make more sounds. If he happens to tap on his highchair or the side of the crib, you tap on the side of the crib, then wait and give him a turn to tap again. With one- to two-year-olds, you might tap on a xylophone and then hand the child a wand to take a turn. You might ring a bell or shake a rattle. You might roll a ball back and forth between you. Many infant games such as Peek-a-Boo and Pat-a-Cake foster turn taking (Kumin, 1994). With an older child, you might blow bubbles or play a game in which there are turns such as Candyland or Go Fish. It is beneficial to mark the turns—baby's turn or Sheila's turn, mommy's turn or daddy's turn. Use hand over hand assistance to help the child go through the actions until he can independently take his turn.

## REQUESTING/PROTESTING

At any specific moment, a baby may have different reasons for communicating. The most common reason is to request something. He may be crying to request his bottle or to refuse a bottle, or he may reach toward you because he wants you to continue making that funny face. She may pick up her hands high over her head because she wants to be picked up out of the crib, or she may coo and gurgle because she is satisfied and warm and dry after finishing her bottle and being changed.

How does a baby protest? Does she cry or flail her body and try to push something away? Why does she protest? Does she prefer warmth, and push away things that are cold? Does she protest at bath time? One of the things that we are looking for is whether certain sensory messages are uncomfortable. It is possible that she is having difficulty with processing some types of sensation, and that can be worked on through sensory integration therapy. Protesting empowers the child. Responding to the baby's protests helps foster communicative intent.

## SOCIAL COMMUNICATION

Infants and toddlers with Down syndrome are socially responsive (Roizen, 2001). Most early communication attempts are nonverbal and interactive; they are either facial expressions and body movements such as smiling or pointing or sounds such as cooing, laughing, crying, or grunting. Early social communication usually consists of gestures and body movements that are used to interact with others. Waving hello and bye-bye, blowing kisses, and shaking your head *yes* and *no* are examples of social communication. The exciting part for the child is that these communication attempts are easily understood by most people. So, when the child waves bye-bye, he gets an enthusiastic response from all those around him.

## PREREQUISITE SKILLS FOR LANGUAGE

The prerequisite skills for language are *visual skills, auditory skills, tactile skills, imitation skills, motor skills, cognitive skills,* and *referential knowledge.* According to research, there is an organized hierarchy of sensory integration levels. The child progresses from tactile skills to visual skills, then to auditory skills, and only then is ready to master language and cognitive skills (Ayres, 1980).

Tactile, visual, and auditory skills help us along the pathway to speech and language (Ayres and Mailloux, 1981). They help us learn sounds and words and enable us to set up feedback loops between the eyes, ears, mouth, lips, tongue, and jaw and the brain. Once these feedback loops are established, we can feel if speech sounds and words look right, sound right, and feel right to us.

## Attentional Skills

Attention means being able to focus in on a person, object, or event. In infants, we observe this skill early as the infant focuses in on his parent's face and as he listens attentively to sounds in his environment (Kumin, 1994).

## Visual Skills

The visual skills on which language learning is built are visual reception, reciprocal gaze, attending, visual tracking, and referential gaze (Kumin, 1994).

Visual Reception.    Visual reception is the ability to use the sense of vision, that is, a combination of sight and the ability to understand what you see. Physicians recommend early vision examination by a pediatrician or ophthalmologist to check for vision problems (Cohen et al., 1999, Roizen et al., 1992).

Reciprocal Gaze.    Reciprocal gaze is eye contact; I look at you and you look at me. Because of low muscle tone and visual difficulties, it may be necessary to provide more support for the child's head and neck and to compensate for any visual problems. Children with Down syndrome are successful at learning reciprocal gaze. This skill is the basis for learning speech and language by observation and watching, as well as for eye contact in later conversation.

Attending.    For learning language concepts, the child needs to be able to visually attend to an object—to look at it for a prolonged period of time. So once the child can look at you, look at an object, and follow a moving object, you want to keep him looking and prolong the time that he looks at an object.

Visual Tracking.    This skill is sometimes called visual pursuit. It is the ability to follow an object as it moves and to track it with your eyes. It is a skill that helps the infant learn about the world around her.

Referential Gaze.    Referential gaze means that the baby focuses in on an object. In the beginning, the baby may simply look at the object. Responding to the child's lead, you can then label the object. In the second phase, shared gaze, the baby follows another person's line of gaze, and pays attention to whatever that person is looking at. Other terms used to describe this skill are *joint gaze, shared focus, joint attention,* and *visual regard*. Referential gaze is the basis for learning the names of objects. When a child can focus on an object, can explore the object, and has mastered object permanence (this object is a "thing"), he or she is ready to learn the word for the object.

## AUDITORY SKILLS

The auditory skills that are prerequisites to language are auditory reception, auditory attending, increasing the time that the child attends to sound, sound localization, and auditory integration.

AUDITORY RECEPTION.    Children with Down syndrome are at increased risk for hearing loss. It is essential to have the pediatrician and the audiologist monitor hearing on a regular basis and treat any hearing problems (Cohen et al., 1999, Roizen et al., 1994, Shott, 2000). Some kinds of tests can be used to test infants within the first week of life. Otitis media with effusion (OME), inflammation of the middle ear with fluid buildup behind the eardrum, is the most common problem related to hearing. The fluid interferes with sound transmission, and the result is a conductive hearing loss that is fluctuating. It is difficult for infants and toddlers to learn to listen and to attend to sounds when they sometimes can hear the sounds and other times cannot (Roberts and Medley, 1995).

AUDITORY ATTENDING AND INCREASING AUDITORY ATTENDING TIME. When it is confirmed that a child is able to hear environmental and speech sounds, practice in listening or "attending" to sounds can begin. Music and tapes of familiar sounds, See 'n'Say toys and other musical toys, and musical games with hand movements are helpful. The goal is to lengthen the time that the child attends to sounds.

SOUND LOCALIZATION.    Sound localization is the ability to turn toward a sound source when you hear the sound, that is, to locate the sound source. This skill can be taught, as long as the child has adequate hearing. A good technique to help a child learn to localize is to sit in a swivel chair. Have a friend or sibling ring a bell, or start an audiotape out of the child's view. Say, "Do you hear that bell?" Then, swivel the chair, and look directly at the source of the sound. "There's the bell." Then have the person ring the bell again within the child's sight to reinforce the connection between the bell and the sound. Practice sound localization for short periods many times during the day (Kumin, 1994).

AUDITORY INTEGRATION.    Auditory integration is the ability to organize and interpret auditory stimuli including sounds, speech, and music. Some children with Down syndrome have difficulty with auditory integration; others do not. The difficulty may be seen in a variety of situations including difficulty tolerating loud sounds, difficulty focusing on more than one speaker at a time, and difficulty listening to a conversation when there is background noise.

## TACTILE SKILLS

The sense of touch is very important to infants. It not only helps them establish attachments to people and objects, but also provides a means for exploring their world. The infant has many more nerve endings in the oral area than in the fingers, so it makes sense that the infant explores objects with his mouth. As the infant explores, he sets up feedback loops that help him integrate information about the objects he is touching. Young children may enjoy exploring texture or may be very sensitive to touch and not want to touch or be touched (this is known as tactile defensiveness).Tactile skills can be worked on in early intervention through sensory integration therapy (Ayres, 1984).

## IMITATION SKILLS AND MOTOR SKILLS

There are many opportunities to teach and practice imitation, and imitation is a skill basic to learning speech sounds and words. Practice should begin with motor imitation and progress to body imitation, oral motor imitation, and imitation of speech sounds.

## COGNITIVE SKILLS

The cognitive skills that are basic to language development are *object permanence, cause and effect,* and *means-end knowledge.*

OBJECT PERMANENCE. This is the understanding that an object still exists even though it cannot be seen. We know that a child understands object permanence when a child searches for a hidden toy or when he throws toys over the side of the highchair and then looks for them. This is an important precursor to labeling with speech or signs, because if you do not have the concept that objects have permanence, labeling objects does not make sense.

CAUSE AND EFFECT. Cause and effect is learning that every action has a result or consequence. Children who are learning about cause and effect love to turn light switches on and off and watch the instant result. This is a skill that is closely related to communicative intent (Kumin, 1994).

MEANS-END. Means-end is the understanding that a plan of action is needed to accomplish a goal. For example, if a beach ball is in front of the television, it needs to be pushed away in order to see the television. Creating sentences (an expressive language skill) and certain strategies for communication are based on this cognitive skill.

REFERENTIAL KNOWLEDGE.   Referential knowledge is the ability to make the connection between the object and the linguistic label, that is, between the ball and the word *ball*. Visual skills such as referential gaze and cognitive skills such as object permanence are the basis for this ability.

## PREREQUISITE SKILLS FOR SPEECH

Prerequisite skills for speech include respiratory skills, feeding skills, tactile skills, imitation skills, oral motor skills, motor planning skills, and sound production skills. Speech is a secondary function overlaid on the structures and movements used for breathing and feeding.

### RESPIRATORY SKILLS

When we breathe, we inhale and exhale, but speech is spoken on exhalation only. When we are speaking, we need to use about 90% exhalation and only 10% inhalation. Crying and babbling, as well as breathing exercises give the infant practice in prolonging exhalation.

### FEEDING SKILLS

Feeding uses many of the same structures and movements that are used for speaking, although the neural substrates for feeding and speech are different. Feeding gives the child practice in muscle movement and coordination. Children with Down syndrome may have difficulty with feeding because of low muscle tone, inability to form a seal with the lips, difficulties with jaw or tongue control, and increased tactile sensitivity or tactile defensiveness (Kumin and Bahr, 1999). Speech-language pathologists or occupational therapists can work on feeding as part of the child's early intervention program.

### TACTILE SKILLS

Exploring toys with the mouth provides feedback information so that the child develops the feel of the tongue, lips, and jaw moving. Massage and brushing the teeth and gums with a toothette or a soft toothbrush can help the child explore different feelings of touch. The goal is to stimulate placement of the tongue and lips, as well as develop feedback loops.

### IMITATION SKILLS

Early imitation is usually motor imitation, such as banging a xylophone or moving a toy car. The goal of imitation for speech is to help the child move from motor imitation to sound imitation.

## Oral Motor Skills

Central hypotonia is common in infants and young children with Down syndrome (Roizen, in press). Many of the difficulties seen in speech intelligibility are due to low muscle tone and weak lip, tongue, and palate muscles. The goal is to help the child improve muscle strength and control in the oral area. This can be done with stimulation and with imitation. Nuk exercisers may be used. Using a mirror to provide visual feedback is very effective.

## Motor Planning Skills

When the child practices oral movements, and sets up feedback loops for how movements feel, templates are developed in the brain that help the movements become almost automatic. This practice is helpful for all children with Down syndrome. Some children have difficulty with motor planning for speech, known as verbal dyspraxia, which will not be evident until later in development.

## Sound Production Skills

The first sound that the infant makes is usually a crying sound. As the child develops, he will begin to make a wider array of sounds. Laughing, grunting, cooing, popping, screeching, and raspberry sounds are early sound productions. When the child begins to produce strings of sounds, for example, babababa, mamamama, this is known as babbling. In early babbling the child appears to like the feel of the sounds, whereas in later babbling the child begins to narrow her sound production to the sounds of her native language. As the child progresses, she will begin to have what sounds like mini-conversations using jargon. This demonstrates understanding of the rhythm and inflection of the language; she knows the song of the language, but still has to learn the words. The child will also begin to imitate and echo words. This is the final prespeech stage. It means that the child is almost ready to begin to use spoken words.

## Transitional Communication Systems

The child with Down syndrome is ready to communicate well before he or she is able to speak. Some children have mastered all of the pragmatic and language prerequisites and are ready to use language to communicate 2–3 years before they are ready and able to use speech. Speech is the most complex communication system because it relies on muscle strength and coordination and accurate movement of the articulators. Transitional communication systems enable the child to communicate before he is able to use

TABLE 29.I. EARLY INTERVENTION SPEECH AND LANGUAGE PROGRAM

### I. Pragmatic/Language Level
A. Communicative intent _____

B. Turn-taking _____

C. Engaging _____

D. Requesting _____

E. Protesting _____

F. Social communication _____

### II. Sensory Input/Integration Skills
A. Visual skills _____

B. Auditory skills _____

C. Tactile skills _____

D. Imitation skills _____

E. Motor skills _____

### III. Cognitive/Linguistic Skills
A. Object permanence _____

B. Cause and effect _____

C. Referential knowledge _____

### IV. Prespeech Skills
A. Respiration _____

B. Feeding skills _____

C. Tactile skills _____

D. Imitation skills _____

E. Oral motor skills _____

F. Motor planning skills _____

G. Sound production skills _____

### V. Transitional System/Assistive Technology Needs
A. Sign language _____

B. Communication board _____

C. High-tech communication system _____

D. Assistive listening devices _____

E. Other _____

### VI. Referrals Needed

| | | | |
|---|---|---|---|
| Ophthalmologist | _____ | Otolaryngologist | _____ |
| Feeding Specialist | _____ | Audiologist | _____ |
| Sens. Integration Spc | _____ | Psychologist | _____ |
| Special Educator | _____ | Occup. Therapist | _____ |
| Pediatrician | | Neurologist | _____ |
| Physical Therapist | _____ | Other | _____ |

speech. It cuts down on frustration and allows the child to continue to make progress in vocabulary development and other areas of language when he is not yet physiologically and developmentally ready to use speech (Kumin, 1994). The most frequently used transition system is Total Communication, in which speech and sign are used simultaneously by the adult communication partner, while the child uses sign language to communicate. Signed Exact English, a language in which the signs are basically a translation of English, and American Sign Language, which has its own grammar and word order, are the most frequently used language systems. Communication boards with pictures, words, or symbols may also be used. For children who have much to communicate but have difficulty learning sign language, a computer-based communication system that uses synthesized speech can be used. These transitional communication systems are not mutually exclusive. The child might be using signs for "juice" but also use magnets with pictures of apple and grape juice on the refrigerator door to indicate which juice he wants.

It is important that, whatever transition system is used, the language concepts taught are those that are meaningful for the child, that is, those messages that he really wants to communicate. The system must be functional for the child to get his needs met and make his wants known. In this way, the transition communication system greatly diminishes the frustration felt by a child who cannot communicate with his environment. Research has shown that using sign language helps the child's vocabulary grow, and helps language develop (Acredolo and Goodwyn, 1996). Children with Down syndrome as young as 8–12 months can effectively learn signs and use sign language.

## Conclusion

The early intervention program can teach the prerequisite skills for language and speech. A checklist of skills that can be included in early intervention for speech and language can be found in Table 29.1. Early intervention can help the child develop sensory input skills, associative skills, and oral motor output skills that will form the basis for speech and the cognitive and experiential learning skills that will form the basis for language.

## References and Resources

Communicating Together Newsletter/Workshops, P.O. Box 6395, Columbia, MD, 21045-6395; phone: 410-995-0722 subscription newsletter for parents and professionals devoted to speech and language in children with Down syndrome and information on workshops for parents and professionals.

Acredolo L, Goodwyn S (1996): Baby Signs. Chicago, IL: Contemporary Books.

Ayres A J (1980): Sensory Integration and the Child. Los Angeles, CA: Western Psychological Publishers.

Ayres J, Mailloux Z (1981): Influence of sensory integration procedures on language development. Am J Occup Ther 35:383–390.

Cohen W et al. (1999): Health Care Guidelines for Individuals with Down Syndrome (Down syndrome preventive medical check list). Down Syndrome Medical Interest Group. Down Syndrome Q 4:1–26.

Kumin L (1994): Communication Skills in Children with Down Syndrome—A Guide for Parents. Bethesda, MD: Woodbine House (1-800-843-7323).

Kumin L (1999): Comprehensive speech and language treatment for infants, toddlers, and children with Down syndrome. In: Hassold TJ, Patterson D (eds.), Down Syndrome: A Promising Future, Together. New York: Wiley-Liss, pp 145–153.

Kumin L, Bahr DC (1999): Patterns of feeding, eating, and drinking in young children with Down syndrome with oral motor concerns. Down Syndrome Q 4:1–8.

Kumin L, Goodman MS, Councill C (1991): Comprehensive communication intervention for infants and toddlers with Down syndrome. Infant-Toddler Intervention 1:275–296.

Roberts JE, Medley L (1995): Otitis media and speech-language sequelae in young children: Current issues in management. Am J Speech-Language Pathol: J Clin Pract 4:15–24.

Roizen NJ (in press): Down syndrome. In: Batshaw ML (ed.), Children with Disabilities (5th ed.). Baltimore, MD: Paul H. Brookes Publishers. Note: Book is not yet paginated.

Roizen NJ, Mets MB, Blondis TA (1994): Ophthalmic disorders in children with Down syndrome. Dev Med Child Neurol 36:594–600.

Roizen NJ, Wolters C, Nicol T, Blondis T (1992): Hearing loss in children with Down syndrome. Pediatrics 123:S9–S12.

Shott SR (2000). Down syndrome: Common pediatric ear, nose, and throat problems. Down Syndrome Q 5:1–6.

# Maximizing Speech and Language in Children and Adolescents with Down Syndrome

## Libby Kumin, Ph.D., CCC-SLP

Children and adolescents with Down syndrome are at high risk for speech and language difficulties based on anatomic, physiological, and cognitive factors (Kumin, 1994, 1999). There is a high incidence of speech and language problems, particularly in the areas of intelligibility of speech and conversational skills. Speech is an overlaid function on the same structures and movements used for the biological functions of respiration, self-regulation, and feeding. Speech is an output system, dependent on well-functioning sensory input systems such as hearing, vision, and touch. Even before the child is speaking, it is possible to work in early intervention on oral motor skills, sensory input and integration skills, and cognitive skills that provide the foundation for speech and language development. As the young child begins to process information from his environment, there are many techniques that can be used in treatment and at home to facilitate speech and language development. In the preschool years, the focus should be on learning concepts and on expanding vocabulary and social interactive language skills. In children of school age, there is an opportunity to focus on school-based language so that children can make progress in school subjects. In adolescence, there is a need to plan for transitioning into the world of work (Kumin,

*Down Syndrome*, Edited by William I. Cohen, Lynn Nadel, and Myra E. Madnick.
ISBN 0-471-41815-3    Copyright © 2002 by Wiley-Liss, Inc.

1999). At all stages, there is a need to be proactive in evaluating and treating communication difficulties.

What is an effective speech and language treatment program? A program is effective if it is meeting an individual's needs and helping that person reach his or her goals. Although all treatment plans must be individualized, there are some general concepts that underlie effective speech and language treatment programs.

1. Families and professionals must be partners in speech and language treatment.

Communication is an activity of daily living. Speech, language, and communication are best learned and practiced in daily life. But there are specialized methods for teaching children with Down syndrome to speak. Through a family-centered comprehensive speech and language treatment program, families are taught the tools that they need to help their child (Kumin et al., 1996) Families have many opportunities to observe their child's communication difficulties. Families can provide feedback relating to the child's interests and activities and can help prioritize the communication goals that will have maximum impact on the child's daily life. Speech and language treatment is only valuable if the skills learned carry over into real-life use, into the classroom, the home, and the community. Families, teachers, and friends can provide the support for the child to ensure that there is practice in real life. They can provide ongoing feedback so that the speech language pathologist knows whether the treatment methods are effective or need to be modified.

2. Comprehensive evaluation leads to an individualized comprehensive treatment plan.

Speech and language treatment must be individualized. There is no one pattern of speech and language characteristics or development for children with Down syndrome. For example, children with Down syndrome have been reported to say their first words from 9 months to 11 years of age, and combining two words has been reported from 18 months to 12 years. A detailed profile of the communication strengths and challenges for an individual child at a particular time leads to the development of an appropriate treatment plan. If the child is in an ongoing treatment program, subsequent evaluation can occur, as diagnostic therapy, on a continuing basis. If the child is not enrolled in treatment, speech, language, and oral motor progress should be monitored on an annual basis.

3. All children and adolescents need systems that will enable them to communicate effectively throughout life.

For most children with Down syndrome, speech will be their primary communication system. But a child with Down syndrome may not be developmentally ready to speak until ages 2–4 or even older. Until the time he is able to use speech, he needs a system that will enable him to communicate with his environment (Kumin, 1994). That might be sign language or a communication board or a computer-based language system. For the older child or adolescent who is very difficult to understand, a communication system to assist speech intelligibility or to substitute for speech may be needed. This is known as augmentative or alternative communication (AAC). At different times in the life cycle, an individual may need to supplement speech to aid understanding.

4. There is a basic relationship among input-association-output systems.

Speech and language development is based on hearing language in the environment. Sensory inputs from auditory, visual, tactile, kinesthetic, and proprioceptive systems enable infants and toddlers to learn about the objects and people in their environment. The associative areas of the brain enable infants to make sense out of what they see and hear in the environment and to connect sounds and symbols with people, objects, and events.

Speech is an output system that is based on sensory input, tactile input, oral motor muscle strength, precision and coordination, and associations between symbols and referents that form the basis for language. Children who have difficulty with being touched around the mouth or on the tongue, or who have difficulty with suck-swallow-breath coordination or with chewing different food textures are at high risk for having difficulty developing the sensory, tactile, and motor bases for speech (Kumin and Bahr, 1999). When these difficulties are addressed early through feeding therapy or sensory integration therapy, there is a positive benefit for speech development. For speech, the output system, to function well, hearing, vision, and touch must function well.

5. There is no one pattern of communication strengths and weaknesses for children with Down syndrome.

Some children have more difficulty with sound discrimination and phonological awareness. Others have difficulty with motor planning for speech. Some children have hypernasality, while others do not. Some older children and adolescents develop stuttering problems, while others do not. Although many children have problems in speech intelligibility, the factors contributing to the difficulties in being understood vary from child to child. Some children speak in single words, whereas other children have long conversations.

The most common risk factors that we see in infants and toddlers with Down syndrome that directly influence speech and language development are low muscle tone in the oral motor area, including the lips, tongue, and jaw (Kumin and Bahr, 1999), relative macroglossia (Desai, 1997), and otitis media with effusion (Roizen et al., 1992) resulting in fluctuating hearing loss. Because there is no one communication profile, there is no one treatment plan. Treatment should be individually designed to meet all of the communication needs of the child.

> 6. Most children with Down syndrome have more advanced receptive language skills than expressive language skills. Expressive language and speech problems lead many professionals to underestimate the intelligence and capabilities of children and adolescents with Down syndrome.

Children with Down syndrome have more difficulty with speech and language development than they experience in other areas of early development (Miller, 1988). Speech and expressive language are more involved than receptive language skills (Miller et al., 1999). At all ages, children with Down syndrome understand more than they can say. They learn through the visual channel more easily than through the auditory channel (Buckley, 1996), so reading will often be easier than listening. Reading instructions may be easier than following oral instructions in class.

When we compare an individual child's skills across linguistic areas, namely, phonology, semantics, morphosyntax, and pragmatics, it is rare for the child to be functioning at the same level in all four linguistic areas. Typically, the child with Down syndrome is more advanced in vocabulary (semantics) (Miller, 1988, Kumin et al., 1998) and social interactive language skills (pragmatics) and has more difficulty with phonology (the sound system) and morphosyntax (grammar, structure, word endings, etc.) (Fowler, 1995). Reading and writing (via word processors) may be easier for the child than speaking and may serve as pathways to improve overall language and communication skills (Buckley, 1996).

Expressive language and intelligibility problems lead professionals to underestimate intelligence and capabilities. When you ask a child a question, and he or she does not respond with a clearly framed, grammatically correct, well-articulated response, it is easy to assume that the child is not able. When children have open mouth posture, drooling, and low muscle tone in their lips, tongue, and cheeks, with subsequent difficulties in intelligibility, it is easy to underestimate their abilities. The danger is that the child will not be provided with opportunities that will help him reach his potential. Look beyond the speech abilities. Parents can request that their child be given a speech and language battery and a nonverbal intelligence test to separate out expressive language abilities from intelligence level.

7. Legislation and the educational model form the major basis for service delivery. An educational model addresses only part of the communication difficulties.

Legislation beginning with Public Law 94-142 and continuing through the current Public Law 105-17, IDEA 97, has resulted in funding sources for special education and speech-language pathology services through the local educational agency (LEA). Under the legislation, speech-language pathology services are provided, at no cost to the family, but are based on educational communication needs and are heavily focused on language, rather than speech (Kumin, 1998, 2001). Feeding therapy, oral motor therapy, and speech intelligibility treatment are often not viewed as needed to help the child make progress in the regular education curriculum. Comprehensive Down syndrome centers, university clinics, hospitals, and private practitioners can provide speech-language pathology services. But, for many families, cost is a major factor and the educational settings, because they can provide free services, are the largest speech language pathology service providers for children from birth to 21 years of age.

8. A remediation treatment model is *not* effective for children and adolescents with Down syndrome. A proactive treatment plan is needed.

The IEP is based on a remediation model. For each area in which the child will receive services, the IEP must document the child's present level of performance, annual goals, and short-term objectives, including how progress will be measured and benchmarks. Generally, present performance and progress are measured by test results, and test scores must indicate delays and deficits to qualify for services. When a child makes progress and reaches the objectives stated in the IEP plan, new objectives may be developed or the child may no longer be eligible for services. For children with Down syndrome, there are a multitude of risk factors for difficulties in the areas of speech and language. A prevention model will enable us to treat the child proactively, before the difficulties, for example, low muscle tone, are evidenced in speech. A prevention model is used medically to treat recurrent ear infections with fluid buildup, through the use of tubes or a prophylactic antibiotic regimen. In physical therapy, treatment starts early to help children progress to walking. But in speech-language pathology services based in schools, families are still being told to come back when their child is talking or to come back at some specific time, for example, age 3 or 5 years. We need to be proactive. We need to develop databases so that we know what is typical for children with Down syndrome. We also need to develop speech and language treatment guidelines for children with Down syndrome so that we can better target when to evaluate and how to most effectively treat their speech and language problems.

## SPEECH TREATMENT PROGRAM PLAN

A comprehensive speech treatment plan should consider all of the factors that are affecting speech output. If the underlying problem is muscle tone, strength, and coordination, an exercise program should be included in the treatment plan. Exercises need to be done regularly to make a difference; therefore, a home treatment program in which oral motor exercises can be done on a daily basis is essential.

Sometimes children have difficulty with motor planning. This is known as developmental apraxia of speech. In these children, we will see difficulty in saying long words, sound reversals and leaving out syllables, more difficulty as the phrase or sentence gets longer, and inconsistency in production. One time they can say the sound, word, or sentence easily, and at other times, they struggle and grope for the sounds and just cannot say the same word, sentence, or phrase (Kumin and Adams, 2000). The treatment programs for apraxia focus on gradually increasing the length of the sound sequences. The child may start with vowels, progress to consonant-vowel sequences such as /ma/ and then go on to longer and more complex words. Frequent practice is part of an apraxia program. We don't know the incidence of developmental apraxia of speech in children with Down syndrome, but we do know that it affects speech intelligibility in some children with Down syndrome. When a child has a speech evaluation, the speech language pathologist should test for developmental apraxia of speech.

A comprehensive speech intelligibility evaluation can determine the need for speech treatment in many areas including:

*articulation:* how the child produces the sounds of speech

*phonological processes:* sound patterns such as leaving off final sounds

*loudness:* is the speech too loud, too soft or inappropriate?

*resonance:* is there excessive nasality because of palate muscle weakness or does the speech sound "stuffed like a cold" because of allergies or swollen tonsils and adenoids?

*rate:* is the speech too fast, too slow, or inconsistent?

*prosody:* the rhythm of language. Does the child's speech sound animated with varied pitch and melody or is it monotone?

*fluency:* is the speech dysfluent? Is there stuttering and struggle?

Language and auditory factors also impact on the intelligibility of speech and may need to be targeted in treatment. Pragmatics is the study of language in use—real everyday communication. Often, if the child does not look at the speaker, this will affect the communication interaction. The pragmatic and language skills that affect speech can be targeted in therapy. If the child is having difficulty with hearing speech, he may need an assistive listening device or a system that will amplify speech in the classroom. If people are having great difficulty understanding the child's speech, an augmentative communication system should be considered. Table 30.1 presents a checklist for developing a comprehensive speech treatment plan for children and adolescents with Down syndrome.

TABLE 30.1. Comprehensive Speech Treatment Program Plan for Children and Adolescents with Down Syndrome

A comprehensive treatment plan for an individual with Down syndrome may include any of the following as needed.

I. **Exercise Programs**
   A. Oral motor muscle strengthening
   B. Intervention for feeding problems
   C. Intervention for tongue thrust/swallowing problems

II. **Muscle Programming and Coordination Level**
   A. Intervention for developmental apraxia of speech
   B. Intervention for oral apraxia

III. **Speech Production Level**
   A. Articulation therapy
   B. Treatment for phonological processes
   C. Treatment for volume and loudness
   D. Voice therapy
   E. Resonance therapy
   F. Rate control
   G. Prosody treatment
   H. Fluency therapy

IV. **Pragmatic/Language Level**
   A. Treatment for nonverbal factors
   B. Language skills that impact on intelligibility
   C. Communication interactions in school/workplace

V. **Assistive Technology Needs**
   A. Augmentative communication for classroom use
   B. Augmentative communication for general use
   C. Assistive listening devices

VI. **Supports and Modifications Needed**

VII. **Referrals Needed**

| Psychologist | Otolaryngologist | Feeding Specialist | Other |
| Audiologist | | Neurologist | |

TABLE 30.2. COMPREHENSIVE LANGUAGE TREATMENT PROGRAM PLAN FOR CHILDREN AND ADOLESCENTS WITH DOWN SYNDROME

I. **Receptive Language Skills**
   A. Language comprehension
   B. Auditory processing skills
      1. Following directions
      2. Language of instruction
   C. Vocabulary/Semantics
      1. Language of curriculum
      2. Language of daily living
   D. Morphosyntax

II. **Expressive Language Skills**
   A. Vocabulary usage
      1. Increasing vocabulary skills
      2. Divergent language skills
      3. Convergent language skills
      4. Language of curriculum
   B. Morphosyntax
      1. Increasing MLU
      2. Increasing complexity of language output

III. **Pragmatics Skills**
   A. Social interactive skills
      1. Family
      2. Peers
      3. Teachers and other familiar adults
      4. Unfamiliar adults
   B. Communication activities of daily living
   C. Classroom routines
   D. Conversational skills
   E. Requests
   F. Clarification strategies/Repairs

IV. **Language Literacy Skills**
   A. Reading proficiency
   B. Reading comprehension
   C. Narrative discourse

V. **Assistive Technology Needs**
   A. Augmentative communication for classroom use
   B. Augmentative communication for general use
   C. Assistive listening devices

VI. **Supports and Modifications Needed**

VII. **Referrals Needed**

| Special Educator | Otolaryngologist | Psychologist | Audiologist |
| Reading specialist | Neurologist | | Other |

## LANGUAGE TREATMENT PROGRAMS: MAXIMIZING LANGUAGE SKILLS IN SCHOOL AND AT HOME

A comprehensive language treatment program should address the child's needs in several areas:

- Treatment should consider the child's strengths and challenges in different channels. For example, does he have more difficulty with expressive language than receptive language? Does he need help with language literacy skills?
- Treatment should also consider the child's relative strengths and difficulties in various areas of language. Does the child have more difficulty with grammar than vocabulary? Does she use language for social interactions effectively?
- A treatment plan should also address language needs for school. Can he follow directions in class? Does he need help with the language of the curriculum, that is, the language in the texts and the worksheets for specific subjects (Kumin, 2001)?
- A comprehensive language treatment plan should consider what kind of assistive technology, modifications, and services (such as classroom aides) the child will need to succeed in class (Kumin, 2001). IDEA 97 states that the need for assistive technology must be considered at each IEP planning meeting.

For adolescents, from age 14 on, speech and language should be part of the transition plan and should include emphasis on:

1. educational language needed for school;
2. any communication difficulties impacting behavior;
3. social interactive language; and
4. speech and language needs for the future, including communication in work settings and community living.

Table 30.2 presents a checklist for developing a comprehensive language treatment plan for children and adolescents with Down syndrome.

To plan an effective treatment program, we may need to know more about the physical or psychological factors affecting speech and language for an individual. In that case, referrals can be made to the psychologist, feeding specialist, audiologist, reading specialist, special educator, otolaryngologist, or neurologist. For most children and adolescents with Down syndrome, the primary source of speech and language services is the school speech language pathologist. The IEP is the planning document for school-based speech and language services.

## WRITING EFFECTIVE IEPs

Public Law 105-17 (IDEA 97) begins with the assumption that special education is a support service for children to help them progress in the least restrictive environment, namely, the regular education classroom. Speech therapy is generally defined as a related service. Related services

> means transportation, and such developmental, corrective and other supportive services (including speech-language pathology and audiology services) . . . as may be required to assist a child with a disability to benefit from special education, and includes the early identification and assessment of disabling conditions in children.

Mastering the regular education curriculum always involves language, the language of the curriculum, the language used to teach, and the language that children need for tests and projects to demonstrate that they have learned the material (Kumin, 2001). The criteria for choosing communication goals and objectives are based on several factors. The first is *functionality*, that is, is this a skill that the child needs to learn? Will learning the skill benefit the child? Another factor is *practice opportunities*, that is, will the child have many opportunities to practice the skill in school and at home? The teacher, specialists, and family all want to help the child generalize the skill to different situations. Another consideration is *age appropriateness*, that is, is this goal at the child's level based on his mental and/or chronological age?

The team will write the IEP communication goals, objectives, and benchmarks based on the individual child's needs. Goals are general, and objectives are more specific. They are sometimes referred to as short-term goals. Benchmarks state the schedule and the measures that will be used for judging progress. For each goal, objectives or benchmarks need to be written.

Some examples of goals during the school years are:

- To improve vocabulary
- To follow multistage school directions
- To improve oral motor muscle strength and coordination
- To increase the mean length of utterance (MLU) in conversational speech

## WHEN SHOULD SERVICES BE PROVIDED?

The IEP must include a statement of the scheduling and frequency of services. The schedule should be based on the child's individual needs, not on a general formula of what is provided to children with Down syndrome. It is a violation of the statutes of IDEA 97 and the IEP process for a representative of the IEP team to say "We provide 20 minutes of speech therapy twice weekly in groups for children with Down syndrome."

## WHERE SHOULD SERVICES BE PROVIDED?

The IEP should specify where services are to be provided. The language in IDEA 97 seems to suggest that special education and related services should be provided in the regular education classroom. The statement on inclusion by the American Speech-Language-Hearing Association suggests that speech-language pathology services may be provided in the classroom, in a separate pull-out setting, in the community, at home for early intervention services, or through consultation with the teacher (not direct service), in other words, that the services may be provided in a variety of settings. According to the American Speech-Language-Hearing Association, what is important is that the location of the services match the child's needs (American Speech-Language-Hearing Association, 1996).

## WHAT SHOULD THE IEP FOR SPEECH-LANGUAGE PATHOLOGY INCLUDE?

The speech-language pathology IEP should contain:

- statement of child's present communication skills
- annual goals
- short-term objectives or benchmarks and criteria to measure progress
- tests used
- services to be provided
    - intensity of service
    - frequency of service
    - length of each session
- communication plan for home to school

IDEA 97 specifies that home to school communication plans can be written into the IEP. The IEP can include specific plans for how communication will occur between teachers and related services personnel and others in school and between the school and home.

The IEP plan can also include the need for a home program with follow-up activities to be completed at home and with information sent to the parents on a regular (daily, weekly) basis.

In addition to helping to reinforce the speech and language goals at home, in what other ways can parents help to maximize speech and language skills? Communication happens all of the time. For communication situations that repeat often, such as greetings, telephone messages, requesting information, and ordering in restaurants, parents and children can rehearse scripts and then practice the communication in the real-life situation. To work on vocabulary, word games such as Pictionary and Scattergories can be used. To work on following instructions, games such as Twister and Simon Says can be used. Using recipes and doing crafts activities can provide practice in following written instructions. Throughout the day, in many different situations, there are opportunities to help children and adolescents develop and practice speech and language skills.

## REFERENCES AND RESOURCES

Communicating Together Newsletter/Workshops, P.O. Box 6395, Columbia, MD, 21045-6395; phone: 410-995-0722; subscription newsletter for parents and professionals devoted to speech and language in children with Down syndrome and information on workshops for parents and professionals.

American Speech-Language-Hearing Association (1996): Inclusive practices for children and youths with communication disorders: Position statement and technical report. ASHA 38 (Suppl. 16):35–44.

Buckley S (1996): Reading before talking: Learning about mental abilities from children with Down's syndrome. Paper presented at the University of Portsmouth Inaugural Lectures, May 9, 1996.

Desai SS (1997): Down syndrome: A review of the literature. Oral Surg Oral Med Oral Pathol 84:279–285.

Fowler AE (1990): Language abilities in children with Down syndrome: Evidence for a specific syntactic delay. In Cicchetti D, Beeghley M (eds.), Children with Down Syndrome: A Developmental Perspective. Cambridge: Cambridge University Press, pp 302–328.

Fowler AE (1995): Linguistic variability in persons with Down syndrome: research and implications. In Nadel L, Rosenthal D (eds.), Down Syndrome: Living and Learning in the Community. New York: Wiley-Liss, pp 121–131.

Kumin L (1994): Communication Skills in Children with Down Syndrome: A Guide for Parents. Bethesda, MD: Woodbine House.

Kumin L (1996): Speech and language skills in children with Down syndrome. Ment Retard Dev Disabil Res Rev 2:109–116.

Kumin L (1999): Comprehensive speech and language treatment for infants, toddlers, and children with Down syndrome. In: Hassold TJ, Patterson D (eds.), Down Syndrome: A Promising Future, Together. New York: Wiley-Liss, pp 145–153.

Kumin L (2001): Classroom Language Skills in Children with Down Syndrome: A Guide for Parents and Teachers. Bethesda, MD: Woodbine House.

Kumin L, Adams J (2000): Developmental apraxia of speech and intelligibility in children with Down syndrome. Down Syndrome Q 5:1–8

Kumin L, Bahr DC (1999): Patterns of feeding, eating, and drinking in young children with Down syndrome with oral motor concerns. Down Syndrome Q 4:1–8.

Kumin L, Councill C, Goodman M (1998): Expressive vocabulary development in children with Down syndrome. Down Syndrome Q 3:1–7.

Kumin L, Goodman M, Councill C (1996): Comprehensive communication assessment and intervention for school-aged children with Down syndrome. Down Syndrome Q 1:1–8.

Laws G, Buckley SJ, Bird G, MacDonald J, Broadley I (1995): The influence of reading instruction on language and memory development in children with Down's syndrome. Down's Syndrome Res Pract 3:59–64.

Miller JF (1988): Developmental asynchrony of language development in children with Down syndrome. In Nadel L (ed.), Psychobiology of Down Syndrome. New York: Academic Press.

Miller JF, Leddy M, Leavitt LA (1999): Improving the communication of people with Down syndrome. Baltimore, MD: Paul H. Brookes.

Roizen NJ, Wolters C, Nicol T, Blondis T (1992): Hearing loss in children with Down syndrome. Pediatrics 123:S9–S12.

# LIBERATION FROM TRADITIONAL READING AND MATH TEACHING METHODS AND MEASUREMENTS

## PATRICIA LOGAN OELWEIN, M.ED.

[Author's Note: The methodology is based on methods developed in the Down Syndrome Programs, University of Washington, 1971–87.]

It is liberating to know that students with Down syndrome (DS) are generally very capable of becoming literate (defined as having the ability to construct meaning from symbols) and mathematicians (defined as those who make meaningful use of numbers). It is equally liberating to know that there are specific methods for teaching reading and math to children with Down syndrome—specialized methods that take into consideration their learning differences and individual needs. Also, it is just as liberating to be free from measuring their success in reading and math by the standards and goals developed for children who do not have learning differences.

It was the mother of Alex, a 16-year-old who has Down Syndrome, who expressed to me the freedom she felt after reading a chapter I wrote on individualizing reading for each child's abilities and needs and measuring reading success by the degree to which reading benefits the student (Oelwein, 1999). Her only regret was that she had not been liberated years earlier from the bondage of grade-level reading goals for Alex. It would have saved her a lot of anguish and frustration. And if it had saved her anguish and frustration, think of what it would have done for Alex! It is easy to look

*Down Syndrome*, Edited by William I. Cohen, Lynn Nadel, and Myra E. Madnick.
ISBN 0-471-41815-3   Copyright © 2002 by Wiley-Liss, Inc.

back and wish that you had done things differently—that you had had the information that you have now. I knew Alex and his mother when he was just starting his elementary school years, but I did not have the same information, experience, insight, and perspective that I have now.

## A New Perspective: Readers with Down Syndrome as Overachievers

Follow-up data from the University of Washington (Oelwein, 1988) and Macquarie University (Buckley, 1985) Down syndrome programs had revealed that adolescents (mean age, 14.5) and children (mean age, 8 years) with Down syndrome read above their mental ages by 2 and 2.2 years respectively. Although I viewed these data as being very positive and labeled these children as having a talent for reading and encouraged parents and educators to tap into this valuable talent, grade-level scores and lack of progress in basal or grade-level readers continued to be a concern. An apparent "plateau" at the 2nd, 3rd, or 4th grade level and lower scores on reading comprehension than on word recognition were seen as major problems. It was not until I was studying the data of Fowler et al. (1995) for adults that I had my epiphany: *Readers with Down syndrome are overachievers in reading and remain overachievers even into adulthood.* This was true regardless of their grade-level reading score. Their data revealed what "came out in the wash," and it was very positive.

The study of Fowler et al. reported data on the performance of 33 adults with DS (17–25 years of age) on three reading measures (word attack, word identification, and comprehension) and four cognitive measures (PPVT-R, TACL-R, K-ABC, and arithmetic). Subjects were placed in reading groups (novice, emerging, developing, and skilled) based on their word attack skills. These data showed that, for all four reading groups, on each of the three reading measures, the mean reading scores were *higher* than the mean general ability scores (K-ABC). The greatest discrepancy was observed in the *skilled* reading group (*n* = 5) in word attack skills. The mean age equivalent *word attack skills* score for these readers was *8.9 years higher* than the mean *general ability* score; however, the mean *comprehension* score was only *1.3 years above* the *general ability* score (word attack skills, 16 years; comprehension, 8.4; general ability, 7.1). The *developing* readers (*n* = 6) showed the greatest discrepancy to be in word identification skills, achieving an age equivalent score in *word identification skills 3.1 years above* the mean *general ability* score. The mean age equivalent *comprehension score* for these readers was *1.5 years above* the mean *general ability* score (word identification 9.3 years; comprehension, 7.7; general ability 6.2).

Although these young adults may appear to be stuck—or appear to have plateaued—on a reading level, they are still reading and comprehending at a higher level than their general ability. They are fulfilling their reading potential to the degree that it is useful to them. It is of little value to be able to sound out words at the 11th grade level when your comprehension is at the 3rd grade level, as was the case of the skilled readers. What is of value is the ability to *use* reading skills—no matter how meager they are—as powerful tools in building competencies that lead to greater independence. Students have not plateaued in competencies. They have not plateaued in learning. They have not plateaued in reading. Reading will improve with constant, meaningful use, and any improvements in reading scores are *fringe benefits*. The *real benefits* are the gains in becoming more competent in more and more domains, which leads to gains in general ability—and we do not need a test to determine this. We are liberated from the bondage of striving for higher grade-level scores.

If typical children were reading *a year higher* than their mental age/grade level, they would be considered "overachievers," and their teachers would be given bonuses for doing such a great job. Parents of these children would be feeling very smug, and, chances are, they would be spreading the good news—"little Johnny is above average"—just like all the children in Lake Wobegon! And "above average" is exactly what the *lowest* mean reading score—in *comprehension*—was for the 33 adults in the Fowler et al. study: *one year higher* than the mean general ability score (range, 0.6 year higher for the novice readers to 1.5 for developing readers). And it gets better. The average of the overall means for the three reading measures (word attack, word identification, and comprehension averaged together) is 1.9 years— *almost two years higher* than their general ability age. The overall mean general ability age was 5.9 years (range, 5.0 for novice readers to 7.1 for skilled readers), but these readers were reading as though their general ability age was 7.8 years.

It is difficult to determine which comes first, the chicken or the egg, the general ability or the reading. But I am compelled to venture to suggest that the skilled readers' general ability score was higher, at least in part, because of the competencies they gained through the *use* of their reading—rather than the reverse argument that their higher reading scores were the *result* of their higher general ability score. I will also venture to suggest that the higher comprehension and word identification reading scores were obtained and maintained through *practical use* of reading rather than through instruction in the technicalities of reading.

Instead of setting goals for vertical growth (higher reading levels), where the *end product* for the student is proficiency in technical reading skills, I advocate setting goals for horizontal growth, where the student applies reading abilities to more and more uses and the *end product* is increased competence. The student's success in reading is measured by how it *benefits* him or her in building competencies and independence, which will result in improving quality of life, self-confidence, and self-esteem.

## CITIZENS, SQUATTERS, AND ALIENS

Christopher Kliewer (1998) followed 10 students with DS for two years. He found that two definitions of literacy emerged: (1) developmental—where the *end product* was grade level reading skills; and (2) functional (my term, his definition)—where literacy was regarded as "the construction of shared meaning in specific contexts" (p. 167). The *end product* was communication—constructing meaning from symbols.

In classrooms where the *developmental* approach was held dear, children with DS were at a disadvantage and appeared intellectually incompetent. In classrooms where *functional* literacy was respected and accepted, children with Down syndrome were valued as intellectually competent. It was the teacher's attitude rather than the child's performance that made the difference. Intellectual competence or incompetence was in the eyes of the beholder.

Kliewer observed a stratified literate social structure emerge in the classrooms where the developmental view of literacy was held sacred (or, as I would say, staffed by intellectual snobs). This structure included *all* students in the classroom (non-DS as well as DS). There was the privileged class—the *Citizens*—who conformed to the expectations of the developmental programs. The Citizens had opportunity for full curricular participation in increasingly complex concepts and information. Next were the *Squatters*—students who progressed in the developmental program only partially and at a reduced rate. The Squatters participated in remedial practice on low-level concepts and subskills. And last were the *Aliens*—students who were unable to progress in the developmental program. The Aliens were separated from the literate community and were considered cognitively incompetent. They were not expected to read. They were not seen as symbolic beings.

I have had the opportunity to observe many Squatters and Aliens during my 29 years of serving children with Down syndrome. These are usually the children with one-on-one instructional assistants who have not been trained in providing individualized, specialized, systematic instruction but are generally left to their own devices having received only minimal training. They do the best they can with what they know and generally try to lead the Squatters through the paces of the classroom curriculum that has been modified. When an Alien is in their charge, their primary purpose seems to be preventing the Alien from disturbing the classroom teacher and the Citizens (and managing the student's "behavior management" program) and trying to put the Alien through the paces of packaged special education programs. These students are seldom able to succeed in any academics to the extent that they can apply their academics to developing competencies, and, for all practical purposes, they remain illiterate and basically incompetent, dependent on others to get them through the day and keep them safe.

## ILLITERACY IN PEOPLE WITH DOWN SYNDROME: THE GREAT INTERNATIONAL TRAGEDY

I find illiteracy among people with Down syndrome a tragedy—one that is international in scope. Fowler et al. (1995) estimated a 60% illiterate rate among people with DS. If this is true for the U.S., where reading is generally a part of the curriculum for students with DS and where most schools *try*, worldwide, I would expect the illiteracy rate to be much higher. This is a great waste of human potential and resources that are generally allotted for the student's education. Just think of what it would be like to go through school and not be able to read—to never have a text book, to never be able to take notes, to never be able to look up information that you forgot, and never be able to follow written directions. You are expected to learn and remember through verbal instruction. *And your short-term verbal memory is your weakness! And your strength is visual memory.*

Recent advances in technology have made it possible to study the brain. Wang (1996) cites magnetic resonance imaging studies that show the actual physical difference in the brains of adolescents with Down syndrome that can explain weaknesses in verbal tasks and verbal short-term memory skills and relative strengths in visual-motor skills. Nash (1997) reports remarkable new discoveries about the typical development of the brain. As early as 12 weeks after conception the development of the brain has begun with a frenzy of brain activity. It continues after birth, with the production of trillions of connections between the neurons—many more than it can possibly use. And, starting at around 10 years of age or earlier the brain starts to eliminate connections (synapses) that are seldom or never used and preserves only those that have been transformed by experience. By age 18 the brain has declined in plasticity but increased in power—the power of those strong synapses that are the result of what was learned *thoroughly— and used often.* The potential has been developed, and the individual is ready to fly with it!

How can children with Down syndrome build these strong synapses if the sensory input—the first step in the learning process—is verbal and the differences in their brain are such that they have difficulty processing and therefore remembering and using the information? It's a worldwide hijacking of synapses!

## METHODOLOGY: THE GREAT INTERNATIONAL BREAKTHROUGH

Language, the *symbol system* we use to communicate with, is necessary for the formation of thought. This symbol system is available via both auditory and visual stimuli. People with Down syndrome often have difficulty comprehending and processing verbal language—verbal words exist for only an instant and cannot be retrieved. In addition, they often have difficulty *using* verbal language and find sign language (visual-motor symbol system) a powerful tool that better enables them to connect with others. But sign language is just the beginning of their liberation from being held prisoner by the differences in their brains. Just as a person who is blind is liberated by an education that is specialized to meet his/her special needs, so is the person with Down syndrome. Reading, or comprehending meaning from written symbols, is a relative strength for most people with DS, and they can learn to read at least to the level that it is useful to them. And, if they are taught to *use* this reading to communicate with others and to facilitate learning in all domains, this reading will set them free from the bondage of their learning differences. They can become *Citizens!*

The first step is to respect the child and his learning differences—the same respect that you would have for the person who is blind. We cannot ignore inability to see and teach him as though his blindness did not exist. We cannot ignore the learning differences in the person with Down syndrome and teach her—and have expectations of her—as though they did not exist. We cannot just *expose* her to an education designed for children who do not have learning differences and never teach her anything *thoroughly*, building only weak synapses that die off because of lack of use, never to return.

Specialized teaching methods that respect the student's learning differences exist. They are simple, easy to use, inexpensive, and very effective (and lots of fun!). The catch is that the *instructor* has to make the investment in time to read, study, and make materials. She cannot implement the methods with only *exposure*. She needs to *thoroughly* learn the method, one step at a time (work-study—learn on the job) and to understand the whole process to be successful—bits and pieces are not enough. I have written a book on teaching reading (Oelwein, 1995) that gives step-by-step guidelines on this specialized method, and, currently, I am writing a book on teaching math using the same basic method.

I have been a consultant with a program in Saudi Arabia since 1991. The goal was to develop a model program for educating people with Down syndrome from infancy to adulthood. This competency-based program has reached its goal and demonstrates specialized, individualized, and systematic instruction at all levels. It is a sight to behold! A dream come true! It really works! But it did not happen over night.

There were growing pains. The first problem was challenging behaviors. As I was struggling to teach the methodology, the teachers were *insisting* on behavior management strategies. They said that they could not teach when their students were misbehaving. They wanted me to help them get the behaviors under control so they could teach. They could not even *think* about methodology. They *knew* what the problem was, and it was the students' *disruptive behaviors* that interfered with their teaching.

I was trying to convince the teachers that these behaviors were primarily communication behaviors. The students were communicating that the curriculum did not match their needs and the teaching method did not match their learning differences—*it did not make sense to them*. I assured them that most of these challenging behaviors would disappear when their educational needs were met. They would learn how to meet these needs by teaching the students to become more competent in communication and managing their own behavior. To try to eliminate these undesirable communication behaviors and not replace them with desirable behaviors would be futile.

First, we needed to determine what competencies the students had and what competencies they needed and then teach the skills necessary for meeting these competencies—in a way that made it *feasible* for students to learn them. I kept stressing to the teachers that I was not concerned about the students' behaviors, but rather *their* behaviors. (*They*—the teachers— were *my* students!). If they changed their behaviors and used the specialized teaching methods that I was trying to teach them, and if they stopped trying to teach by lecturing, most of the undesirable behaviors would be replaced by desirable behaviors as the students became more competent.

It did take a while—learning is a gradual process—but they caught on, and the students are now, for the most part (always exceptions), competent managers of their own behavior and are very accomplished students—connecting with their environment using desirable means of communication and reaching their potential. And, needless to say, the teachers are skilled as well. (Watching the classroom is like watching a ballet to me! All the ballerinas know just what to do and when and where to do it in the beautiful set with user-friendly décor and props.)

After the program was falling into place, an experienced teacher joined the teaching staff. As I was going through the steps of teaching reading, she was skeptical. She said that she had taught children with Down syndrome to read, and she had not used that method. I explained to her that some children with Down syndrome were capable of learning to read by any number of methods, but for most, this was the most effective method. This method made it *feasible* for some children with DS to learn to read, and this was the method consistently used throughout this model program. (In short, she had to use it.)

This teacher was excellent, a quick learner who took to the method like a duck to water. After 2 years, she left the school to become the principal of another school. During my last visit she told me that she taught her teachers my method and told them that they *had* to use it for just 3 weeks. After 3 weeks, they could go back to their old method, if they chose to. She said that she had never had a teacher go back to their old way. Once teachers have experienced such success, they never go back. That typewriter just does not cut it after you learn to use the computer!

## MAKING IT EASIER TO HAVE DOWN SYNDROME

Thomas, at age 13, had impressive reading and math skills when he entered middle school, and he was following a modified curriculum. He tried hard and was doing his best. But his best was not good enough. The work was too hard. He observed how easy it was for his classmates. He became depressed. He told his mother that he did not want to have Down syndrome any more. He said that it was *just too hard* to have Down syndrome. He wanted to be *rid of it!*

His parents could not make the Down syndrome go away, but they could work on making it easier for him to have Down syndrome. Instead of struggling through as a Squatter with the *schoolwork* as the *end product*, he needed a curriculum that made him a Citizen with *competencies, citizenship (and fun)* as the *end product*. His Down syndrome entitles him to the privilege of an Individualized Education Program—a curriculum designed to match *his needs and abilities*. He does not have to fit into a program that was designed to meet the needs of students who do not have Down syndrome—in which he does not learn anything *thoroughly*—just endless paper and pencil work that provides only exposure to information that is generally useless to him. Who wouldn't be depressed? Even the President of the United States takes the oath to perform his duties "to the best of my ability." We need not ask more of our children with Down syndrome—when "to the best of my ability" fails to be good enough to perform the "duties" designed for typical children.

Few children with Down syndrome will tolerate programs that do not meet their needs and abilities. The less competent students express their intolerance with challenging behaviors, and the more competent students, such as Thomas, express their intolerance verbally (an important learned competency) and often become depressed when we fail to respond to their anguish. Life is not good for them. We want to change that. They are people who deserve and have earned a good life. We have the methodology to make it better. We just need to put out the effort to learn it—and implement it.

## MATH: MORE LIBERATION

When I let it be known that I was planning to write a book on teaching math, parents and teachers started asking about math ability and achievement in children with Down syndrome. Parents often perceived their child as being an accomplished reader but a struggling mathematician. They also wanted to know "how far" a person with Down syndrome could go in math—what the expectations were.

I did not know the answers to their questions, only impressions based on observations. My general impression was that reading was the stronger subject of the two, although I had observed some children with Down syndrome who I consider to be very competent mathematicians. But because I was planning to write a book on teaching math, I decided that I should have data rather than assumptions. First, I took a look at the math scores that Fowler et al (1995) provided as a cognitive measure alone with the reading scores. Then I distributed a questionnaire to parents and teachers to gather information concerning skills, needs, and attitudes.

## Age-Equivalent Scores

When I compared the math scores to the general ability scores reported for the 33 young adults in the Fowler et al. study, I was pleasantly surprised. The mean age-equivalent arithmetic score for the group was 6.7 years (range, 9.0 for skilled readers to 5.7 for novice readers), and their mean general ability age was 5.9 (range, 7.1 for skilled readers to 5.0 for novice readers). These adults and adolescents with DS appear to be "reaching their potential" in math and exceeding it, qualifying them as *overachievers in math* as well.

The reading comprehension scores, which I consider the best cognitive measure of the reading scores, were very close to the arithmetic scores— reading comprehension, 6.9 years, arithmetic, 6.7—only 0.2 year different. Therefore, the mean scores show that these young adults had only a 0.2-year difference between reading comprehension and math scores. The skilled readers were the only group that actually scored higher on arithmetic (9.0 years) than on reading comprehension (8.4 years).

If you are thinking that this is not the case with your child—that her reading skills are much more advanced than her math skills—then you most likely are right. Remember that these were mean scores of individuals who were 17 or older, and these were the scores that had "come out in the wash." They had had much longer to achieve these levels than your child has. It has been my experience that once a child with DS "catches on" to reading, and it becomes a very useful tool, there is no stopping her. She makes rapid progress. However, in math the progress is generally slower, but I believe that students generally learn the math essential to keeping pace with their need for math in daily life. Students often get "hung up" on math skills that they do not understand and for which they have no practical use. They become trapped in developmental programs designed for students who do not have learning differences.

I have known children who spent the school year working on "borrowing and carrying," only to return the following fall to start all over again and struggle through another year of borrowing and carrying. Remember the pruning of the synapses that Nash reported—skills that are not useful to the student are lost. It is much more important to teach her the essential math she needs to become competent in all domains. I have a little test for the value of math skills, grade-level scores, and math courses. If you have to *tell* others (brag) that the student can do the task, or has achieved a level, or has taken the course, for others to *know* what she has accomplished, the "achievement" is most likely of little or no value to the student. On the other hand, if you have to *tell* others that the student is "poor" in math for them to be *aware* of her weakness, then the student most likely has the math skills that serve her well. (Perhaps she just became hung up on borrowing and carrying.) Pretend that there is a gag rule on, and you cannot tell anyone about your child's accomplishment or lack of accomplishments in math. When you practice such a rule, I would expect your child to become the best mathematician she can by performing "to the best of her ability."

The math skills that are useful will be apparent by the student's behavior in everyday life. She will be competent in many areas that use math. Competent at playing games, keeping score, and determining who won. Competent at making purchases. Competent at arriving and leaving on time. Competent at cooking, washing clothes, and planting seeds. Competent at managing her own diet and fitness program. Competent at using the microwave, stove, TV, VCR, and calculator. Competent at dressing for the temperature. Competent at writing checks and balancing her checkbook. Competent at driving a car and staying within the speed limit.

I am not impressed when I am told that a student took algebra when she is 40 pounds overweight. I am *very* impressed when a student can manage her own fitness program—diet and exercise—and stay trim and fit. She has achieved what many Americans who are skilled in advanced math find it very difficult or impossible to achieve. I want students to have real value from the resources that have been allotted to them. Advanced math, where the only value is the status of having taken the course, is too costly—not only in time and resources, but also in the child's self-esteem.

Few children with DS can get through traditional math courses without a great deal of difficulty, and few would choose to take the course on their own. Self-esteem comes from setting goals and reaching them. If, however, the *student* sets the goal to take the course, and she experiences little difficulty and feels accomplished, then the course has value to her. And if this is the case for your child, then your child most likely does not need special programming—and she does not need liberating. She is where she wants to be and her self-esteem is intact.

For all parents whose children do experience difficulty with nonessential math, I hereby liberate your child from math tasks that are not useful to her and from striving for grade-level accomplishments.

## THE SURVEY: WHAT YOU TOLD ME ABOUT YOUR CHILDREN

A questionnaire was distributed through the Down syndrome list service, parent groups, conferences, special needs teachers and supervisors, and, in some cases, through personal contact. Ninety-nine usable questionnaires were returned. Those lacking important information, such as the student's age, were discarded. About half (46) were from countries other than the U.S., Canada, The Netherlands, and the United Kingdom (most of these from Northern Ireland).

Students were grouped according to age: primary (5–8 years old, $n = 26$); elementary (9–11 years old, $n = 38$); secondary (12–21 years old, $n = 35$). The individual ages most represented were 10 years (18) and 11 years (13). There were only three subjects over 16 years of age. Approximately 46% were female and 54% male. (Sex data was available for only 70 subjects.)

The younger the child, the more time he or she was served in inclusive classrooms: 93% primary; 63% elementary; and 57% secondary. Forty-two percent of the students generally received their math instruction in the regular classroom, taught by an instructional assistant; forty-five percent were in the special education classroom taught by the special education teacher. Over half (54%) of the primary group received their instruction from the regular education teacher in the regular classroom.

Forty-eight percent were using no "published" math program but were systematically taught. Twenty-eight percent were in the same program as their typical classmates, eight percent without accommodations and twenty percent with accommodations. Only 18% were in published special education programs.

Now, for all you parents who want to compare your child's math skills to those in this sampling of skills, here goes. (Note that with 99 subjects, in most cases the percentage and number are the same.)

ROTE COUNTING. Seventeen percent could rote count (say numbers in sequence) to 10 only (8 primary; 5 elementary; and 4 secondary). Sixteen percent could rote count to 20 only (3 primary; 9 elementary; and 4 secondary). Thirty-two percent could rote count to 100 (5 primary; 11 elementary; and 16 secondary). Five percent could rote count to 500 and higher (1 primary; 4 secondary). Fifteen percent could not yet rote count to 10 (6 primary; 8 elementary; 1 secondary).

COUNT AND STATE QUANTITY. Twenty-two percent of students could count objects with quantities up to 10 and state the quantity (9 primary; 8 elementary; 5 secondary). Thirty five percent could do this task to 20 (8 primary; 13 elementary; 14 secondary). Thirteen percent could do this task to 100 (1 primary; 4 elementary; 8 secondary). And 2% (2 secondary) could do the task to 1000. Twenty-four percent (8 primary; 12 elementary; 4 secondary) did not do this task to 10.

READ NUMERALS, PRESENTED RANDOMLY. Twenty-nine percent could read numerals 1 through 10 when these numerals were presented in random order (13 primary; 12 elementary; 4 secondary). Fourteen percent could read numerals 1 to 20 (3 primary; 6 elementary group; 5 secondary). Twenty-five percent could read numerals to 100 (6 primary; 10 elementary; and 9 secondary). Fifteen percent could read numerals to 1000 (1 primary; 2 elementary; 12 secondary). Six percent could read numerals greater than 1000 (1 primary; 1 elementary; 4 secondary). Only 3 (1 primary and 2 elementary) students did not read numerals to 10.

WRITING NUMERALS.   Eleven percent could write numerals 1 to 10, on dictation (2 primary; 7 elementary; 2 secondary). Eighteen percent could write numerals 1 to 20 (4 primary; 8 elementary; 6 secondary). Twenty-eight percent could write numerals 1 to 100 (7 primary; 8 elementary; and 13 secondary). Seven percent could write numerals to 1000 (1 primary; 2 elementary; and 4 secondary). Six percent, all from the secondary group, could write numerals greater than 1000. Twenty-nine percent did not write numerals 1 to 10 (12 primary; 13 elementary; 4 secondary).

RELATIVE VALUE OF NUMBERS.   Fifteen percent could compare two numbers and select the one with the greater value from 1 to 10 (6 primary; 4 elementary; and 4 secondary). Eleven percent could perform the task to 20 (7 elementary; 4 secondary). Six percent could perform the task to 50 (3 primary; 2 elementary; and 1 secondary). Ten percent could do the task to 100 (1 primary; 3 elementary; 6 secondary), and ten percent could do the task to numbers greater than 1000 (1 primary; 9 secondary). Almost half, 47%, could not do this task to 10 (15 primary; 21 elementary; 11 secondary).

ADDITION.   Forty percent could add numbers with one digit (10 primary; 17 elementary; 13 secondary). Eighteen percent could add numbers with two digits (1 primary; 10 elementary; 7 secondary). Fifteen percent could add numbers with three digits (2 primary; 2 elementary; 11 secondary). Twenty-six percent (13 primary, 9 elementary, 4 secondary) did not add one-digit numbers.

Forty-eight percent used objects to add and subtract (14 primary; 21 elementary; 13 secondary). Forty-one percent used a calculator (2 primary; 12 elementary; 27 secondary). Thirty-two percent used a number line (5 primary; 15 elementary; 12 secondary. Other methods used were Touch Math (21%) and math facts (11%).

PRACTICAL USES OF MATH.   Seventy-seven percent used math in games; 42% kept score; 54% told time; 58% used the calendar; 42% made purchases (some indicated "with help"); 33% followed a schedule; 38% cooked; 30% used the TV remote; 11% programmed the VCR; and 8% used the thermometer.

Like/Dislike Math.   An impressive 73% percent responded that their child or student *liked math* (19 primary; 30 elementary; 23 secondary). Only 27% reported that their child or student *disliked math* (7 primary; 8 elementary; 12 secondary).

Successful/Unsuccessful in Math.   Seventy-one percent responded that they considered their child or student successful in math at his/her ability level (19 primary; 29 elementary; 22 secondary). Of this 71%, 43% attributed their child's success to good instruction and programming; 36% to home tutoring; 21% to inclusion; 7% to natural ability.

Some people responded that their child was both successful and unsuccessful in math—it depended on the child's mood, time of day, etc. Therefore, 58% checked unsuccessful. Of these, 40% attributed their child's lack of success to lack of ability; 35% to poor instruction and programming; 5% to lack of inclusion; and 9% to fear failure of subject.

Did the student plateau?   A very impressive 78% reported that their child or student had not plateaued. Of the 22% that reported that their child or student had plateaued, the ages of the perceived plateaus were at ages 6, 7, 10, 11, and 16 years old. Others responded with a "level"—2 at level one; and 1 at level two. One reported that their child was "stuck on five."

Math Skills Most Helpful.   When asked, "What math skill do you think would be most helpful to your child?" 65% responded that money/shopping skills would be most helpful; 37% telling time; 26% adding and subtraction; 22% practical use/life skills; and 8% basic math. Other "most helpful" skills were measuring, numbers, multiplication/division, calendar/schedule, calculator, relative value of numbers, counting, conservation, problem solving, weighing, math facts, 1:1 correspondence, games, number line, estimations, sequencing, fractions, more/less, and rounding off.

## Essential Math In A Capsule

In my upcoming book, *Teaching Math to Children with Down Syndrome*, I explain how to teach children with DS essential math to meet their individual needs. For this chapter, I am providing you with the sequence that I recommend for teaching this essential math.

Cognitive Concepts: Prepare the Child for Numbers.   Preschool children should be prepared for math by enriching play experiences and activities that provide practice using math concepts and vocabulary—without numbers. Therefore, I recommend starting with cognitive concepts that build the foundation for numbers. These concepts include quantity (more/less, few/many), weight (heavy/light), height (tall/short), size (big/little), volume (full/empty), temperature (hot/cold), time (before/during/after), age (baby/child/adult), distance (near/far), and speed (fast/slow).

Children learn to use this vocabulary, these general modifiers, as they learn the concepts. For example, the *big* papa bear, the *medium-sized* mama bear, the *little* baby bear. They need no numbers to describe the bears. The *relative* size of each bear is apparent—Papa is the biggest, then there is Mama, and next is Baby Bear. Providing the weight, height, and measurements of each bear would be meaningless. *Numbers*, however, are *specific* modifiers. They tell us exactly *how* big, full, cold, old, or tall something is. Our use for numbers grows as our cognition develops, and we have a need for the specific modifiers. If we so choose, "Once upon a time" becomes "March 18, 1947 at 8:12 a.m."

Young children have little need for specific modifiers. Their need is to understand and use the general modifiers. These concepts should be embedded in all aspects of every child's life, such as selecting a sock that fits his foot (with a choice of his or Daddy's). Play activities should be designed to reinforce these concepts—block play, puzzles, art projects, copying patterns, stories, active and dramatic play and rote counting (for exposure at first)—all contribute to understanding and using these concepts. And, for most children with DS, these concepts need to be taught systematically with visual illustrations. They do not generally "just pick it up" from the environment. And if they do, they frequently do not have the language to use these concepts in communicating with others.

Start with 1, 2, 3.   Go slowly and be aware of exactly what concept you are teaching and teach it thoroughly. Have activities and games planned for each stage of learning: acquisition, practice to fluency, transfer and generalization. Start with 1:1 correspondence to 3. When she masters this, continue with the following concepts: counting objects to 3; reading numerals to 3; matching quantity to each numeral taught (1, 2, and 3); select specific quantities on cue; write numerals 1, 2, and 3; adding sums to 3; subtracting remainders to 2; putting numerals in order to 3; putting set cards in order to 3; comparing quantities (more/less); and relative value to 3. In other words, be sure that the student has a thorough understanding of 1, 2, and 3 and can use these numbers and quantities daily. This accomplished, do the same all the way to 5. After mastering numbers to 5, add one number at a time, building on and practicing what the student has learned, until she has mastered numbers 1 to 10.

I consider mastery of these numbers (1–10) the first milestone. The next will be reading numbers and using the number line to add and subtract to 20. The third milestone is mastering the sequence of numbers to 100. This involves reading and writing the numbers, finding numbers on the number charts, using the number chart to determine relative value (who won the game), and simple addition and subtraction. The fourth milestone is to teach the student to count by fives and tens to 100. And all along the way, these concepts are taught, practiced, and used throughout the day in their natural context.

After mastery of these useful core concepts, continue to teach the student to *use* these numbers and concepts *as the need arises*—playing games, keeping score, charting her own data, calculating percentages and averages (using a calculator and formula), following a schedule, telling time, counting money, cooking, using the remote control, and endless other things.

The secret (which I wish wasn't such a secret) is to provide a *use* for the skills she has. It is through the useful practice that she will maintain math skills and grow. And, *as the need arises*, additional concepts, such as fractions, place value, and decimals, can be taught. You have a long time to teach her the math she needs at each stage of her life. When there is a need and your child does not have the ability to meet that need, provide her with accommodations—a means to compensate. Even rocket scientists have been known to have accountants to complete their income tax.

## SUMMARY

Most children with Down syndrome have the ability to become literate mathematicians. However, most have learning differences that require specialized, systematic, and individualized instruction to reach this potential. Reading and arithmetic scores generally exceed their general ability score, classifying them, in my opinion as "overachievers" in these areas. Goals in reading and math should be based on the use of and the need for the skills needed to build competencies and independence. Parents and teachers should be liberated from grade-level measurements and be free to focus on developing competencies—competencies for Citizens.

## REFERENCES

Buckley S (1985): Attaining basic educational skills: Reading, writing, and number. In: Lane D, Stratford B (eds.), Current Approaches to Down's Syndrome. New York: Praeger.

Fowler AE, Boherty BJ, Boynton L (1995): The basis of reading skills in young adults with Down syndrome. In: Nadel L, Rosenthal D (eds.), Down Syndrome: Living and Learning in the Community. New York: Wiley-Liss.

Kliewer C (1998): Citizenship in the literate community: An ethnography of children with Down syndrome and the written word. Exceptional Children 64(2):167–180.

Nash JM (1997): Special report: Fertile minds. Time 149(5):48–56.

Oelwein PL (1988): Preschool and kindergarten programs: Strategies for meeting objectives. In: Dmitriev V, Oelwein PL (eds.), Advances in Down Syndrome. Seattle, WA: Special Child Publications.

Oelwein PL (1995): Teaching Reading to Children with Down Syndrome: A Guide for Parents and Teachers. Bethesda, MD: Woodbine House.

Oelwein PL (1999): Individualizing reading for each child's ability and needs. In: Hassold TJ, Patterson D (eds.), Down Syndrome: A Promising Future, Together. New York: Wiley-Liss.

Wang PP (1966): A neuropsychological profile of Down syndrome: cognitive skills and brain morphology. Ment Retard Dev Disabil Res Rev: Down Syndrome 2(2):102–108.

Watkins RV, Bunce BH (1996): Natural literacy: Theory and practice for preschool intervention programs. Topics Early Childhood Spec Educ 16(2):191–212.

# TURNING THE VISION INTO REALITY

# TURNING THE VISION INTO REALITY

## ANDREA LACK, M.S.W., C.S.W.

## WHAT IS THE VISION . . . WHAT IS THE REALITY?

### INTRODUCTION

Simply stated, the vision for people with Down syndrome is that they be included in all aspects of family, school, work, social, recreational, and community life. Also as part of this vision, individuals with Down syndrome would be provided with the same opportunities as those who were not born with this genetic condition.

The reality? This is not the current state of affairs for the majority of people with Down syndrome in the United States. Individuals with Down syndrome and their families are often forced to advocate to receive these very things—things that are taken for granted by the majority of American citizens.

Although we have come a long way toward reaching these visions for people with Down syndrome, this nation has yet to see the full inclusion of individuals with disabilities in its communities. We have yet to offer the same opportunities afforded to most others, even at the beginning of the twenty-first century. That is not to say we are not on the road to making these visions a reality. Change is possible with leadership, collaboration, understanding, skill, and commitment to action. It is, after all, these ingredients that led to the Education for All Handicapped Children Act in 1975

*Down Syndrome*, Edited by William I. Cohen, Lynn Nadel, and Myra E. Madnick.
ISBN 0-471-41815-3   Copyright © 2002 by Wiley-Liss, Inc.

(currently the Individuals with Disabilities Education Act), deinstitutional-
ization in the 1980s, the passage of the Americans with Disabilities Act in
1990, and the Ticket to Work and Incentives Improvement Act of 1999. These
visions *can* be realized.

## THE VISION

People with Down syndrome want to be accepted. They want to be included.
They wish to be provided with choices and opportunities. People with Down
syndrome have goals and dreams. They want their desires to be recognized
and their needs to be met. They want to be heard and given the same respect
as everyone else. They wish to speak for themselves and not let others speak
for them. Individuals with Down syndrome are living, breathing, thinking,
feeling people, and they want to be treated as such. Individuals with Down
syndrome want the same quality of life as everyone else.

Imagine if you were in high school and were forced to study and spend
time with classmates with whom you did not have anything in common.
Imagine if, on graduating from high school, you were told you would be
working in a job cleaning tables when what you really wanted to be doing
was going to college. Imagine if it was assumed that you would live at home
with your parents when you were 30 years old, even though you wanted
your own apartment. What if you wanted to go shopping, but your job
wages were too low for you to afford a new shirt; or if you wanted to work
but to do so would jeopardize your health care benefits? Or what if you
wanted to spend private time with your significant other, but you did not
have any place to go?

These are just a few examples of some of the limitations placed on people
with Down syndrome. The reasons for these include discrimination, stereotypes, prejudice, fear, and ignorance. These barriers, in combination with
economics and inadequate social support systems, have an enormous impact
on the ability of the visions for people with Down syndrome to be realized.

We asked the National Down Syndrome Society's Self-Advocate Advisory Board (a group comprised of teens and adults with Down syndrome
who want to make a difference for themselves, their friends, and future gen-
erations) the following question: "What are your goals, visions, and dreams
for the future?" Their answers, not surprisingly, were not much different
than those you would expect from a group of nondisabled teens and adults.
One self-advocate from New Hampshire wished to graduate from her local
high school and attend college; another young man from California wished
to live in his own home; another from Ohio wanted to own her own business; and another from New Jersey wanted to have friends.

A National Down Syndrome Society survey of parents and family
members about their visions for their children with Down syndrome indicated similar goals—the opportunity for their children to be educated in

their neighborhood school; access to employment and job training; the ability for their children to make friends and socialize; and the choice for their adult children to decide with whom to live and where (NDSS, 2000).

The visions of the individuals with Down syndrome and the visions the parents have for their children do not seem very different. And these visions are not very different from those of anyone you might ask in the general population.

These goals are all attainable. We owe it to individuals and their families to provide them with the opportunities to achieve their goals. With the appropriate supports, attitudes, commitment, and courage—to succeed and to fail—they can achieve these goals. After decades of few to no expectations of the abilities of people with Down syndrome and systematic repression of any vision they or their parents may have had for them, they deserve opportunities to develop, grow, and achieve in all aspects of their lives.

## THE REALITY

Life for individuals with Down syndrome in the United States is better than ever before. Today, people with Down syndrome have the legal right to be included in regular classroom settings with their nondisabled peers. Babies with Down syndrome have the right to early intervention, which will provide them with individualized services designed to help them develop to their fullest potential. Today, people with Down syndrome are receiving quality medical care; much is understood about specific medical concerns of people with Down syndrome, leading to more effective screening and treatment. Today, people with Down syndrome are living on average until age 55 and beyond; and people are integrating nutrition and wellness into their daily routines and taking more control over their own lives. Today, people with Down syndrome are living in their own homes or supported living arrangements and are leading more active and fulfilling lives through work and participation in community activities.

Much is being done in the areas of research, education, advocacy, employment, housing, and health care and in other areas, to help improve the lives of individuals with Down syndrome. However, although the overall status of people with Down syndrome and other disabilities has improved, there is still a wide gap between those with disabilities and those without disabilities.

Two-thirds of the people with disabilities in our society are unemployed, and those who are working generally make less than their nondisabled counterparts (NIDRR, 1998). More than 100,000 people with mental retardation are on waiting lists for housing in the community (The Arc et al., 2001). According to the New Freedom Initiative of President George W. Bush, 71% of people without disabilities own homes, but fewer than 10% of those with disabilities do; 1 of 5 adults with disabilities has not graduated from high school, compared with less than 1 of 10 adults without disabilities. Today, four out of five students leaving our nations secondary schools enroll in post-secondary education, yet very few colleges accept students with disabilities in their programs, denying them the enormous benefits of a college degree; and computer usage and Internet access for people with disabilities is half that of people without disabilities (Bush, 2001).

There are many reasons for these disparities, but the bottom line is that people with Down syndrome are not always treated equally. They are not always accepted for who they are. They do not always have access to the same schools and jobs as everyone else. They must work harder to prove themselves and are given fewer opportunities to do so. In essence, individuals with Down syndrome are often forced to alter their dreams, adapt their goals, and be confined by the limitations society continues to place on them.

There are approximately 54 million people with disabilities in the U.S. (LaPlante and Carlson, 1996), more than 4 million of whom have been categorized as having either mental retardation or a developmental disability (NHIS, 1994–1995), and 350,000 of whom have Down syndrome (NDSS, 2001). Individuals with disabilities as a whole make up 20% of the population, one of the largest minority groups in this country. Even so, they continue to be discriminated against. Legislation designed to end segregation, discrimination, and the exclusion of individuals with disabilities exists; however, the laws are not always implemented.

## HISTORICAL PERSPECTIVE: REFLECTIONS ON THE PAST

To look ahead, it is important to first look to the past to better understand where we are today and where we wish to go in the future.

Down syndrome did not "officially" receive its name from British physician John Langdon Down until 1866; however, there is evidence that Down syndrome existed much earlier in history. Before the twentieth century and into the early part of the 1900s, babies born with Down syndrome did not live beyond the age of nine, with little to no stimulation, medical attention, or opportunities to develop. Because of advances in health care and the discovery of antibiotics, people with Down syndrome were then living on average until age 20. Today, the average life expectancy of a person with Down syndrome is age 55, with many living beyond that age.

Not too long ago in the twentieth century, new parents were automatically told by health care professionals to put their infant with Down syndrome into an institution. The child would never walk, talk, read, or think; the child would not be able to relate to parents or family; and the child would remain a drain on the family financially and emotionally. In other words, having a child with Down syndrome was not accepted by society at large.

It was not until the 1950s and 1960s that parents began to challenge these preconceptions on the parts of the health care professionals whom they believed had all the answers. It was parents such as these that led the beginning of the Down syndrome movement—the movement to bring their babies home and provide all the love, support, and opportunities that they would give any one of their other children.

Throughout the history of the movement, parents have been the primary change agents for their children with Down syndrome. Some made a difference by challenging existing views or systems, thereby paving the way for others that followed. Many formed parent support groups as an organized, grassroots effort to make a difference in their communities. Yet others formed statewide or national coalitions or groups to make an impact on a larger scale. All of these made significant contributions that have led to changes over the past several decades.

These parents did not do it alone; they sought the help of professionals from various disciplines, friends, legislators, and others along the way. Together, they were responsible for the passage of numerous laws designed to protect and ensure the rights of individuals with disabilities. It is this legislation, among other activities, that has helped to shape and improve the current state of affairs for people with Down syndrome.

## THE CURRENT STATUS OF PEOPLE WITH DOWN SYNDROME

The current status of people with Down syndrome is much improved, with so many more resources, services, and opportunities. People with Down syndrome are being seen less as a category and more as individuals—individuals who have unique talents, interests, abilities, and dreams. The relatively recent movement towards "People First" language has contributed to this change in attitude, emphasizing that it is the person rather than the condition, that is, "my child with Down syndrome" rather than "my Down syndrome child." Although seemingly subtle, this shift in language has had an impact on the expectations for, and assumptions made about, that person.

Another major shift over the last decade has been the emergence of the self-advocacy and self-determination movements. Organizations such as *People First* and *Self-Advocates Becoming Empowered* were founded by individuals with disabilities to encourage and teach people with disabilities to speak out for what they believe in. They acknowledge the ability and rights of all people to let their voices be heard. Given the opportunities and supports, individuals with Down syndrome are able to be contributing members of society. This is a significant advance from the beliefs and attitudes of not too long ago.

Self-determination is a relatively new concept that enables individuals with Down syndrome to have greater control over their lives. Based on the core principles of freedom, authority, support, and responsibility, self-determination provides people with disabilities choice and control in the areas of housing, employment, benefits, and socialization. There are a number of model programs that are currently adopting the philosophy and implementing the practice of self-determination.

The more opportunities people with Down syndrome are given, the more they are able to achieve. Today, people with Down syndrome are musicians, writers, dancers, singers, actors, public speakers, advocates, business owners, homeowners, husbands, wives, and much more.

Today, parents and family members, as well as the individuals with Down syndrome, have the right to be active participants in developing and monitoring education plans. They are an integral part of the Individual Family Service Plan (IFSP) and Individualized Education Plan (IEP) teams.

Even with all the legislation in place, the enhancement of programs and services, and the improvement in available opportunities, there are still barriers in place that prevent individuals with Down syndrome from living the life they deserve. Some of these challenges are a result of economic limitations, others a result of attitudinal barriers.

There are more housing options available for adults today; however, there remains a daunting wait list in many areas of the country. There are more employment opportunities outside the traditional sheltered workshop than ever before, but there is a shortage of adequately trained job coaches to support the worker with Down syndrome and limited funding to hire the coaches long term. There are more students with Down syndrome fully included in regular classroom settings; however they are not necessarily supported in the classroom and do not necessarily have teachers who understand or are willing to make the necessary accommodations. There are more people with Down syndrome living independently or semi-independently today, but they often face a higher degree of social isolation. There is much more practical information available now; however not everyone has access to it. There have been more efforts to eliminate stereotypes through education and public awareness, yet slang words like "mongoloid" and "retard" are still in our vocabulary.

Clearly, there is still so much that can—and must—be done to enable individuals with Down syndrome to realize their visions.

## FORWARD THINKING: WHAT DOES THE FUTURE HOLD FOR INDIVIDUALS WITH DOWN SYNDROME?

### IDENTIFYING VISIONS

At the National Down Syndrome Society's 2000 National Conference in Washington, DC, the theme was *Visions for the 21st Century*. More than 500 conference attendees, consisting of parents and family members, teens and adults with Down syndrome, educators, physicians, speech, physical, and occupational therapists, psychologists, nurses, social workers, and other service providers, were encouraged to share their visions for the future for people with Down syndrome. "Vision Surveys" and "Vision Cards" were distributed, working groups in the areas of Education, Research, Advocacy and Self-Advocacy were held, and informal networking led to identifying a number of different visions.

These are some of the visions that were expressed: inclusion that *really* works; no limits on expectations in the classroom; getting services paid for by Medicare; financial assistance for support services not tied to parental income; Mom and Dad could die without worry; options; great jobs and independent living with social activities; support to single parents; support in supported employment; and much, much more (NDSS, 2000).

## IDENTIFYING NEEDS

The messages are clear—changes need to be made if any or all of these visions are to be realized. Changes need to be made in schools, housing, employment, health care, insurance, support services, benefits, transitioning, and family support. Changes will not happen automatically. They require parents, family members, and other interested individuals to become involved in the movement. With 350,000 individuals with Down syndrome in this country and the hundreds of thousands of parents, siblings, relatives, and friends, so much could be accomplished if everyone took just one small step toward making change.

To meet some of the goals and visions for people with Down syndrome, we need to: include individuals with Down syndrome in the process; support the individuals, their families and the professionals who serve them; not stop at getting legislation passed, but continue until it is implemented; begin the process of transitioning early on; ensure choice, with the opportunities to fail and to succeed; learn and exercise creative problem solving when faced with challenges, and learn to think "outside the box"; allow adults with Down syndrome to remain in control of their own lives; reach out to those who for whatever reason do not reach out to us; continue to support research to gain a greater understanding of various aspects of Down syndrome, to help improve lives; empower people; appreciate and celebrate cultural diversity; work together, listen to one another and learn from one another; acknowledge that there are no guarantees; and see people for the individuals they are.

We also need to be open to sharing information rather than spending limited time and resources reinventing the wheel; knowing when to provide support and understand when to foster independence; emphasizing the use of computers, the Internet and assistive technology, all of which provide greater access to information and enable barriers to be broken down; providing opportunities to follow dreams, to grow, to learn and develop; educating the public about Down syndrome to gain acceptance and promote community inclusion; taking risks, which ultimately will lead to growth; keeping our own fears and biases in check so that they do not interfere with the lives of others; and finally, believing in our own ability, and that of others, to make a difference.

## CONCLUSION

It may seem as though some of the visions are unattainable, but then again, 25 years ago the thought of having students with Down syndrome included in regular classrooms, learning and socializing with nondisabled students, must have seemed like a pipe dream.

All it takes is a vision and a willingness to try. As Margaret Mead once said, "Don't think a small group can't change the world. Indeed, it's the only way it has ever happened." It is a small group of parents, professionals, and concerned citizens who have the ability to change the world for people with Down syndrome. It was these very groups of people that created the reality that we live in today. Although by no means ideal, the world for people with Down syndrome is constantly changing and improving. It is up to us to turn these visions into reality.

## REFERENCES

AAMR (1992): Mental Retardation: Definition, Classification, and Systems of Support (9th ed.). Washington: American Association on Mental Retardation.

Bush GW (2001): New Freedom Initiative. Washington: The White House.

Hassold TJ, Patterson D (eds.) (1999): Down Syndrome: A Promising Future, Together. New York: Wiley-Liss.

LaPlante M, Carlson D (1996): Disability in the United States: Prevalence and Causes, 1992. Washington: U.S. Department of Education, National Institute on Disability and Rehabilitation Research.

Nadel L, Rosenthal D (eds.) (1995): Down Syndrome: Living and Learning in the Community. New York: Wiley-Liss.

NDSS (2000): Shaping the Vision for the 21st Century Survey. New York: National Down Syndrome Society.

NHIS (1994–1995): 1994, 1995 National Health Interview Survey. CD-ROM Series 10, Nos. 9 and 10c. SETS Version 1.21a. Washington: U.S. Government Printing Office.

NIDRR (1998): Centers of Excellence Announced. Washington: U.S. Department of Education, National Institute on Disability and Rehabilitation Research.

The Arc, AAMR, AAUAP (2001): People with Mental Retardation and Related Disabilities are Waiting for Housing in the Community. Washington: The Arc.

# Index

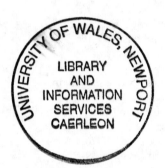

UNIVERSITY OF WALES, NEWPORT
LIBRARY
AND
INFORMATION
SERVICES
CAERLEON

But here this is, the book you're reading.

Obviously.

Your book—it's started now, it's touched and opened, held. You could, if you wanted, heft it, wonder if it weighs more than a pigeon, or a plimsoll, or quite probably rather less than a wholemeal loaf. It offers you these possibilities.

And, quite naturally, you face it. Your eyes, your lips are turned towards it—all that paleness, all those marks—and you are so close here that if it were a person you might kiss. That might be unavoidable.

You can remember times when kissing has been unavoidable. You are not, after all, unattractive: not when people understand you and who you can be.

And you're a reader—clearly—here you are reading your book, which is what it was made for. It loves when you look, wakes when you look, and then it listens and it speaks. It was built to welcome your attention and reciprocate with this: the sound it lifts inside you. It gives you the signs for the shapes of the names of the thoughts in your mouth and in your mind and this is where they sing, here at the point where you both meet.

Which is where you might imagine, might even elicit, the tremble of paper, that unmistakable flinch. It moves for you, your book, and it will always show you all it can.

And this is when it needs to introduce you to the boy.

This boy.

This boy, he is deep in the summer of 1974 and

1

by himself and cutting up sharp from a curve in the road and climbing a haphazard, wriggling style and next he is over and on to the meadow, his purpose already set.

No, not a *meadow*: only scrub grass and some nettles, their greens faded by a long, demanding summer and pale dust.

So it's simply a field, then—not quite who it was in its spring.

A field with an almost teenager live inside it.

He is, taken altogether, a taut thing and a sprung thing, free and also rattled with being free, and there is no particular path across this field, but the boy knows his way and heads for its most distant border. Hands quick, feet quicker, plimsolls and a washed-out yellow shirt, shorts that are greyish and fawnish, that have a torn pocket at the back. His clothes are too small and yet also slack in a way that suggests he is both longer and leaner than when they were bought. He is running as if pursued.

Ahead of him, the air shrugs with afternoon heat, distorts—he likes this. He mainly likes uncertain and changeable things—they seem to offer more chances for comfort, success. And sometimes they're all that he gets so he has to make the best of them.

His footfalls jar, drum, as he drives into a harder and harder pace, fists lifting as high as his throat, head back. He is as brown as all the island's children, dark from months of swimming, running, rowing, scrambling, months of bicycles and horses, little boats, months of hoarding stones and noting birds and of the pleasures in simple exhaustion. The boy's expression is currently thin and fierce. At a distance, it isn't easy to judge if this comes from effort, or emotion.

2